# Pediatric Amplification: Enhancing Auditory Access

**Editor-in-Chief for Audiology**
Brad A. Stach, PhD

**Core Clinical Concepts in Audiology**
*Series Editor*
Brad A. Stach, PhD

***Basic Audiometry***

*Acoustic Immittance Measures: Basic and Advanced Practice*
Lisa Hunter, PhD, FAAA, and Navid Shahnaz, PhD, Aud(C)

*Speech Audiometry*
Gary D. Lawson, PhD, and Mary E. Peterson, AuD

*Basic Audiometry Learning Manual*
Mark DeRuiter, MBA, PhD, and Virginia Ramachandran, AuD, PhD

*Pure-Tone Audiometry and Masking*
Maureen Valente, PhD

***Electrodiagnostic Audiology***

*Otoacoustic Emissions: Principles, Procedures, and Protocols*
Sumitrajit Dhar, PhD, and James W. Hall III, PhD

*Objective Assessment of Hearing*
James W. Hall III, PhD, and De Wet Swanepoel, PhD

***Cochlear Implants***

*Programming Cochlear Implants, Second Edition*
Jace Wolfe, PhD, and Erin C. Schafer, PhD

*Cochlear Implant Patient Assessment: Evaluation of Candidacy, Performance, and Outcomes*
René H. Gifford, PhD

*Objective Measures in Cochlear Implants*
Michelle L. Hughes, PhD, CCC-A

***Balance and Vestibular Assessment***

*Electronystagmography/Videonystagmography (ENG/VNG)*
Devin L. McCaslin, PhD

*Vestibular Learning Manual*
Bre Lynn Myers, AuD

***Pediatric Audiology***

*Comprehensive Handbook of Pediatric Audiology*
Richard Seewald, PhD, and Anne Marie Tharpe, PhD

*Foundations of Pediatric Audiology*
Fred H. Bess, PhD, and Judith S. Gravel, PhD

# Pediatric Amplification: Enhancing Auditory Access

Ryan W. McCreery, PhD
Elizabeth A. Walker, PhD

Plural Publishing Inc.

PLURAL PUBLISHING
INC.

5521 Ruffin Road
San Diego, CA 92123

e-mail: info@pluralpublishing.com
Website: http://www.pluralpublishing.com



Typeset in 11/13 Palatino by Flanagan's Publishing Services, Inc.
Printed in the United States of America by McNaughton & Gunn, Inc.



Library of Congress Cataloging-in-Publication Data

Names: McCreery, Ryan W., author. | Walker, Elizabeth, 1976- author.
Title: Pediatric amplification : enhancing auditory access / Ryan W. McCreery, Elizabeth Walker.
Description: San Diego, CA : Plural Publishing, [2017] | Includes bibliographical references and index.
Identifiers: LCCN 2017004149 | ISBN 9781597569927 (alk. paper) | ISBN 1597569925 (alk. paper)
Subjects: | MESH: Hearing Loss—therapy | Hearing Aids | Treatment Outcome | Infant | Child
Classification: LCC RF293 | NLM WV 271 | DDC 617.8/86—dc23
LC record available at https://lccn.loc.gov/2017004149

# Contents

# Preface

The clinical processes related to providing amplification for infants and children have changed rapidly in recent years. The idea that children could be identified with hearing loss at birth and that hearing aids could be provided within the first few months of life seemed unfathomable several decades ago. In the 21st century, we have a new generation of children with hearing loss who have the opportunity to be fit with hearing aids at very young ages and receive quality, family-centered early intervention. The field of pediatric audiology has responded to this new opportunity by developing clinical processes and protocols so that the full potential of these opportunities can be realized. The changes in the population of children who are hard of hearing and the clinical practices that are needed to support them were a major contributing factor to the decision to write this book.

There are a number of excellent book chapters and review articles that cover the topic of providing amplification for infants and children, many of which have been cited in this book. These other resources inspired our efforts to develop an entire textbook that follows not only the clinical processes of providing amplification for infants and children, but also the screening and diagnostic assessment that leads to a diagnosis of hearing loss. An expanded discussion of the use of outcome measure to monitor auditory development and speech perception was included to describe the important steps that occur after the hearing aids are fitted. The inclusion of a chapter on outcome validation led to the inclusion of a specific chapter on assessing children who are under consideration for cochlear implant candidacy. Each component of this textbook seemed to lead to the inclusion of another facet of the pediatric amplification process.

The potential danger in the approach of writing a textbook in this way is that the book could end up being a collection of tangential concepts. Fortunately, at the same time that we were thinking of writing this book, we were also privileged enough to be co-investigators in the longitudinal, multi-center Outcomes of Children with Hearing Loss (OCHL) and Outcomes of School-Age Children who are Hard of Hearing studies. As described by our esteemed colleague, Dr. Mary Pat Moeller, in the Foreword, the scientific framework of those studies served as a natural organizational structure for describing the processes that are related to providing amplification for children. The main goal of providing amplification for children who are hard of hearing is to enhance their auditory access. Over time, we strive to improve their cumulative auditory experience. The theoretical model of cumulative auditory experience not only helped us learn about the areas of risk and resilience experienced by children who are born with hearing loss and use hearing aids, but also provides clinical guidance on the goals and objectives that should guide an evidence-based approach to providing amplification for children.

As will be obvious from the first chapter, these concepts about maximizing auditory experience for children with hearing loss are not novel. These themes are apparent in the pioneering research of Julia Davis and her colleagues at the University of Iowa in the 1970s and 1980s, which was continued by Patricia Stelmachowicz at Boys Town National Research Hospital in the 1990s and 2000s. What is new is our ability to apply these ideas to children at younger ages. Early identification and intervention of hearing loss has the potential for greater impact on language and academic achievement than ever before. We hope that this text provides a comprehensive resource for professionals who serve children who are hard of hearing and their families and caregivers.

# Foreword

Pediatric amplification practices have evolved in a myriad of ways in an era of early identification and advancing hearing technologies. Practicing audiologists serve the youngest of infants and their families, adapt their strategies to meet the children's changing needs as they grow, monitor children's outcomes, and maintain currency regarding the increasing array of technologies that may be applied across children's developmental course to adulthood. All the while, practitioners strive to incorporate the best scientific evidence while individualizing their procedures to the needs of their patients and families. In reality, this can be a tall order. It is challenging to stay current with the burgeoning research literature and the moving target that represents current technology. *Pediatric Amplification: Enhancing Auditory Access* addresses this reality by providing a comprehensive and practical management guide that is elegantly interwoven with theory and supporting research evidence. This volume translates the science into a comprehensive set of resources that readers will find indispensable in their quest to provide evidence-based practice.

The text begins by introducing the reader to the theory of cumulative auditory access, and this foundational theoretical model is expertly integrated throughout subsequent chapters. The authors' clear elucidation of the theory clarifies the essential role that appropriately fit amplification plays in providing children with robust access to linguistic input and developmental opportunities. This theory is immediately backed up with current evidence drawn from an National Institute for Deafness and Other Communication Disorders-funded longitudinal study, *Outcomes of Children with Hearing Loss.* As a co-principal investigator of this project, I had the honor and pleasure of working side by side with the authors of this text, Ryan W. McCreery and Elizabeth A. Walker. Their contributions to the project were immense, and their research and clinical experiences are now expertly distilled in the pages that follow.

The introductory chapter sets the stage for remainder of the book. I expected to learn from reading this work, but I was also inspired by it. Concepts tackled in the introduction will pique interest and motivate readers to want to know the specific research findings and their implications for positively impacting children's outcomes. In the first chapter and throughout the book, concepts are organized in terms of malleable and nonmalleable influential factors—those factors we can directly impact in practice, and those that we may not be able to address head on, but need to consider and influence in indirect ways. This is a useful dichotomy that will provoke readers to think about novel ways to approach old problems.

The subsequent chapters provide comprehensive coverage of the essential topics related to pediatric amplification, including diagnosis of hearing loss, selecting amplification, and verifying hearing aid fittings for children. An entire chapter is devoted to the topic of hearing aid orientation and strategies for enhancing hearing aid use. Given recent evidence demonstrating the challenges of hearing aid use for some infants and young children, readers will find a rich set of evidence and resources to guide their work with families. This is paired with a chapter on evidence and techniques for monitoring auditory outcomes in children, which is essential for determining if hearing aid fittings are bringing about expected outcomes. Also provided are essential strategies for identifying children in need of additional or modified supports at the earliest possible ages. Meredith Spratford joins the primary authors in a discussion of the use of remote-microphone and connective device technologies to enhance cumulative auditory experience. Particularly innovative is the exploration of this topic in a developmental framework, considering the varied applications of technologies from infancy in the home through the young adulthood, when students access a range of electronic media sources. Another chapter is devoted to unique adaptations for special populations. The text concludes with case studies, which allow for application of the concepts presented throughout the book in way that guides both the "art" and the "science" of pediatric practice.

This volume is a treasure trove of resources for pediatric audiologists. The authors uniquely blend developmental theory with current evidence, resulting in considerable motivation and support for the clinical practice recommendations provided. This text will convince readers of the critical importance of best practices and why they matter for children's outcomes. It is a must read for those engaged in pediatric audiology in any arena. It will become a valued resource that guides the effort to promote optimal developmental outcomes for children in this promising era of early service provision.

—Mary Pat Moeller, PhD

# Acknowledgments

This book would not have been possible without the help of individuals at Boys Town National Research Hospital and the University of Iowa, including David Kessler, Kelsey Klein, and Clairissa Mollak. They provided support and assisted in the editing, proofreading, and design of the book. Their input is greatly appreciated.

We also wish to express our appreciation for the staff at Plural Publishing, especially Kalie Koscielak. We owe her thanks for keeping us on schedule and providing positive encouragement throughout the writing process.

We wish to acknowledge the support of the National Institutes of Health (NIH) National Institute for Deafness and other Communication Disorders (NIDCD) for supporting the research that helped to develop the framework for this book.

Above all, we would like to express our gratitude to our spouses and children, who supported and encouraged us, in spite of the time spent away from them while we wrote this book. We could not do any of this without you.

# Acknowledgments

# Contributors

**Ryan W. McCreery, PhD**
Director, Center for Audiology
Director, Audibility, Perception and Cognition Lab
Boys Town National Research Hospital
Omaha, Nebraska

**Meredith Spratford, AuD, CCC-A**
Staff Research Audiologist
Boys Town National Research Hospital
Omaha, Nebraska
*Chapter 7*

**Elizabeth A. Walker, PhD**
Assistant Professor
Department of Communication Sciences and Disorders
The University of Iowa
Iowa City, Iowa

*We dedicate this book in memory of Julia Davis, who was a pioneer in the field of pediatric audiology. Her seminal publication,* "Our Forgotten Children: Hard of Hearing Pupils in the Schools," *sought to inform research and clinical service provision for children who are hard of hearing.*

*We also dedicate this book in honor of Mary Pat Moeller and J. Bruce Tomblin, principal investigators on the "Outcomes of Children with Hearing Loss" study. They have mentored us, inspired us, and cheered us on throughout our careers. We are continuously grateful for their support and leadership.*

# 1

# An Introduction to Cumulative Auditory Experience

*Ryan W. McCreery and Elizabeth A. Walker*

## INTRODUCTION

The recent implementation of universal newborn hearing screening and early diagnosis and intervention in many countries around the world creates an opportunity for a brighter future for children who are deaf or hard of hearing. Hearing loss is the most frequently occurring congenital condition identified at birth. Decades of evidence have documented the negative developmental consequences that occur when a child's access to sound is limited. Fortunately, hearing technologies and family-centered early intervention have shifted the landscape of service provision for children who are deaf or hard of hearing, leading us to expect that language delays can be minimized or prevented altogether. In the following chapter, we will provide an overview of the concept of *cumulative auditory experience*: how hearing loss affects development by limiting access to sound over time. We will discuss the following topics in detail:

- The effects of early identification and intervention of hearing loss on developmental outcomes over time
- The role of hearing aids in enhancing auditory experience in children
- Clinical strategies for maximizing auditory experience in children with hearing loss

Our goal in this introductory chapter is to provide a theoretical foundation for the model that will serve as the basis for the rest of the text.

## THE EFFECTS OF HEARING LOSS ON DEVELOPMENT IN CHILDREN

Congenital or prelingual hearing loss affects development by reducing access to acoustic cues needed to fuel the development of speech and language. Language development is driven by perceptual experiences and interactions with other people that begin even before a child is born.

Studies have shown within a few hours of birth, newborns show clear preferences for their mother's voice over others (DeCasper & Fifer, 1980; Mehler, Bertoncini, Barrière, & Jassik-Gerschenfeld, 1978), suggesting that formative auditory experiences begin in the womb. Cross-linguistic studies have indicated that young infants' preferences for sounds in their primary language over speech sounds from other languages emerge within the first few months of life (Werker & Tees, 1984). This process of increasing sensitivity for the acoustic cues in their native language provides infants with early tools to learn new words and to develop a system of language (Werker & Yeung, 2005). Learning to communicate is driven by language input from the child's environment and occurs as soon as the child can hear prenatally. For the child who is hard of hearing, this early auditory experience may be reduced or eliminated.

In children who have hearing loss at birth or acquire it early in the process of developing language, language learning can be significantly interrupted, though the prospects for children who are deaf or hard of hearing have improved immensely over the last century. Early descriptions of deafness in children focused primarily on children with severe or profound hearing loss and limited residual hearing, which was equated to sensory deprivation (Myklebust, 1960). In those early years, the lack of early identification and intervention programs meant that children who were deaf or hard of hearing faced substantial delays in communication development, which often cascaded into academic and social problems during school age. Given the limited residual hearing and auditory access associated with profound hearing loss, such significant language development problems were not surprising.

Perhaps more surprising was the fact that nearly any amount of hearing loss was found to impact the emergence of speech and language abilities. Children with milder degrees of hearing loss were not as well studied as their peers with severe and profound degrees of hearing loss, but even early investigations found that milder degrees of hearing loss could be quite disruptive to development. For example, one of the first investigations of vocabulary and reading ability in a cohort of children with hearing losses ranging from mild to profound found that children with hearing loss experienced delays in language and reading abilities compared to peers with normal hearing, even for mild or moderate losses (Hood, 1949). This observation ran against the prediction that the amount of disruption in communication development might be easily predicted by the child's degree of hearing loss. Further pioneering work by Julia Davis and her colleagues helped to reveal the developmental challenges faced by children with mild or moderate hearing losses. In one of many studies authored by Davis, Elfenbein, Schum, and Bentler (1986), Davis challenged the idea that the developmental effects of hearing loss were entirely predictable based on the child's degree of hearing loss. As Davis wrote:

> The data indicate that it is not possible to predict hearing-impaired children's language or educational performance on the basis of degree of hearing loss alone, whether the measure used is a pure-tone average or one of speech reception and/or recognition. Therefore, the assumption that the greater the hearing loss the more severe the language and educational deficits is not supported by these data . . . (p. 51)

Davis had identified that while the child's degree of hearing loss was one potential factor in predicting developmental outcomes, there were many other aspects related to children and their environment at play that could be pivotal in helping to guide intervention. The prevailing assumption at the time, which was that children with the most significant degrees of hearing loss might be at the greatest risk, led to an intense focus on developing interventions for children with the greatest degrees of hearing loss, including cochlear implants. Less emphasis was placed on children with mild and moderate degrees of hearing loss who wore hearing aids, based on the assumption that milder degrees of loss would not lead to significant problems in communication development. This focus prompted Julia Davis to refer to children with mild-to-moderate hearing loss as "Our forgotten children."

The amount of research about the effects of hearing loss on children with milder degrees of hearing loss has increased since Davis's influential work, but the idea that mild or moderate hearing loss is not a major threat to development is persistent. For example, Ching and colleagues (2013) found no advantage for early amplification for children with mild-to-moderate hearing loss and concluded:

> . . . most of the children with hearing aids at the time of assessment had a mild or moderate loss. Perhaps the auditory stimulation these children received unaided was sufficient to enable development of the auditory cortex, such that when hearing aids were later provided, the children were able to make just as good use of the signals received as children who received their hearing aids earlier. (p. 548)

The clear implication of this statement is that children with mild-to-moderate hearing loss have sufficient residual hearing without amplification to provide a foundation for auditory development and learning. However, examining only the potential advantages related to the timing of amplification clearly ignores the influence of factors such as how well the child's hearing aids restore audibility for speech, how often the child is wearing his/her hearing aids, and the type of intervention or environment to which the child is exposed. As is discussed in the next section of the chapter, some of the limited effects of the timing of amplification in recent research is likely related to the fact that most children who are hard of hearing receive amplification within the first few months of life (Holte et al., 2012). The shift to lower ages of hearing aid fitting before and after the implementation of universal newborn hearing screening is shown in Figure 1–1. This is a contrast to early research where the average age of identification was over 2 years of age (Moeller, 2000). As a result, research has shifted toward the other factors, in addition to the timing of amplification that could affect developmental outcomes in children who wear hearing aids.

Subsequent research has attempted to quantify the impact of child- and family-specific characteristics, timing and quality of early intervention, hearing aid effectiveness, and language environment to name just a few. In the following sections, the features that have been identified in research as the most influential associates of development in children who are deaf or hard of hearing are discussed. In particular, a recent theoretical perspective, known as the model of cumulative auditory experience, is highlighted. The model of cumulative auditory experience includes multiple facets of the child's auditory abilities, their environment, and intervention, in an attempt to enumerate the quality and quantity of a child's auditory experience over time. Clinicians can use their knowledge of these factors to guide families in important clinical decisions regarding the types of interventions that might be most successful for the children that they serve.

## MALLEABILITY

There are two broad categories of features that have been identified as influencing developmental outcomes in children who are deaf or hard of hearing: malleable and nonmalleable factors. Malleable factors are any aspects of the child, his or her environment, or interventions that can be changed with minimal effort. One example of a malleable factor that receives considerable emphasis throughout this text is the audibility of speech provided by the child's hearing aid. Speech audibility from a hearing aid is malleable in the sense that if a child comes into the clinic with a hearing aid that is not providing an adequate amount of audibility for their degree of hearing loss, the audiologist can adjust the hearing aid to maximize the child's access to speech. A number of other malleable factors have been shown to influence developmental outcomes in children.

In contrast, nonmalleable factors are features related to the child, their environment, or interventions that cannot be modified easily. One example of a nonmalleable factor is the socioeconomic status of the child's family. Low family socioeconomic status can have negative effects on development for children who are otherwise typically developing, and represents an additional risk for developmental delays in children who are hard of hearing. Sadly, the socioeconomic status of the family cannot be easily modified through intervention. Changes in socioeconomic status at the level of individual families are difficult to

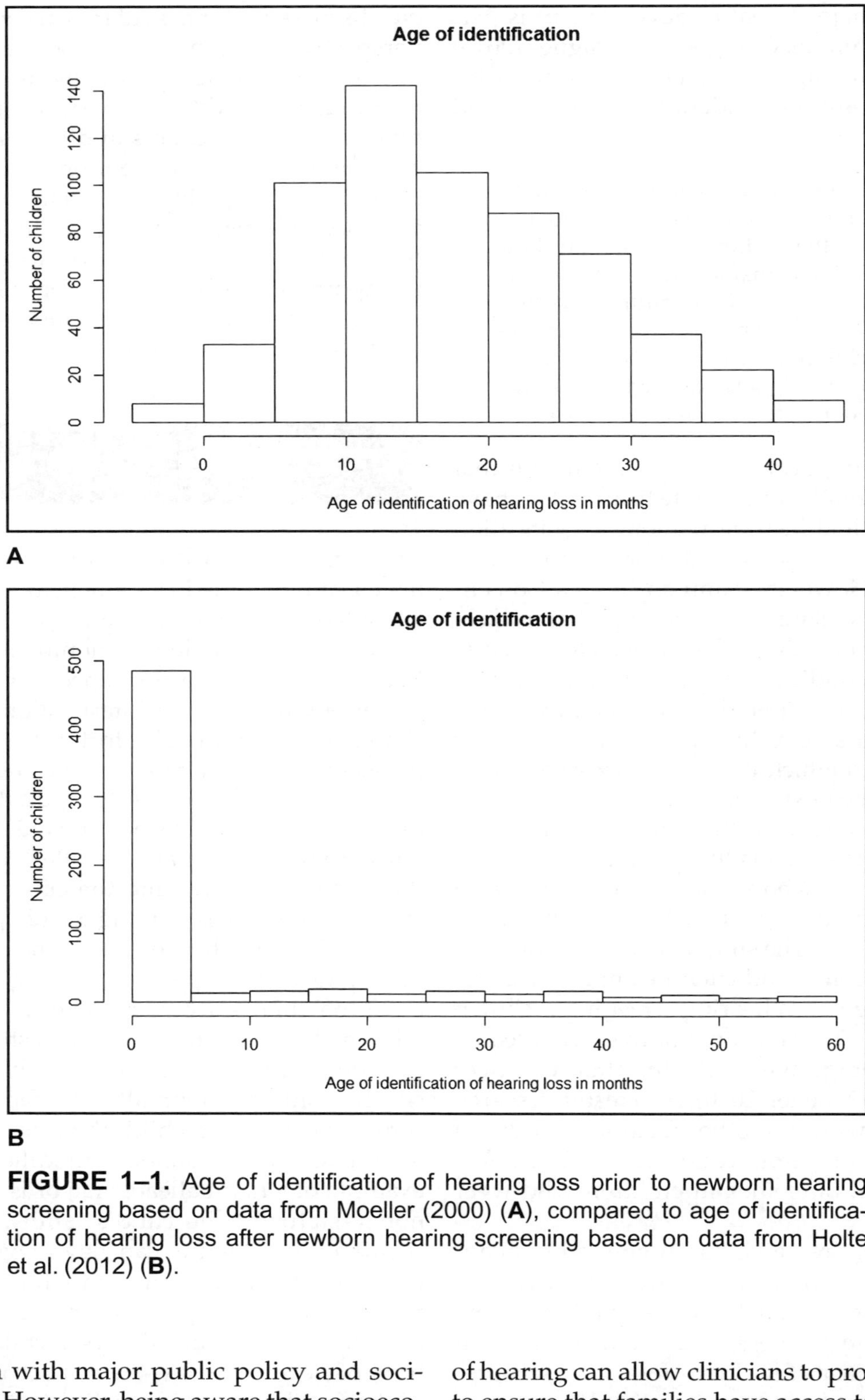


**FIGURE 1–1.** Age of identification of hearing loss prior to newborn hearing screening based on data from Moeller (2000) (**A**), compared to age of identification of hearing loss after newborn hearing screening based on data from Holte et al. (2012) (**B**).

achieve even with major public policy and societal changes. However, being aware that socioeconomic status is a potential risk factor for additional developmental concerns in children who are hard of hearing can allow clinicians to provide supports to ensure that families have access to intervention services for their children. Nonmalleable factors may not be directly modifiable, but clinicians should be aware of these factors so that they can assess the risk for developmental delays related to these factors.

Malleable and nonmalleable factors also may interact in ways that have important clinical implications. The audibility of speech sounds through the hearing aid use has both malleable and nonmalleable influences. For example, Figure 1–2 displays the relationship between audibility and degree of hearing loss for children who are fit to the Desired Sensation Level (DSL) (Scollie et al., 2005) multistage algorithm, which is a popular hearing aid prescriptive approach for children.

As the child's degree of hearing loss increases, the amount of audibility that is prescribed, and that can be provided, decreases. This relationship exists because of how sensorineural hearing loss affects the listener's dynamic range. The dynamic range of hearing is defined as the difference between the listener's hearing thresholds and the level where loudness discomfort occurs. As hearing loss increases, the listener's thresholds increase, but the sound level where loudness discomfort occurs remains relatively stable and can even become less for some listeners. The net effect is that the dynamic range of hearing, which can span 100 dB in listeners with normal hearing, can be reduced to only 20 to 30 dB in listeners with severe or profound sensorineural hearing loss. The child's degree of hearing loss, therefore, is a nonmalleable factor that places constraints on the amount of audibility for speech that can be prescribed and achieved with amplification. However, aided audibility also has an important malleable aspect. Providing a hearing aid fitting that closely approximates prescriptive targets for the child's degree of hearing loss allows audiologists to provide consistent audibility. The nonmalleable facet of audibility related to the degree of hearing loss can by mitigated by the malleable aspect related to how closely the hearing aid is fit to prescriptive targets. In one study, the amount of variability in aided audibility related to how well the hearing aids were fit was equal to the amount of variability related to degree of hearing loss in a large group of children who wore hearing aids (McCreery, Bentler, & Roush, 2013). An understanding of malleable and nonmalleable factors that are associated with developmental outcomes in children who are deaf or hard of hearing is an essential foundation for understanding why children who are hard of hearing exhibit such a wide range of developmental outcomes. The model of cumulative auditory experience that is the key framework of this text incorporates both malleable and nonmalleable factors in an attempt to create a model that reflects the realities of providing clinical services to children who wear hearing aids. The interactions between these factors must also be considered, as the effects of hearing loss on development in children are inherently complex and multivariate. The interactions, in particular, may be important to discuss with families to avoid overly simplistic conclusions about a child's potential for development.

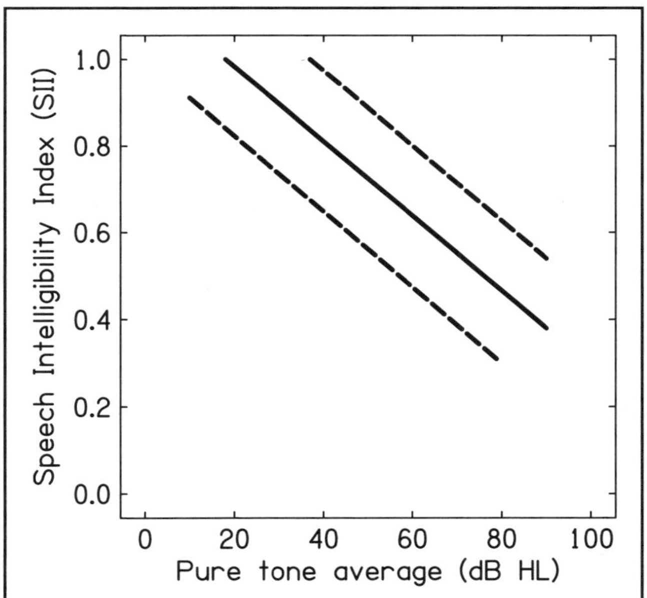


**FIGURE 1–2.** Aided audibility as a function of degree of hearing loss for children fitted to the Desired Sensation Level (DSL) algorithm, based on data from McCreery et al. (2013).

## Nonmalleable Factors

As noted in the previous section, nonmalleable factors are any characteristics of the child, environment or intervention that cannot easily be modified. Nonmalleable factors have been widely studied because they are often easy to measure or document. An exhaustive discussion of nonmalleable factors that affect developmental outcomes in children who are deaf or hard of hearing is beyond the scope of this clinically focused overview, but particular attention will be given to nonmalleable factors that could influence clinical interventions. The child's degree of hearing loss, the age of identification/hearing aid fitting/intervention, socioeconomic status, presence of additional disabilities aside from hearing loss, and gender are all nonmalleable factors that have been reported in previous studies.

### *Degree of Hearing Loss*

As already noted in earlier sections of this chapter, the degree of hearing loss has been an effective predictor of developmental outcomes in children who are deaf or hard of hearing in some studies. Even a lay person with limited experience working with children who are deaf or hard of hearing might make the intuitive prediction that children who have more hearing loss would experience greater impact on their development than peers with less hearing loss. However, the pattern of data in the research literature has not always confirmed this prediction. Children with greater degrees of hearing loss have had poorer outcomes in speech and language than peers with milder degrees of hearing loss in some studies (Ching et al., 2010; Ching et al., 2013; Fitzpatrick, Crawford, Ni, & Durieux-Smith, 2011; Fitzpatrick, Durieux-Smith, Eriks-Brophy, Olds, & Gaines, 2007; Hood, 1949; Sininger, Grimes, & Christensen., 2010; Tomblin, Oleson, Ambrose, Walker, & Moeller, 2014; Tomblin et al., 2015; Wake, Hughes, Poulakis, Collins, & Rickards, 2004; Yoshinaga-Itano, Coulter, & Thomson, 2000 Yoshinaga-Itano, Sedey, Coulter, & Mehl, 1998), but not in others (Davis et al., 1986; Gilbertson & Kamhi, 1995; Moeller 2000). Similarly, children who have more significant degrees of hearing loss also show greater deficits in speech recognition compared to peers with less hearing loss (Blamey et al., 2001; Davidson & Skinner, 2006; McCreery et al., 2015). This apparent inconsistency across studies can be confusing for parents and caregivers of children who are deaf or hard of hearing, who may expect that their child with mild hearing loss might develop typically or that their child with profound hearing loss might not be able to communicate using spoken language.

There are many reasons why degree of hearing loss by itself is not a singular predictor of development in children who are deaf or hard of hearing. Degree of hearing loss is often represented as a single number, such as the pure-tone average, which is the arithmetic mean of the audiometric thresholds at 500 Hz, 1000 Hz, and 2000 Hz (and sometimes 4000 Hz additionally). In some cases, degree of hearing loss is represented by the broad semantic categories of mild, moderate, severe, or profound. Attempting to reduce hearing down to a single number or category will mean that there are often significant individual differences between children who have similar pure-tone averages or the same degree of hearing loss. Children with similar pure-tone averages can have varying configurations of hearing loss that could impact their access to speech in different ways, as shown in the example in Figure 1–3.

Additionally, degree of hearing loss reflects unaided hearing, when most children who are deaf or hard of hearing will spend most of their day using hearing aids or a cochlear implant. Children with cochlear implants are an interesting example of how the effect of degree of hearing loss has changed over time. In some recent investigations, children with cochlear implants have more favorable developmental outcomes compared to peers with hearing aids (e.g., Ching et al., 2013), despite having severe or profound degrees of hearing loss. For this reason, many researchers include measures of aided hearing, including aided audibility for speech and aided speech recognition abilities in addition to estimates of unaided hearing when attempting to evaluate risk for developmental delays in children with hearing loss.

Finally, evidence from children who have mild or unilateral hearing loss (which is discussed in greater detail in Chapter 9) suggests that even minimal disruptions in audibility can have an impact on communication development. A paper from Walker et al. (2015) included three groups of children with similar degrees of mild hearing loss: full-time hearing aid users, part-time hearing aid users and children who did not use amplifi-

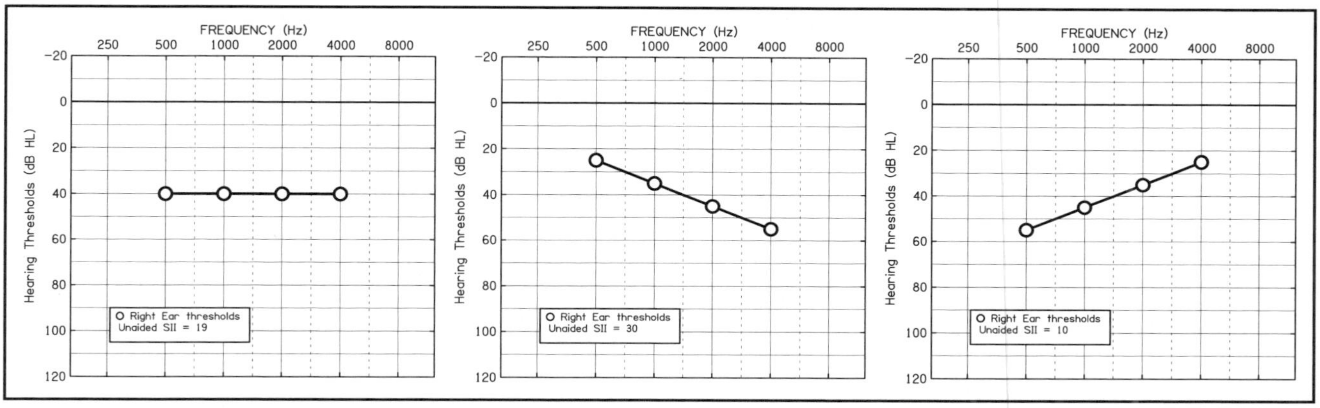


**FIGURE 1–3.** Three audiograms with the same pure-tone average (PTA) can have very different effects on the audibility of speech. Note the differences in the unaided Speech Intelligibility Index (SII) across the examples for children who have a PTA of 40 dB HL.

cation. Despite having similar degrees of hearing loss, the children who did not wear amplification or receive early intervention services had poorer speech and language outcomes in several specific domains compared to the part-time or full-time hearing aid users. This demonstrates not only that even mild hearing loss can affect developmental outcomes, but also that degree of hearing loss does not adequately reflect the factors related to amplification and intervention that could also influence developmental processes in children who are deaf or hard of hearing.

### *Age of Identification/Hearing Aid Fitting/Intervention*

Over the last two decades, questions about the timing of intervention for children who are deaf or hard of hearing have been conducted to evaluate the need for universal newborn hearing screening and early intervention programs. Many early studies contrasting developmental outcomes for children with different timing for identification and intervention were based on opportunistic samples in areas where universal newborn hearing screening and early intervention programs were implemented at varying times in the same hospital or educational areas. The sequential implementation of newborn hearing screening and early intervention programs created naturally occurring early- and later-identified groups of children who were otherwise very similar. In one of the first studies to evaluate questions about timing of early identification and intervention, Yoshinaga-Itano and colleagues (1998) found higher language quotients for children who were enrolled in early intervention before 6 months of age, compared to children who were enrolled in early intervention at later ages. This finding of improved language outcomes has been replicated in numerous studies subsequently (Calderon & Naidu, 1999; Kennedy et al., 2006; Moeller, 2000; Sininger et al., 2010) and expanded to long-term reading outcomes as children get older (Pimperton & Kennedy, 2012; Pimperton et al., 2016).

Like degree of hearing loss, however, there are also exceptions that have not found similar advantages for early identification and intervention (Ching et al., 2013). Additionally, many of the studies contrasting early- and later-identified children who are deaf or hard of hearing have been criticized for a lack of true random assignment (Nelson, Bougatsos, & Nygren, 2008). Another challenge in more recent studies is that the ages of identification, fitting of hearing aids, and early intervention are occurring more uniformly early. For example, one recent longitudinal study found that 76% of children who were hard of hearing were identified through newborn hearing screening and the median age at hearing aid fitting was just 7 months of age (Holte et al., 2012). With early identification becoming more consistent, the ability to document the advantages for early identification over a shrinking group of late-identified children becomes more difficult. Furthermore, late-identified children in the sample (Walker et al., 2014) tended to have milder degrees of hearing loss or were more likely to have passed universal newborn hearing screening. In these cases, children may have periods of normal auditory experience or better audibility, compared with cohorts of children who were later identified in previous studies. These early periods of auditory experience may help to minimize the effects of later identification, compared to previous cohorts of children who were later identified and had hearing loss from birth.

A critical point is that the diminishing effect of age of identification in more recent studies should not be taken as evidence that early identification and intervention for children who are hard of hearing is not important. Establishing early auditory experience provides auditory stimulation during sensitive periods for language and brain development (Garcia-Sierra et al., 2011; Sharma, Dorman, & Kral, 2005). Children with mild hearing loss who received early intervention and amplification were found to have better language outcomes in some domains than peers with mild hearing loss who did not receive these services (Walker et al., 2015). These results suggest that providing early and consistent auditory experience can be important, even in cases where hearing loss might have a minimal impact of auditory access. Furthermore, lowering the age of identification has allowed researchers and clinicians to focus on other explanatory variables that could influence developmental outcomes in children who are deaf or hard of hearing. This progress has raised new questions about how auditory experience in children who are deaf or hard of hearing can be quantified, beyond the degree of hearing loss and age of identification.

### *Socioeconomic Status*

Children who are raised in homes with limited economic resources are at greater risk for a wide range of developmental concerns including language, cognitive, behavioral, and academic difficulties, compared to peers who are raised in more economically advantaged homes (see Bradley & Corwyn, 2002, Hoff, 2006, or Bornstein & Bradley, 2014 for review). The role of socioeconomic status in child development is controversial and has been widely studied because of the implications for targeted intervention and public policy. Socioeconomic status has been measured in research studies using a wide range of metrics, including the mother or father's level of educational achievement, family income, access to free or reduced school lunch programs, or the parent's employment status. The developmental disadvantages faced by children who are raised in poverty are likely related to a wide range of sources, some of which are listed in Table 1–1. Additional discussions of the effects of socioeconomic status are briefly discussed in this chapter's section on the child's linguistic environment as a malleable factor in the development of children who wear hearing aids.

Children who are hard of hearing from low socioeconomic status homes face additional risks to their development beyond those faced by peers with higher socioeconomic status (Ching et al., 2013; Tomblin et al., 2014). For example, Ching and colleagues reported that global language outcomes were more favorable for children with mothers who had at least a college degree when compared to children with mothers who had not finished a high school education. The findings from Ching also point to other factors that are potentially confounded with socioeconomic status that might influence development. Children from lower socioeconomic status backgrounds also had later ages of identification and later ages of hearing aid fitting than peers from higher

**Table 1–1.** Developmental Risks for Children with Low Socioeconomic Status

| |
|---|
| Low parental academic attainment |
| Neighborhood and environmental factors |
| Poor nutrition |
| Reduced school quality |
| Parental mental health |
| Educational opportunity |

*Source:* Adapted from Yoshikawa, H., Aber, J. L., & Beardslee, W. R. (2012).

socioeconomic status backgrounds. This relationship demonstrates that children who are hard of hearing and who are also from lower socioeconomic status backgrounds are likely to face challenges related to timely access to services that may impact their outcomes over the longer term. Other studies have found that children from lower socioeconomic backgrounds may be more likely to be lost to follow-up or documentation after universal newborn hearing screening (Liu, Farrell, MacNeil, Stone, & Barfield, 2008) and are less likely to have consistent hearing aid use during early childhood (Walker et al., 2013). Each of these differences could create additional challenges for optimal development in children who are hard of hearing.

Differences in developmental outcomes related to socioeconomic status are considered nonmalleable because the efforts to alter economic conditions require societal changes. Without major reforms in social and economic policies at the governmental level, large gains in outcomes related to improving overall socioeconomic status are not likely to occur. A more realistic approach to managing the influences of socioeconomic status is to provide consistent early access to services and support for families who may have limited economic means. Recognizing that families with limited economic means will face greater challenges in accessing care and intervention for their children can help clinicians to provide greater support in those cases. Specific examples related to enhancing hearing aid use in children from economically disadvantaged backgrounds are reviewed in greater detail later in the book.

### *Additional Disabilities*

Approximately 40% of children who have hearing loss also have an additional condition that could affect their development (Gallaudet Research Institute, 2008). Developmental evaluations of children who have hearing loss reveal that 68% have a developmental concern besides speech or language (Wiley, Arjmand, & Dixon, 2011). While any developmental condition can co-occur with hearing loss, some of the most frequently occurring are general cognitive delays, motor or oral motor disorders, vision problems, and autism spectrum disorders (Meinzen-Derr, Wiley, Grether, & Choo, 2010). Figure 1–4 shows the distribution of additional disabilities from one study of development in children with hearing loss.

Some longitudinal studies of children who are hard of hearing have purposefully excluded children who have additional disabilities to focus on the effects of hearing loss (e.g., Tomblin et al., 2015). Other studies have attempted to recruit cohorts of children that better represent the general population of children with hearing loss by including children with additional disabilities (e.g., Ching et al., 2013), but the results, unsurprisingly, show that children with hearing loss who have additional disabilities have poorer outcomes than peers with hearing loss who do not have additional disabilities. Considerable variability in outcomes is often noted among the group of children with hearing loss and additional disabilities and often overlaps the distribution of children with hearing loss without additional disabilities (e.g., Wiley, Jahnke, Meinzen-Derr, & Choo, 2005). This overlap between groups is not surprising, given the fact that children with widely varying diagnoses and severity of additional disabilities are often grouped together in these types of analyses. Even if a large number of children with the same additional diagnosis (autism, for example) could be recruited, the amount of variability in developmental outcomes within that diagnosis can make generalizations about the additional effect of that specific diagnosis extremely difficult.

General findings that children with hearing loss plus additional disabilities do more poorly than their peers who have hearing loss alone are not generally informative for clinicians or parents who must make decisions about the best intervention to maximize each child's potential. Instead of generalizations provided by research studies, the development of a specific intervention plan that addresses the child's specific strengths and needs is important. Examples include positioning the head of a child with significant motor delays in such a way that does not limit the ability to wear hearing aid, or providing adaptations to help children with motor delays insert and remove their hearing aids and change the batteries. The goals of increasing auditory access and experience do not change for children who have additional

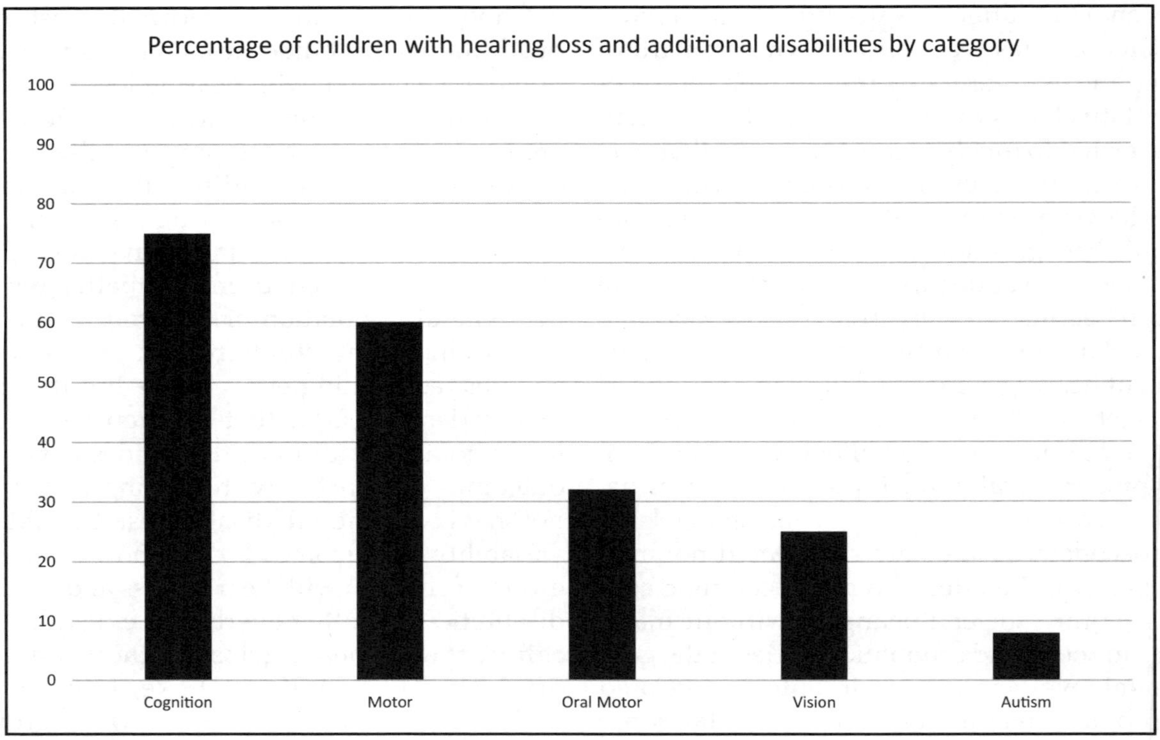


**FIGURE 1–4.** The distribution of additional disabilities for a sample of children with hearing loss based on data from Meinzen-Derr et al. (2010).

disabilities along with hearing loss, but the way in which those services are provided may need to be individually adapted to better suit the child.

### *Gender*

Differences in developmental outcomes for children with hearing loss based on gender have been reported in the literature, with the general trend that girls have more favorable language outcomes than boys (Ching et al., 2013). In general, it is important to acknowledge the potential for these differences, but also to put them into the context of potential confounding factors that may provide plausible mechanisms between girls and boys. For example, boys may be more likely than girls to have hearing loss with an additional disability (Meinzen-Derr et al., 2010). Differences in general language development between girls and boys have also been reported among typically developing preschool children (Huttenlocher, Haight, Bryk, Seltzer, & Lyons, 1991). These differences are not attributed to biological differences between girls and boys in terms of language acquisition, but rather differences in how parents and caregivers talk to and interact differently with boys than girls. Clinicians should be aware of the potential for differences based on gender, but also understand that these differences are quite small in practice and should not be cited as a reason why a child is experiencing considerable delays in language abilities.

### *Summary of Nonmalleable Factors*

There are multiple nonmalleable factors shown to influence development in children who are hard of hearing. Much of the earliest research focused on nonmalleable factors, as they are easy to document and collect as part of the research studies. The downside to nonmalleable factors is that they cannot be easily altered through intervention, which could lead to a sense that such factors are deterministic, meaning that the course of development for children with certain characteristics cannot be altered. The deterministic view of nonmalleable factors should be avoided because recent research has shown that malleable factors can have as much, if not more, influence on developmental outcomes in children who are hard of hearing. Nonmalleable factors are important to consider for identifying children who may be at additional risk for developmental delays or who may need customized or targeted early intervention services.

## Malleable Factors: Quantifying Cumulative Auditory Experience

With earlier and more consistent identification of hearing loss, there is still considerable variation in language and other developmental outcomes in children who are deaf or hard of hearing (Ching et al., 2013; Tomblin et al., 2014; Tomblin et al., 2015). If variability in outcomes is still present in children who have early identification, what are the other potential factors that influence outcomes? An investigation by Ching and colleagues (2013) found that children who are deaf or hard of hearing with additional disabilities, greater degrees of hearing loss, or those who came from economically disadvantaged homes, or who had English as a second language in the home, had poorer outcomes than peers without disabilities, milder degrees of hearing loss, or from economically advantaged backgrounds, where English was the primary language spoken in the home. While these factors are important for our understanding of the developmental effects of hearing loss and designing interventions to target populations that could be at the greatest risk for challenges, none of these factors are easily modifiable by parents or clinicians. This led other researchers to examine aspects of the child's hearing aids and environment that affected outcomes, but could be more easily targeted for intervention.

A recent investigation, led by Mary Pat Moeller and Bruce Tomblin and a team of multidisciplinary researchers (Moeller, Tomblin, and the Outcomes of Children with Hearing Loss collaboration, 2015) attempted to document a wide range of factors that could be influential in the development of children with mild to severe hearing loss. This study, Outcomes of Children with Hearing Loss (OCHL), provided the central framework for this textbook and the clinical intervention strategies that will be presented. Moeller, Tomblin and their colleagues operated under the theory that the auditory experiences of children who are deaf or hard of hearing shape their development, in addition to the nonmalleable factors that affected outcomes in previous studies. The factors that they identified that could be targeted by intervention were: (1) the degree to which speech sounds are audible through the child's hearing aids, known as aided audibility, (2) the duration and consistency of hearing aid use, and (3) the quality and quantity of linguistic input in the child's environment. Each of these factors combines to influence outcomes in children who are deaf or hard of hearing, as depicted in Figure 1–5. Children with greater aided audibility for speech, longer and more consistent hearing aid use, and higher quantity and quality of linguistic input from parents or caregivers were predicted to have better developmental outcomes than peers with poorer aided audibility, less consistent hearing aid use, or limited quantity or quality language environments. An overview of each component of the cumulative auditory experience is provided in the sections that follow.

### *Audibility for Speech*

Because the primary negative developmental consequences of hearing loss occur as the result of the loss of access to the acoustic cues that comprise communication, it is perhaps not surprising that the extent to which access can be restored with amplification might be an important factor in optimizing these outcomes with amplification. However, the influence of audibility specifically has only recently been considered as a potential contributing factor to a child's auditory experience. As noted above, much attention in previous research had been paid to the child's degree of hearing loss as a predictor of outcomes. There are several reasons why unaided hearing alone would not be expected to predict the extent of a child's access to their auditory environment or be a strong predictor of outcomes. For children

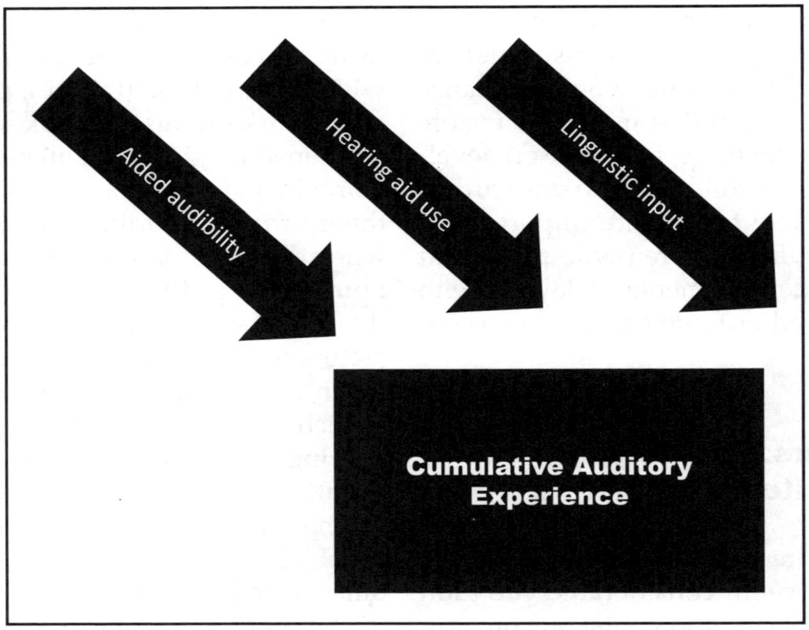


**FIGURE 1–5.** The factors that contribution to cumulative auditory experience in children who wear hearing aids are (1) aided audibility for speech, (2) consistent hearing aid use, and (3) the quantity and quality of linguistic input.

who wear hearing aids, measures of unaided hearing, such as the child's better-ear pure-tone average from the audiogram, simply do not reflect how much the child can hear with amplification. It is generally the case that the amount of aided audibility that can be provided decreases as the degree of hearing loss increases, but significant individual variability in audibility for children with the same better-ear pure-tone average has been reported, primarily due to differences in the quality of the hearing aid fitting (McCreery et al., 2013). As noted above, the predicted pattern of worsening outcomes as degree of hearing loss increases has been observed in some studies (Sininger et al., 2010; Tomblin et al., 2015), but not in others (Wake et al., 2004). The introduction of early cochlear implantation for children with severe and profound hearing losses has also improved outcomes for children with the greatest degrees of unaided hearing. For these reasons, aided audibility is thought to be a more representative metric of the amount of access that a child has to their auditory environment, as it not only takes into account the child's degree of hearing loss, but also how well hearing aids are fitted.

Aided audibility is quantified most often using the Speech Intelligibility Index (SII) ANSI S3.5-1997, R2007), which is a standardized method of estimating the amount of speech that is audible to the listener. The SII is based on the long-term average speech spectrum (LTASS) and the listener's hearing thresholds from the audiogram converted to dB SPL. The LTASS represents the average energy as a function of level and frequency for speech averaged over time. Examples of the effects of increasing degrees of hearing loss on audibility can be observed in Figure 1–6. The SII is based on the idea that different frequency regions of the speech signal, known as bands, contribute different amounts of information to our understanding of speech.

Limited audibility will have a greater impact on speech understanding and development if it occurs for frequency bands that carry more speech information. For example, the frequencies between 500 to 2000 Hz contain more than half

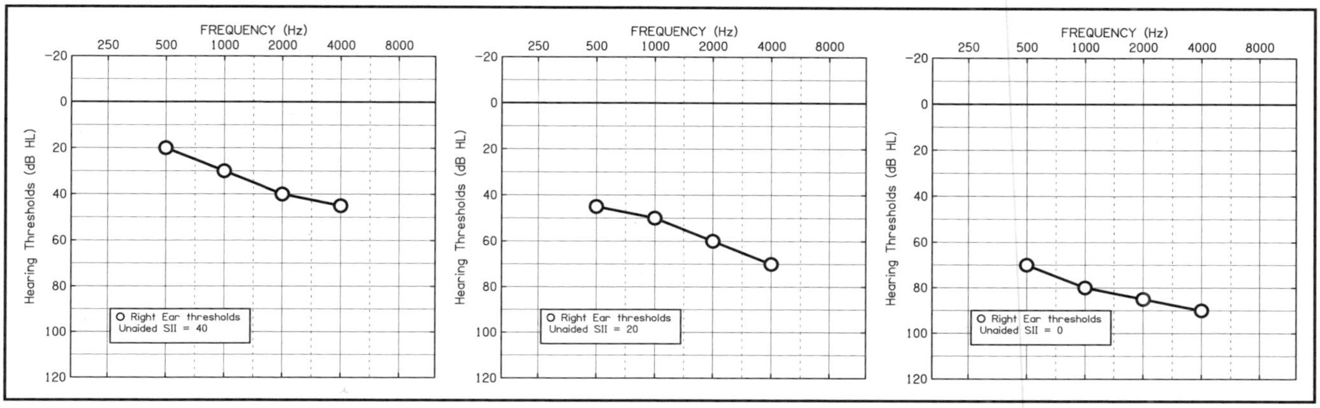


**FIGURE 1–6.** The degree of hearing loss has an influence on the unaided audibility for speech. Note that the unaided SII decreases as the degree of hearing loss increases from Panel A to Panel B to Panel C.

of the information needed to understand speech, and thus, these frequency bands are assigned greater weighting in audibility calculations. Loss of audibility in the frequency range from 500 to 2000 Hz will have a greater negative effect on audibility than loss of audibility at lower or higher frequencies. To calculate the SII, the proportion of the LTASS that is above the listener's audiometric threshold is calculated for each discrete frequency band. The audibility of each band is then multiplied times the importance factor for each band, which is a number designed to reflect the relative importance of that frequency band to speech understanding. The weighted audibility estimates for all of the frequency bands are added together to estimate audibility. The resulting SII is a number between 0 and 1, where 0 represents that none of the LTASS is audible to the listener and 1 represents full audibility of the entire LTASS.

The SII can be expressed in several different ways for clinical applications. If the SII is measured with an unamplified LTASS, the resulting estimate of audibility is known as an unaided SII. If the SII is measured with an LTASS that has been amplified through a hearing aid, the estimate of audibility is known as the aided SII. The SII is most often calculated for an average speech input, which is usually assumed to be the level of speech for an average talker who is one meter away. The resulting level for average speech without background noise is 60 or 65 dB SPL. The audibility for average speech is often based on these assumptions of listening in quiet and facing the talker of interest at a reasonable distance. Infants and children often communicate with conversational partners in background noise or at greater distances, so the actual amount of audibility that a child might have in a given listening situation in their daily life is likely to vary somewhat from this estimate. Additionally, infants and young children may experience nonstandard listening configurations that lead to better audibility than would be predicted from one meter away, including being cradled by a parent or held on the hip in close proximity to their parent or caregiver. In later chapters, tools to estimate the impact on audibility of these nonstandard listening situations experienced by children are reviewed. Despite the variance in audibility across different listening situations, the use of average speech in quiet gives a standardized comparison for estimating audibility for speech that can be consistently applied. In later chapters, the use of alternative assumptions for estimating audibility is discussed in greater detail.

Aided audibility is often measured as part of the hearing aid verification process. In these cases, the LTASS is measured either in the child's ear canal or in a coupler designed to mimic the characteristics of the ear canal. The amplified measurements of speech are compared to the listener's thresholds from the audiogram to calculate the aided SII. Most clinical verification equipment has the capability to automatically estimate aided and unaided audibility, which makes audibility easy to document for clinicians without having to understand or apply the underlying calculations. Aided audibility should be documented periodically as the child grows and develops to maintain the child's access over time. The process of hearing aid verification is discussed in greater detail in Chapter 4.

As a component of the model of cumulative auditory experience, aided audibility is considered to represent more than simply the child's access to the average LTASS. The benefits of good aided audibility are not only important for understanding speech, but are thought to reflect the amount of auditory experience that children are likely to accumulate over time when wearing their hearing aids. To analyze the effects of audibility over time, Tomblin and colleagues (2015) used longitudinal growth curve analyses to measure the impact of aided audibility on language development between 2 and 6 years of age. Interestingly, the effects of degree of hearing loss in the study were predictable and constant across the age range. Specifically, language ability followed an orderly pattern where language abilities decreased as degree of hearing loss increased and this relationship was consistent between 2 to 6 years of age. After taking into account the effect of degree of hearing loss, a different pattern was observed for the effect of audibility over time, as shown in Figure 1–7.

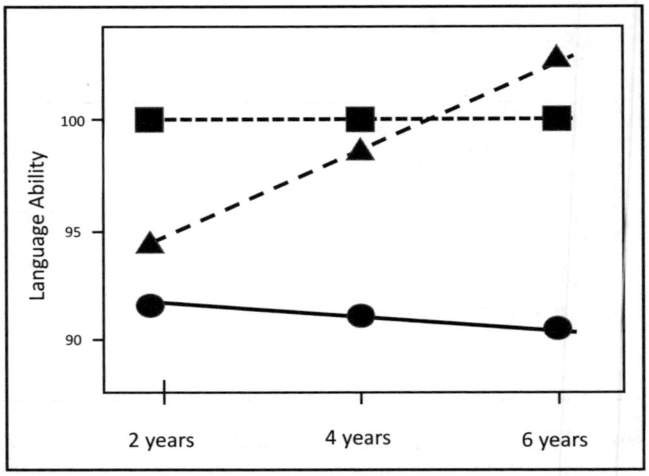


**FIGURE 1–7.** The relationship between aided audibility and language growth functions between 2 and 6 years of age for children in the Tomblin et al. (2015) study. Language standard score is plotted on the *y*-axis with age on the *x*-axis. The line with triangles represents children with the highest audibility improvements with their hearing aids, while the line with circles represents children with the poorest audibility improvement with their hearing aids. The dashed line with square symbols represents the average language scores for children with normal hearing.

At age 2, there were limited differences in language outcomes between children with the largest improvements in aided audibility and their peers with less improvement in aided audibility. By 6 years of age, however, the children with the largest gains in audibility from their hearing aids had made greater progress in language development over time than their peers with less improvement in audibility, resulting in nearly two-thirds of a standard deviation difference at that time point. This pattern suggests that children with greater improvement in audibility with hearing aids are likely to experience greater gains in language over time than peers with poorer audibility.

Aided audibility, therefore, can be used to reflect the child's auditory experiences and access to speech over time in the model of cumulative auditory experience. The pattern also highlights the importance of fitting hearing aids to provide consistent audibility by observing best practices for pediatric hearing aid fitting and verification. However, there are also some important caveats that should be considered related to using aided audibility as a metric for predicting developmental outcomes in children who are deaf or hard of hearing. Because the estimate of audibility is based on an acoustic measurement of speech, there is not a method at present for estimating a child's audibility when using a cochlear implant, because the output of the cochlear implant is electric. Therefore, real-ear acoustic measures cannot be conducted. Methods for generating estimates of audibility based on the aided pure-tone thresholds for listeners with cochlear implants have been proposed, but have not been shown to have the same explanatory power as estimates of aided audibility measured electroacoustically from hearing aids (Bass-Ringdahl, 2010). Furthermore, using the audibility for average speech to estimate difficulties associated with mild hearing loss may be difficult because children with mild hearing loss can have very similar audibility to children with normal hearing, and yet, may still experience deficits in development associated with hearing loss. Finally, as we will discuss in the next section, aided audibility for speech can only be a good predictor of outcomes if children wear their hearing aids. Aided audibility may overestimate developmental abilities for children with limited use of amplification, simply because the aided audibility does not accurately reflect what the child hears on a daily basis.

### *Hearing Aid Use*

Auditory experience of a child is diminished if hearing aids are not worn consistently. One of the first studies to evaluate device use in a group of children with hearing aids and a group of children with cochlear implants found that the children who wear hearing aids were at much greater risk for limited use during early childhood than children who wear cochlear implants (Marnane & Ching, 2015). This is presumably because children with hearing aids often have considerable residual hearing that they can rely on to a limited degree, whereas children with cochlear implants often have limited to no residual hearing without their device. Some studies, based solely on parent report of hearing aid use, suggest that many infants and young children who are hard of hearing are consistent hearing aid users (Ching et al., 2013), but studies that rely on automated data logging values to measure daily use suggest that parents are likely to overestimate hearing aid use time. Also, children with mild to severe hearing loss appear to struggle with hearing aid use. For example, Walker et al. (2015) found that infants average approximately 4.5 hours of hearing aid use per day, which is considerably less than the numbers of hours per day that most infants are awake. Given that the clinical recommendation for hearing aid use for children is often that the device be used for all waking hours (Muñoz et al., 2015), limited hearing aid use may contribute to persistent deficits in communication development for children who are hard of hearing.

If the amount and consistency of hearing aid use over time supports speech and language outcomes in children who are hard of hearing, it should follow that children who were more consistent hearing aid users would have stronger outcomes than peers with more limited hearing aid use, above and beyond the contributions of the child's audibility or degree of hearing loss. This hypothesis was confirmed in the aforementioned study by Tomblin et al. (2015). Again, looking at language development between 2 and 6 years of age, Tomblin and colleagues documented that children who had more than 10.5 hours of hearing aid use per day had language growth trajectories that exceeded those of children with less than 10.5 hours of hearing aid use per day. Further evidence is needed to confirm this effect, but the limited evidence suggests that there could be a requisite amount of hearing aid use that is needed to provide the cumulative auditory experience that children who are hard of hearing need to develop speech and language.

Although there is emerging evidence that hearing aid use is an important factor for predicting linguistic outcomes in children who are hard of hearing, there are also unresolved questions that further research should address. Although the Tomblin et al. (2015) paper found that the trajectories of language development were shallower for children with less than 10.5 hours of hearing aid use, the specific amount of hearing aid use that is necessary to support these developmental processes remains undetermined. Some might argue that the best clinical recommendation might be to suggest to parents that infants and children who are hard of hearing wear their hearing aids for all waking hours. Evidence suggests that few parents, particularly during infancy, can achieve this level of hearing aid use on a regular basis (Walker et al., 2015). Instead it may be more realistic to focus efforts on increasing hearing aid use during highly communicative periods of time to increase the child's exposure to language, rather than issuing blanket recommendations about simply increasing the quantity of time that a child wears their hearing aids. These issues are discussed in greater depth and detail in Chapter 5. Additionally, specific interventions that could be designed to support families in achieving more consistent hearing aid use will also be highlighted. In the next section, we will discuss the importance of the quality and quantity of language that a child is exposed to as the final component of cumulative auditory experience.

### *Linguistic Input*

The final component in the model of cumulative auditory experience put forth by Moeller and Tomblin (2015) is the quality and quantity of linguistic input that children receive. While audibility and hearing aid use are both important prerequisites for communication, children must also be exposed to high-quality linguistic experiences to drive their language and intellectual development. Much of the theoretical basis for this theory comes from the foundational work of developmental scientists Betty Hart and Todd Risley. Hart and Risley (1995) studied the importance of parent-child interactions in the child's development by observing these interactions in the homes of families. The first key finding from Hart and Risley was that differences in language abilities among children from varying socioeconomic backgrounds were associated with differences in the language that parents used to talk to their children. Hart and Risley documented that by four years of age, children from more affluent homes heard 45 million words, while children from the poorest economic backgrounds heard only 13 million words—a gap of over 30 million words. Follow-up studies indicated that the gap in the number of words helped to explain individual differences in language, and later, academic achievement among children in the study. These findings support the notion that differences in the quantity of language that children are exposed to can shape their development and have effects that persist into elementary school years.

The implications for children who have hearing loss are multifaceted. There are several ways in which the quantity and quality of linguistic input to the child could be affected by the child's hearing loss, as depicted in Figure 1–8.

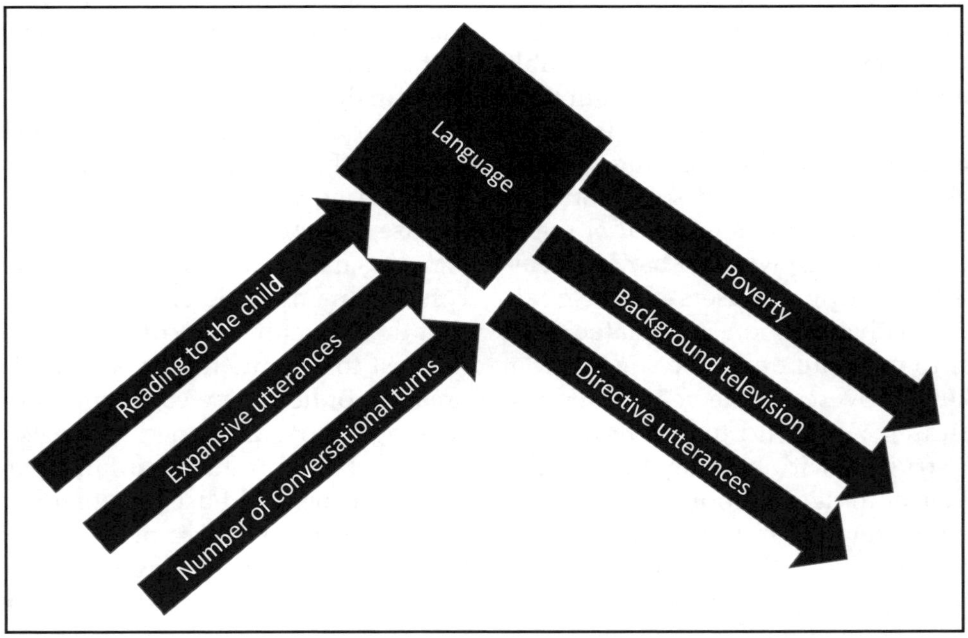


**FIGURE 1–8.** A depiction of the many factors that can influence the quantity and quality of language experience in children who wear hearing aids. Arrows that angle upward represent positive factors. Arrows that angle downward represent negative factors.

First, we expect that children who are deaf or hard of hearing might experience less access to language input, regardless of the quantity or quality provided by caregivers, because of reduced acoustic access to incidental learning. Research studies have shown that overhearing words that are unfamiliar can be a mechanism for learning new vocabulary (Akhtar, Jipson, & Callanan, 2001; Akhtar, 2005). Children who are hard of hearing may have reduced access for soft sounds or sounds originating from a distance, and have shown less ability to learn novel words through overhearing than peers with normal hearing (Moeller, 2010). Secondly, parents are adept at adjusting the level of their language to match that of their child. While this is an important adaptation that parents make automatically, it could also mean that children who have lower language abilities might be exposed to less complex linguistic input than peers with higher language abilities (Ambrose, Walker, Unflat-Berry, Oleson, & Moeller, 2015). The bidirectional nature of the parent's language use and the child's language abilities mean that children who experience delays in communication might experience a confounding effect of limited linguistic input from parents and caregivers who have adapted their communication to match their child's skills. Finally, the socioeconomic gap in exposure to the quantity of words would still be expected to be a factor among children who are hard of hearing, with children who are hard of hearing who have the lowest socioeconomic status experiencing an additional barrier to their language development beyond reduced auditory access.

Recent research has supported the potential for all three of these factors to influence the linguistic environment and language learning in children who are hard of hearing. In one study, Ambrose, VanDam, and Moeller (2014) examined the effect that exposure to electronic media, such as having the television on in the background, had on the linguistic input to a group of children with normal hearing and a group of children with hearing loss. The study used a small body-worn recording device that generated full-day recordings of the child in their home environment. Software was used to analyze the audio recordings to estimate the number of words each child heard and the number of conversational turns with adults. The software was also able to classify the child's auditory environment as containing background noise, including background television or electronic media. Greater number of hours of exposure to background electronic media in the home was associated with lower receptive language outcomes at two years of age. An exploration of the quantity of conversational turns between parents and their children from the automated recording system found that background television reduced the number of conversational turns between parents and children regardless of hearing status. The reduced conversational turns helped to explain the reduced language abilities in children with more background television in their home environments. In this study, there did not appear to be a difference between children with normal hearing and children who were hard of hearing in terms of the quantity of language input from parents overall. Additionally, differences in language input across different levels of socioeconomic status were also not evident. These results further support the link between parent input and language development, but did not support predictions of differential vulnerability for children with hearing loss.

In another study by the same researchers, an experimental task, referred to as the Art Gallery task, was used to observe parent-child interactions. In this task, different pictures are placed around a room. The parents are instructed to take their child to each picture and discuss the picture with their child. The result of the Art Gallery interaction was a structured interaction between the parent and their child that lasted approximately 30 minutes. The study included groups of parents and children with normal hearing and parents and children with hearing loss. The main outcome measures were the number of words and conversational turns in a five-minute sample of the parent-child interaction. However, the researchers also documented the type of interactions parents had with their children. In addition to coding the length of utterances from parents and the number of different words that parents used, parent responses to the child were coded as being directive or more expansive. Directive utterances were used to categorize parent responses that directed the child to do something (e.g., "Say car."). Expansive utterances were used to categorize utterances where parents provided their child with an opportunity to expand on the parent's utterance, such as open-ended questions (e.g., "What do you like about fishing?"). The task was completed at 18 months and again at 3 years of age. Unlike the previous study, parents of children with normal hearing used more words, longer utterances, and fewer directives than parents of children who were hard of hearing. These differences in language input at 18 months of age were predictive of language abilities at 3 years of age.

As noted previously, these results should not be taken as evidence that parents of children who are deaf or hard of hearing are less capable or talk less to their children than parents of children with normal hearing or that they use less complex language on purpose. These group differences between parents of children with normal hearing and parents of children who are hard of hearing likely reflect parents' attempts to adapt their language to match their child's abilities. However, this represents a bit of a chicken or egg problem in terms of determining whether the child's language is driving the parents' responsiveness or the parents' language use is driving the child's language development. In reality, parent-child interactions probably represent a bidirectional interaction, where both the parent's and child's language shape the interaction. Intervention strategies designed to increase the quantity and quality of parent linguistic input may be one way to use intervention to impact the linguistic environments of children who are deaf or hard of hearing in a positive way.

## Interactions Between Malleable and Nonmalleable Factors

Table 1–2 displays a summary of malleable and nonmalleable factors. As noted in the example of the interaction between the child's degree of hearing loss and the aided audibility for speech, malleable and nonmalleable factors can interact in ways that can influence the development of children who are hard of hearing who wear hearing aids. The goal of this interplay between these factors is to demonstrate that these aspects of the child's development do not occur in isolation and can lead to complex patterns of outcomes.

One practical example of how these factors can interact is related to the relationship between age of identification and language outcomes for children who are hard of hearing. Much of the early work to support the implementation of universal newborn hearing screening and early intervention programs was based on research that showed that earlier ages of identification of hearing loss, earlier ages of amplification, and earlier ages of enrollment in early intervention were beneficial to children's outcomes (e.g., Moeller, 2000; Yoshinaga-Itano et al., 1998). This research is highly influential because the results are intuitive and fit with our expectations that if hear-

**Table 1–2.** Summary of Malleable and Nonmalleable Factors That Influence Outcomes of Children with Hearing Loss

| *Malleable Factors* | *Nonmalleable Factors* |
|---|---|
| Aided audibility (McCreery et al., 2013, 2015) | Degree of hearing loss (e.g., Davis et al., 1986; Moeller, 2000; Wake et al., 2004) |
| Consistency of daily hearing aid use (Walker et al., 2013, 2015) | Age of identification/hearing aid fitting/intervention (e.g., Calderon & Naidu, 1999; Pimperton et al., 2016) |
| Quantity and quality of linguistic input (Ambrose et al., 2015) | Socioeconomic status (e.g., Ching et al., 2013; Tomblin et al., 2014) |
| | Additional disabilities (Ching et al., 2013) |
| | Gender (Meinzen-Derr et al., 2010) |

ing loss affects developmental processes, providing intervention at earlier ages will be advantageous over providing intervention at later ages. While early identification and intervention are fundamentally important, overgeneralizing these concepts without considering other potential factors can lead to false conclusions. For example, in the seminal Moeller (2000) paper that demonstrated advantages for children who enrolled in intervention within the first year of life, an interaction was also observed with ratings of parental involvement. Specifically, parents who had higher ratings of involvement showed smaller delays in communication development as the age of enrollment in intervention increased. This demonstrated that some of the effects of later identification could be mitigated through parental involvement. Parents of children who are identified with hearing loss at later ages or enrolled in services at later ages may feel guilty or helpless if the message that earlier intervention is always better is not qualified with the caveat that parental involvement can also be protective against delays. Similarly, Tomblin et al. (2015) reported that children who were identified after 12 or 18 months of age caught up in language development with peers who had earlier ages of identification by age 6, assuming that the later-identified children were provided with well-fit hearing aids that were worn consistently and enrolled in intervention programs. These findings and others highlight the need to consider interactions between malleable and nonmalleable factors when thinking about the variables that influence development in children who are hard of hearing who wear hearing aids.

Nonmalleable factors, such as degree of hearing loss, socioeconomic status, and age of enrollment in intervention, can be discouraging for parents, caregivers, and service providers of children who are hard of hearing, primarily because these factors cannot be easily altered. By considering the nonmalleable factors in conjunction with malleable factors (i.e., providing hearing aids that make speech audible, supporting consistent use, and providing a rich and consistent linguistic environment), professionals and parents can feel empowered to play a positive role in the intervention process for children who have hearing loss. Focusing on those factors that can be influenced by and changed through intervention will provide the best opportunity to maximize development in this population by increasing cumulative auditory experience and understanding the additional factors that can influence those processes.

## CONCLUSION

In this chapter, we have introduced a theoretical foundation for the rest of the text, known as the model of cumulative auditory experience. The model helps to describe how hearing loss negatively affects communication development in children who have hearing loss, and the types of interventions that can be used to minimize those negative effects. Nonmalleable factors such as degree of hearing loss, age of identification, hearing aid fitting, enrollment in intervention, and others, are important for understanding how hearing loss can influence development and for targeting intervention strategies for children who are at the greatest developmental risk. Malleable factors, including the audibility of speech through hearing aids, consistent hearing aid use, and a high-quality language environment, have also been shown to influence developmental outcomes in children who are hard of hearing, but can be targeted for improvement by intervention. Clinicians should also consider potential interactions between malleable and nonmalleable factors because communication development in children who are hard of hearing is inherently complex. The following chapters will provide a clinical framework, starting from the diagnosis of hearing loss, selection and fitting of amplification, maximizing hearing aid use, and documenting outcomes to monitor progress. Additional chapters will provide readers with background in hearing assistance technology and connectivity for children who wear hearing aids, as well as special populations of children with hearing loss, including mild and unilateral hearing loss, and auditory neuropathy spectrum disorder, as well as case examples. The chapters that follow provide a comprehensive clinical approach for incorporating the model of cumulative auditory experience into practice.

## REFERENCES


Akhtar, N. (2005). The robustness of learning through overhearing. *Developmental Science, 8*(2), 199–209.

Akhtar, N., Jipson, J., & Callanan, M. A. (2001). Learning words through overhearing. *Child Development, 72*(2), 416–430.

Ambrose, S. E., VanDam, M., & Moeller, M. P. (2014). Linguistic input, electronic media, and communication outcomes of toddlers with hearing loss. *Ear and Hearing, 35*(2), 139–147.

Ambrose, S. E., Walker, E. A., Unflat-Berry, L. M., Oleson, J. J., & Moeller, M. P. (2015). Quantity and quality of caregivers' linguistic input to 18-month and 3-year-old children who are hard of hearing. *Ear and Hearing, 36*, 48S–59S.

American National Standards Institute (ANSI). (1997). S3. 5–1997. *Methods for the calculation of the speech intelligibility index*. New York, NY: Author.

Bass-Ringdahl, S. M. (2010). The relationship of audibility and the development of canonical babbling in young children with hearing impairment. *Journal of Deaf Studies and Deaf Education, 15*(3), 287–310.

Blamey, P. J., Sarant, J. Z., Paatsch, L. E., Barry, J. G., Bow, C. P., Wales, R. J., . . . Tooher, R. (2001). Relationships among speech perception, production, language, hearing loss, and age in children with impaired hearing. *Journal of Speech, Language, and Hearing Research, 44*(2), 264–285.

Bornstein, M. H., & Bradley, R. H. (Eds.). (2014). *Socioeconomic status, parenting, and child development*. New York, NY: Routledge.

Bradley, R. H., & Corwyn, R. F. (2002). Socioeconomic status and child development. *Annual Review of Psychology, 53*(1), 371–399.

Calderon, R., & Naidu, S. (1999). Further support for the benefits of early identification and intervention for children with hearing loss. *Volta Review, 100*(5), 53–84.

Ching, T. Y., Crowe, K., Martin, V., Day, J., Mahler, N., Youn, S., . . . Orsini, J. (2010). Language development and everyday functioning of children with hearing loss assessed at 3 years of age. *International Journal of Speech-Language Pathology, 12*(2), 124–131.

Ching, T. Y., Dillon, H., Marnane, V., Hou, S., Day, J., Seeto, M., . . . Zhang, V. (2013). Outcomes of early- and late-identified children at 3 years of age: Findings from a prospective population-based study. *Ear and Hearing, 34*(5), 535–552.

Davidson, L. S., & Skinner, M. W. (2006). Audibility and speech perception of children using wide dynamic range compression hearing aids. *American Journal of Audiology, 15*(2), 141–153.

Davis, J. M., Elfenbein, J., Schum, R., & Bentler, R. A. (1986). Effects of mild and moderate hearing impairments on language, educational, and psychosocial behavior of children. *Journal of Speech and Hearing Disorders, 51*(1), 53–62.

DeCasper, A. J., & Fifer, W. P. (1980). Of human bonding: Newborns prefer their mothers' voices. *Science, 208*(4448), 1174–1176.

Fitzpatrick, E. M., Crawford, L., Ni, A., & Durieux-Smith, A. (2011). A descriptive analysis of language and speech skills in 4- to 5-yr-old children with hearing loss. *Ear and Hearing, 32*(5), 605–616.

Fitzpatrick, E., Durieux-Smith, A., Eriks-Brophy, A., Olds, J., & Gaines, R. (2007). The impact of newborn hearing screening on communication development. *Journal of Medical Screening, 14*(3), 123–131.

Gallaudet Research Institute. (2008). *Regional and national summary report of data from the 2007–08 annual survey of deaf and hard of hearing children and youth*. Washington, DC: Author.

Garcia-Sierra, A., Rivera-Gaxiola, M., Percaccio, C. R., Conboy, B. T., Romo, H., Klarman, L., . . . Kuhl, P. K. (2011). Bilingual language learning: An ERP study relating early brain responses to speech, language input, and later word production. *Journal of Phonetics, 39*(4), 546–557.

Gilbertson, M., & Kamhi, A. G. (1995). Novel word learning in children with hearing impairment. *Journal of Speech, Language, and Hearing Research, 38*(3), 630–642.

Hart, B., & Risley, T. R. (1995). *Meaningful differences in the everyday experience of young American children*. Baltimore, MD: Paul H Brookes.

Hoff, E. (2006). How social contexts support and shape language development. *Developmental Review, 26*(1), 55–88.

Holte, L., Walker, E., Oleson, J., Spratford, M., Moeller, M. P., Roush, P., . . . Tomblin, J. B. (2012). Factors influencing follow-up to newborn hearing screening for infants who are hard of hearing. *American Journal of Audiology, 21*(2), 163–174.

Hood, H. B. (1949). A preliminary survey of some mental abilities of deaf children. *British Journal of Educational Psychology, 19*(3), 210–219.

Huttenlocher, J., Haight, W., Bryk, A., Seltzer, M., & Lyons, T. (1991). Early vocabulary growth: Relation to language input and gender. *Developmental Psychology, 27*(2), 236–248.

Kennedy, C. R., McCann, D. C., Campbell, M. J., Law, C. M., Mullee, M., Petrou, S., . . . Stevenson, J. (2006). Language ability after early detection of permanent childhood hearing impairment. *New England Journal of Medicine, 354*(20), 2131–2141.

Liu, C. L., Farrell, J., MacNeil, J. R., Stone, S., & Barfield, W. (2008). Evaluating loss to follow-up in newborn hearing screening in Massachusetts. *Pediatrics, 121*(2), e335–e343.

Marnane, V., & Ching, T. Y. (2015). Hearing aid and cochlear implant use in children with hearing loss at three years of age: Predictors of use and predictors of changes in use. *International Journal of Audiology, 54*(8), 544–551.

McCreery, R. W., Bentler, R. A., & Roush, P. A. (2013). The characteristics of hearing aid fittings in infants and young children. *Ear and Hearing, 34*(6), 701–710.

McCreery, R. W., Walker, E. A., Spratford, M., Oleson, J., Bentler, R., Holte, L., & Roush, P. (2015). Speech recognition and parent ratings from auditory development questionnaires in children who are hard of hearing. *Ear and Hearing, 36*, 60S–75S.

Mehler, J., Bertoncini, J., Barrière, M., & Jassik-Gerschenfeld, D. (1978). Infant recognition of mother's voice. *Perception, 7*(5), 491–497.

Meinzen-Derr, J., Wiley, S., Grether, S., & Choo, D. I. (2010). Language performance in children with cochlear implants and additional disabilities. *Laryngoscope, 120*(2), 405–413.

Moeller, M. P. (2000). Early intervention and language development in children who are deaf and hard of hearing. *Pediatrics, 106*(3), e43–e43.

Moeller, M. P. (2010). Optimizing early word learning in infants with hearing loss. *Audiology Today, 22*, 19–27.

Moeller, M. P., & Tomblin, J. B. (2015). An introduction to the Outcomes of Children with Hearing Loss study. *Ear and Hearing, 36*, 4S–13S.

Moeller, M. P., Tomblin, J. B., & the OCHL Collaboration. (2015). Afterword: Lessons learned about multi-center research collaboration. *Ear and Hearing, 36*, 99S–101S.

Muñoz, K., Olson, W. A., Twohig, M. P., Preston, E., Blaiser, K., & White, K. R. (2015). Pediatric hearing aid use: Parent-reported challenges. *Ear and Hearing, 36*(2), 279–287.

Myklebust, H. R. (1960). *The psychology of deafness: Sensory deprivation, learning, and adjustment*. Oxford, UK: Grune & Stratton.

Nelson, H. D., Bougatsos, C., & Nygren, P. (2008). Universal newborn hearing screening: Systematic review to update the 2001 US Preventive Services Task Force Recommendation. *Pediatrics, 122*(1), e266–e276.

Pimperton, H., Blythe, H., Kreppner, J., Mahon, M., Peacock, J. L., Stevenson, J., . . . Kennedy, C. R. (2016). The impact of universal newborn hearing screening on long-term literacy outcomes: A prospective cohort study. *Archives of Disease in Childhood, 101*(1), 9–15.

Pimperton, H., & Kennedy, C. R. (2012). The impact of early identification of permanent childhood hearing impairment on speech and language outcomes. *Archives of Disease in Childhood, 97*, 648–653.

Scollie, S., Seewald, R., Cornelisse, L., Moodie, S., Bagatto, M., Laurnagaray, D., . . . Pumford, J. (2005). The desired sensation level multistage input/output algorithm. *Trends in Amplification, 9*(4), 159–197.

Sharma, A., Dorman, M. F., & Kral, A. (2005). The influence of a sensitive period on central auditory development in children with unilateral and bilateral cochlear implants. *Hearing Research, 203*(1), 134–143.

Sininger, Y. S., Grimes, A., & Christensen, E. (2010). Auditory development in early amplified children: Factors influencing auditory-based communication outcomes in children with hearing loss. *Ear and Hearing, 31*(2), 166–185.

Tomblin, J. B., Harrison, M., Ambrose, S. E., Walker, E. A., Oleson, J. J., & Moeller, M. P. (2015). Language outcomes in young children with mild to severe hearing loss. *Ear and Hearing, 36*, 76S–91S.

Tomblin, J. B., Oleson, J. J., Ambrose, S. E., Walker, E., & Moeller, M. P. (2014). The influence of hearing aids on the speech and language development of children with hearing loss. *JAMA Otolaryngology-Head and Neck Surgery, 140*(5), 403–409.

Wake, M., Hughes, E. K., Poulakis, Z., Collins, C., & Rickards, F. W. (2004). Outcomes of children with mild-profound congenital hearing loss at 7 to 8 years: A population study. *Ear and Hearing, 25*(1), 1–8.

Walker, E. A., Holte, L., McCreery, R. W., Spratford, M., Page, T., & Moeller, M. P. (2015). The influence of hearing aid use on outcomes of children with mild hearing loss. *Journal of Speech, Language, and Hearing Research, 58*(5), 1611–1625.

Walker, E. A., Holte, L., Spratford, M., Oleson, J., Welhaven, A., & Harrison, M. (2014). Timeliness of service delivery for children with later-identified mild-to-severe hearing loss. *American Journal of Audiology, 23*(1), 116–128.

Walker, E. A., Spratford, M., Moeller, M. P., Oleson, J., Ou, H., Roush, P., & Jacobs, S. (2013). Predictors of hearing aid use time in children with mild-to-severe hearing loss. *Language, Speech, and Hearing Services in Schools, 44*(1), 73–88.

Werker, J. F., & Tees, R. C. (1984). Cross-language speech perception: Evidence for perceptual reorganization during the first year of life. *Infant Behavior and Development, 7*(1), 49–63.

Werker, J. F., & Yeung, H. H. (2005). Infant speech perception bootstraps word learning. *Trends in Cognitive Sciences*, *9*(11), 519–527.

Wiley, S., Arjmand, E., & Dixon, M. (2011). Findings from multidisciplinary evaluation of children with permanent hearing loss. *International Journal of Pediatric Otorhinolaryngology, 75*(8), 1040–1044.

Wiley, S., Jahnke, M., Meinzen-Derr, J., & Choo, D. (2005). Perceived qualitative benefits of cochlear implants in children with multi-handicaps. *International Journal of Pediatric Otorhinolaryngology*, *69*(6), 791–798.

Yoshikawa, H., Aber, J. L., & Beardslee, W. R. (2012). The effects of poverty on the mental, emotional, and behavioral health of children and youth: Implications for prevention. *American Psychologist*, *67*(4), 272–287.

Yoshinaga-Itano, C., Coulter, D. K., & Thomson, V. (2000). The Colorado Newborn Hearing Screening Project: Effects on speech and language development for children with hearing loss. *Journal of Perinatology, 20*(8), S132–S137.

Yoshinaga-Itano, C., Sedey, A. L., Coulter, D. K., & Mehl, A. L. (1998). Language of early- and later-identified children with hearing loss. *Pediatrics, 102*(5), 1161–1171.

# 2

# Diagnosis of Hearing Loss: A Foundation for Pediatric Amplification

*Ryan W. McCreery and Elizabeth A. Walker*

## INTRODUCTION

The first step in providing early amplification for children with hearing loss is diagnosis. Universal newborn hearing screening in many countries can mean that the age of diagnosis of hearing loss can be in the first few months of life. Diagnostic techniques must be available to identify the type, degree, and configuration of hearing loss in order to accurately prescribe amplification, help to determine whether the hearing loss is permanent or temporary, and aid in the search for potential etiologies that may reveal other underlying medical conditions that are associated with hearing loss. Inaccurate diagnosis can delay the provision of amplification and intervention, lead to inappropriate medical recommendations and unnecessary evaluations, as well as create inaccuracies in the prescription of amplification that limit audibility or put the child at risk for over-amplification. In this chapter, the diagnostic process that provides clinicians with high-quality information to proceed with amplification during infancy is reviewed. The process of selecting the appropriate diagnostic tests based on sensitivity and specificity is highlighted. An overview of universal newborn hearing screening programs and the types of hearing loss that they are designed to identify will set a foundation for the types of tests that will be used to diagnose hearing loss for children who fail newborn hearing screening. The appropriate assessments for diagnosis of hearing loss vary based on the developmental age of the child. The diagnostic test battery that includes immittance and otoacoustic emissions is valuable for any age. Auditory brainstem response is discussed as the basis for diagnosis of hearing loss in infants, while developmentally appropriate methods of behavioral assessment will serve as the primary means of determining audiometric threshold in older children. Protocols and guidelines for continued audiological assessment are also important for monitoring changes in hearing over time.

## ASSESSING TEST PERFORMANCE

Decisions about what tests should be used in the process of screening for and diagnosing hearing loss in infants and children should be based on objective data about how well those tests can identify hearing loss. The accuracy of screening and diagnostic tests for identifying a specific condition can be quantified in two dimensions: sensitivity and specificity. Sensitivity is how accurately a test correctly identifies a target condition (i.e., true positives). Specificity, on the other hand, is how accurately a test correctly excludes individuals without the target condition (i.e., true negatives). A good clinical screening or diagnostic test maximizes sensitivity and specificity. It is important to consider that nearly all of the tests used by audiologists to diagnose hearing loss do not have perfect sensitivity or specificity. Thus, clinicians must weigh the impact of false positives, individuals without the condition who are erroneously identified as having the condition by the test, and false negatives, where individuals with the condition are erroneously identified as not having the condition. It is generally agreed that the cost of missing a case of hearing loss has a much larger negative impact than referring a child with normal hearing for further assessment to rule out hearing loss. Thus, many audiological tests have higher false positive rates in order to ensure that the number of false negatives remains low.

Figure 2–1 shows an illustrative example of a specific test designed to identify middle ear dysfunction in children. The population being tested is divided into children with middle ear dysfunction and children without middle ear dysfunction, based on a gold standard test. The gold standard test for any condition is generally the test that is considered the best at diagnosing a specific condition. In the case of the middle ear dysfunction, the gold standard is surgically confirmed middle ear dysfunction. The test performance of the test of middle ear function, 1000 Hz tympanometry, was conducted on a group of children who were about to undergo surgery to place tympanostomy tubes due to chronic middle ear effusion. This allowed the test measure to be conducted immediately before a surgical procedure where the condition of the middle ear could be directly examined under microscopy. Test performance data are only as accurate as the gold standard comparison being conducted. In this example, the test has sensitivity of 0.80, indicating that 80% of the children with middle ear dysfunction were correctly identified as having middle ear dysfunction. The specificity was 0.90, indicating that 90% of the children without middle ear dysfunction were correctly identified as having normal middle ear function by the test. The false positive rate would be the 10% of individuals with normal middle ear function who were identified as having middle ear dysfunction and the false negative rate would be the 20% of

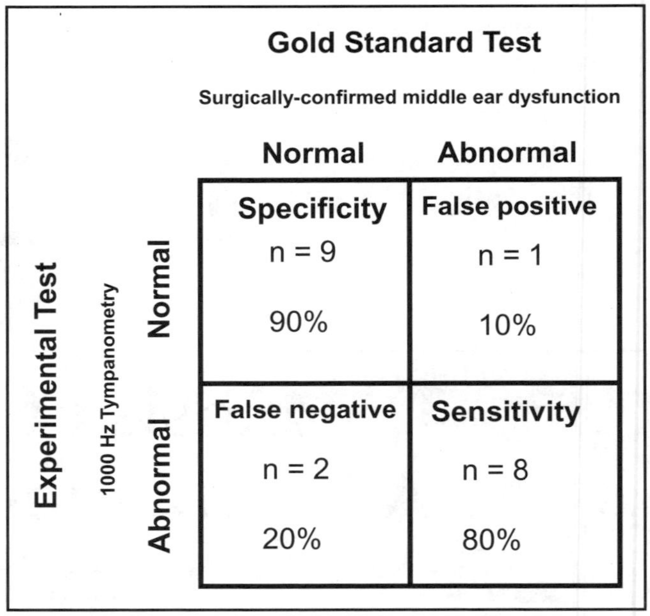


**FIGURE 2–1.** Calculating test performance for a test of middle ear dysfunction. Test performance is determined by comparing the results from any test to a gold standard test.

children with middle ear dysfunction that the test classified as being normal. This example illustrates the trade-offs between sensitivity and specificity.

Test performance data are not only useful in comparing different tests, but also comparing the effects of altering specific test criteria on the accuracy of a test. Figure 2–2 shows test performance data for two specific criteria for a "pass" result on an otoacoustic emissions (OAE) screening. In one case, the individual must have a signal-to-noise ratio of +6 dB between the level of the OAE and the noise floor to pass the test. In the other case, the individual must have a signal-to-noise ratio of +12 dB to pass. The 12 dB pass criterion will have greater sensitivity for detecting hearing loss because most ears with hearing loss will not produce an OAE with that high of an SNR. The data in the figure from Gorga et al. (2002) support that. There are also a portion of individuals with normal hearing who are unable to produce an OAE with a 12 dB signal-to-noise ratio, so that false positive rate for that criterion is higher than for the 6 dB criterion. Generally, changing the parameters of a test to improve the sensitivity will generally have the effect of decreasing specificity. Clinicians must consider the population that is being tested and the desired goals of the screening process when selecting the optimal test criteria that balance sensitivity and specificity.

## METHODS OF UNIVERSAL NEWBORN HEARING SCREENING

The ability to screen hearing in infants within the first few hours of life has dramatically lowered the age that hearing loss can be identified. An understanding of the methods of newborn hearing screening and the types of hearing loss that are likely to be identified by these methods is important for developing diagnostic protocols for diagnosis of hearing loss in infants. In most places, newborn hearing screening is conducted in the hospital by nurses or trained volunteers. The two most frequently used types of assessments for

**Gold Standard Test**

Experimental Test: DPOAE at 4 kHz with 6 dB SNR

| | Behavioral audiogram at 4 kHz: Normal | Behavioral audiogram at 4 kHz: Abnormal |
|---|---|---|
| Normal | Specificity<br>n = 99<br>99% | False positive<br>n = 1<br>1% |
| Abnormal | False negative<br>n = 39<br>39% | Sensitivity<br>n = 61<br>61% |

DPOAE at 4 kHz with 12 dB SNR

| | Behavioral audiogram at 4 kHz: Normal | Behavioral audiogram at 4 kHz: Abnormal |
|---|---|---|
| Normal | Specificity<br>n = 98<br>98% | False positive<br>n = 2<br>2% |
| Abnormal | False negative<br>n = 29<br>29% | Sensitivity<br>n = 71<br>71% |

**FIGURE 2–2.** A comparison of test performance for two different signal-to-noise ratio (SNR) criteria (6 dB at left and 12 dB at right) for distortion-product otoacoustic emissions (DPOAE) for predicting normal behavioral thresholds at 4 kHz. Note that the more stringent SNR criterion does not increase the false positive rate, but does improve the sensitivity for DPOAEs.

universal newborn hearing screening are (1) automated otoacoustic emissions (AOAE) and (2) automated auditory brainstem response (AABR). Both methods have gained acceptance in newborn hearing screening programs based on reasonable test performance and ease of administration.

Both OAE and ABR assessment methods are used in the diagnostic process, but the automated screening versions of these tests are distinctive from the diagnostic versions in several important ways. Screening versions of these tests are automated to avoid the requirement that a trained expert, such as an audiologist, needs to interpret the results of the test. For this reason, both AOAE and AABR equipment have algorithms that automatically determine whether or not the results are consistent with normal hearing, known as a "Pass" result, or cannot rule out the presence of hearing loss, known as a "Refer" result. The automated screening versions of these tests cannot be used to determine the amount or type of hearing loss, only that further diagnostic testing is warranted to rule out the presence of hearing loss. This is an important factor to remember when discussing the results of newborn hearing screening tests with parents, who may assume that a "Refer" result on a newborn hearing screening indicates that hearing loss is certainly present, or even that the child may be deaf. Clinicians must strike a balance between reassuring parents that screening tests are different than diagnostic tests in terms of the conclusions that can be made, but also stress the need for diagnostic assessment if an infant has a "Refer" result in one or both ears.

The AOAE and AABR screening tests also differ from the diagnostic versions in terms of the frequency specificity of the tests. In most cases, the screening tests primarily assess hearing above 2000 Hz to identify significant high-frequency hearing loss, whereas diagnostic versions discussed later in the chapter can assess roughly the same range as the audiogram for an ABR and both mid- and high-frequency hearing for OAE. The consequence of assessing a more limited frequency range for screening assessments is that children with low-frequency hearing loss and regions of normal high-frequency hearing may not be identified through newborn hearing screening programs. This decision to focus on high-frequency hearing regions is based on the fact that most children with significant hearing losses have high-frequency hearing loss (Pittman & Stelmachowicz, 2003). Additionally, sound conduction through the middle ear of infants is less efficient at low-frequencies (Werner, Levi, & Keefe, 2010) and may be more likely to be affected by the presence of middle ear fluid left over from being in the womb (Sanford et al., 2009). Both of these factors related to the middle ear system could lead to false positive screening results (infants with normal hearing identified as having hearing loss) if newborn hearing screening tests included lower frequencies.

Another potential group of children who are not likely to be identified by screening AOAE and AABR assessments are children with mild degrees of hearing loss. Children with mild loss can have present OAEs (Gorga et al., 1997). Most screening AABR equipment sets a test level of 35 dB nHL, which means that children with mild hearing loss can have a "Pass" result on an AABR assessment. As with the frequency range, there were justifications for selecting this level as the cutoff for newborn hearing screening. The first limitation is related to the noise in the test environments where newborn hearing screening is conducted. Unlike standard audiometric tests that are conducted in sound-treated audiometric test booths that meet minimum acoustical standards, newborn hearing screening tests are conducted in hospital rooms, nurseries, and other environments where the noise levels are often considerably higher. These acoustic limitations mean that in some cases, mild hearing loss cannot be easily differentiated from normal hearing.

Furthermore, there is a trade-off between sensitivity, the ability for screening tests to accurately identify children with hearing loss, and specificity, the ability for screening tests to accurately exclude children with normal hearing. Attempts to increase the sensitivity of newborn hearing screening tests to more accurately identify children with mild hearing loss have typically come at the cost of significantly higher false positive rates for children with normal hearing (as noted in the previous section). Whereas some might argue that the risks of mild hearing loss to development warrant the increase in false positive rate, others have argued that having a screening assessment where a large portion of infants with normal hearing fail the test has negative consequences (Bess & Paradise, 1994). Having a large number of infants with normal hearing who fail their hearing screening not only creates unnecessary costs related to follow-up testing and parental worry and anxiety, but also erodes trust and confidence from parents and medical professionals about the accuracy of the test. Thus, the 35 dB HL threshold level that may be the cutoff for newborn hearing screening assessments represents a trade-off between identifying the children with the most significant hearing losses and minimizing the number of infants with normal hearing who receive a "Refer" result.

Even after efforts to balance the sensitivity and specificity of tests used for newborn hearing screening, the number of infants who have a "Refer" result on newborn hearing screening is an order of magnitude larger than the prevalence of hearing loss at birth. Prevalence estimates put the number of infants born with hearing loss in the United States at 1 to 2 per 1000 live births (Joint Committee on Infant Hearing, 2007), but the referral rate for a newborn hearing screening program is considered acceptable at 2 to 3%. In this case, 10 infants with normal hearing will be referred for diagnostic assessment for every one infant with hearing loss. Efforts are currently underway to develop newer protocols that would increase the specificity of universal newborn hearing screening programs without sacrificing sensitivity (Sanford et al., 2009).

## Automated Otoacoustic Emissions

OAEs are sounds that are produced by the outer hair cells of the cochlea when those cells receive incoming auditory stimulation. In infants who are only a few hours old, OAEs can be measured noninvasively by placing a probe in the ear canal. Because most people with normal hearing have measurable OAEs and damage to the cochlear outer hair cells is a common feature for most types of sensorineural hearing loss, OAEs have reasonable test performance when used for newborn hearing screening, with sensitivity values around 0.80 and specificity around 0.90 in infants (Gorga et al., 2002). AOAE tests require no interpretation of results by the person administering the test. The tester simply places the probe in the infant's ear canal, starts the test and waits for the equipment to provide a "Pass" or "Refer" result. Most screening protocols for AOAE assessment require that OAE responses be measured at three out of four test frequencies (usually between 2000–6000 Hz) for an ear to receive a Pass result.

AOAE screening tests have several advantages as a newborn hearing screening tool. As noted above, AOAEs require no formal knowledge of hearing assessment to administer. The tester must only be trained on how to properly insert the probe into the ear safely, and how to start the test. Compared to AABR as a screening test, which is discussed in the next section, the initial cost of equipment and disposable eartips are considerably less for AOAE. Most AOAE equipment costs less than $10,000 and disposable ear tips for the probe are less than $1 per baby. These factors have led many hospitals to adopt AOAE as their primary method of newborn hearing screening.

The relative disadvantages of AOAEs are also important to note. Because OAEs require an eliciting stimulus to travel through the ear canal and middle ear to reach the cochlea and for the emission to travel back through the middle ear and ear canal to be measured by the probe, debris in the ear canal or fluid in the middle ear space can cause OAEs to be absent or reduced, even if a child has normal hearing. Because newborn infants have been in a fluid environment in the womb during gestation, they may have vernix or other debris in the ear canal, as well as fluid in the middle ear space, particularly within the first few hours of birth. This phenomenon leads to a higher failure rate for AOAE screenings conducted closer to the infant's birth that decreases over the first 48 hours of life (Sanford et al., 2009). Internal sources of noise, such as sucking or crying, and external sources of noise, such as other infants crying or room noise, can also affect the ability to measure AOAEs in the newborn hearing screening environment. As a result of these factors, the refer rate for AOAE is higher than it is for AABR screening. The cost savings associated with using AOAE can often be offset by the need for additional diagnostic tests for infants who have false positive results on AOAE tests. Another disadvantage of AOAEs relates to the site of lesion of the hearing loss. Because AOAEs only require function up to the level of the cochlear outer hair cells, infants with neural hearing loss, such as those with auditory neuropathy spectrum disorder, will often pass newborn hearing screening if AOAE is the only assessment that is used.

Overall, AOAE assessment is a frequently used assessment tool in newborn hearing screening programs. Because the incidence of neural hearing loss among babies born into a well-baby nursery is extremely low (Berg, Prieve, Serpanos, & Wheaton, 2011), AOAEs are most frequently used in those cases. In the diagnostic process following a Refer result on an AOAE test, the presence of debris in the ear canal or fluid in the middle ear should be evaluated as a potential contributing factor. Infants with risks for neural hearing loss, including a stay in the Neonatal Intensive Care Unit (NICU) of more than five days or an associated developmental condition affecting the nervous system, should receive follow-up AABR or diagnostic testing due to the risk of late-onset and neural hearing loss.

### Automated Auditory Brainstem Response

The other frequently used assessment in newborn hearing screening programs is the AABR. The ABR differs from OAEs in the fact that ABR is an electrical response to sound that can be measured using small electrodes placed on the head. Brief, high-frequency sounds, known as clicks, are rapidly delivered via earphones to elicit the ABR response. The electrical recordings from the electrodes are averaged over thousands of presentations to minimize the influence of nonauditory electrical activity from the brain and muscles. Using this method, the small changes in voltage that occur at the auditory nerve and brainstem in response to sound can be detected at even the lowest stimulus intensities.

The AABR has been a popular option for newborn hearing screening because of some of the advantages that it has over AOAE assessment. Although not immune to the influence of ear canal debris and middle ear fluid, the fact that the AABR response does not have to travel back through the middle ear to be measured offers a considerable advantage for testing newborns who are likely to have middle ear fluid from being in the womb compared to AOAE. As a result, the refer rate for AABR is generally lower than for AOAE. As noted above, the lower refer rate minimizes the costs of the newborn hearing screening associated with performing follow-up screening or diagnostic assessment on infants with normal hearing who refer on their screening. Unlike AOAE, the AABR screening test is also sensitive to neural hearing losses because it requires an electrical response from the auditory nerve, not only the outer hair cells in the cochlea.

Like AOAE assessment, AABR can be contaminated by noise, but the sources of noise that affect the test will be different. Acoustic noises from the infant or the test environment are less of a factor for AABR than AOAE simply because the response being measured for the AABR is electric and not acoustic. Electrical signals, however, can be negatively affected by much larger electrical signals that are generated by head and neck muscles from movement, as well as electromagnetic interference from large electrical equipment that is often present in hospitals. While these issues can affect AABR assessment, the overall accuracy of the test for identifying hearing loss is high. The ability to detect neural hearing loss, in particular, makes it an ideal test for assessing newborns who are in the NICU, who are at much higher risk for neural hearing loss than children in the well-baby nursery. For this reason, the Joint Committee on Infant Hearing (2007) recommends that AABR screening be used for infants who are in the NICU for more than five days, as AOAE screening might miss neural hearing loss conditions by only testing up to the level of the cochlear outer hair cells.

## FOLLOW-UP AFTER A "REFER" RESULT ON NEWBORN HEARING SCREENING

When an infant does not pass their newborn hearing screening, the next steps may vary depending on the follow-up protocol in the locality where the infant was tested. Infants may receive rescreening in the hospital where they were born as an outpatient. In some areas, infants who do not pass newborn hearing screening are referred to their primary care doctor to repeat the screening assessment. This approach has gained popularity because many infants do not pass the newborn hearing screening because of the persistence of fluid in the middle ear space shortly after birth. Some localities require that an infant who fails an inpatient hearing screening must be referred to an audiologist for assessment. Repeating the screening test within the first two weeks of life may help to minimize unnecessary costs associated with diagnostic assessment. In cases where rescreening is conducted, the number of rescreening attempts should be minimized and infants who do not pass rescreening should be directly referred to an audiologist for diagnostic assessment. To minimize the potential for the infant to be lost to follow-up, some localities will refer an infant for diagnostic testing directly after failing newborn hearing screening without a rescreening attempt. This approach may be less cost effective because most infants who are referred from newborn hearing screening do not have hearing loss, but it can minimize the amount of time between not passing the screening and identification of hearing loss, and thus reduce the likelihood that the family will not return for an appointment.

## DIAGNOSTIC TEST BATTERY FOR IDENTIFYING HEARING LOSS IN INFANTS

As noted in the discussion about test performance, none of the audiological tests that are currently available have both perfect sensitivity and specificity. Such tests are unlikely to be developed, simply because there are always trade-offs between these parameters. As an alternative to developing a test with perfect test performance, Jerger and Hayes (1976) introduced what is known as the Cross-Check principle. The Cross-Check principle relies on multiple tests to confirm the diagnosis of hearing loss in infants, rather than a single test. The effectiveness of this approach has been noted in previous studies where the sensitivity and specificity of multiple tests together is often higher than a single test alone (e.g., Sanford et al., 2009). The use of multiple tests in the infant hearing assessment battery maximizes the likelihood that the correct type, degree, and configuration of hearing loss will be identified in a timely manner, so that the amplification process can begin.

In infants, the Cross-Check principle means that there should be an assessment of the outer, middle, and inner ear, as well as the auditory nerve. Different combinations of test results can help to identify the type of hearing loss as conductive, sensorineural, or mixed, which can be an important determination for management. Outer ear assessment is an otoscopic evaluation of the ear canal. Middle ear assessment relies on immittance measures, including tympanometry, acoustic stapedial reflexes, and/or wideband middle ear reflectance. Evaluation of the inner ear relies on OAEs. The status of the auditory nerve and estimates of behavioral thresholds to determine the degree and configuration of hearing loss are estimated from ABR or auditory steady-state response (ASSR) measures. Using this combination of measures provides an excellent starting point for the amplification process, as well as details that will be helpful in medical and genetics evaluations about the etiology of the hearing loss.

### Otoscopic Examination

Ensuring that the ear canal is free of debris through visual inspection is an important first step for diagnostic assessment of hearing at any age. Although cerumen is not often a major concern during the first few weeks of life, infants may have residual birthing debris in their ear canals. The audiologist should visualize both ear canals with an otoscope prior to inserting probes or earphones for any type of testing. Debris may become impacted or block the delivery of sound through the transducer, leading to false positive or unreliable results on other diagnostic tests.

Otoscopy may be used in older children and adults to visualize the condition of the tympanic membrane and middle ear. In infants, the small size of the ear canal prevents adequate lighting of the ear canal and visualization of the tympanic membrane can be challenging without the use of a microscope (Rogers, Boseley, Adams, Makowski, & Hohman 2010). When performed by otolaryngologists using pneumatic otoscopy to pressurize the ear canal to help visualize the dynamics of the tympanic membrane, otoscopy was as effective as tympanometry in identifying middle ear dysfunction in infants and young children (Toner & Mains, 1990). Neither microscopy or pneumatic otoscopy is routinely used by audiologists to assess the condition of the tympanic membrane, particularly in infants. Therefore, the main purpose of otoscopic evaluation by audiologists during infancy is to ensure that the ear canal is clear to permit further assessment, not to detect middle ear dysfunction. As children get older and their ear canals grow, otoscopy may be valuable in identifying gross abnormalities of the tympanic membrane, including large perforations, acute otitis media, tympanostomy tubes, or exostoses (bone growth) of the ear canal that could affect diagnostic testing. The identification of middle ear dysfunction as part of the comprehensive diagnostic assessment will primarily be based on acoustic immittance measures.

## Acoustic Immittance

The presence of middle ear dysfunction related to fluid or negative pressure behind the tympanic membrane can not only contribute to hearing loss, but can also negatively affect the accuracy of other tests used to assess hearing. Between 2 to 12 months of age, approximately 91% of infants will have at least one episode of otitis media (Paradise et al., 1997). As is discussed in the section on threshold estimation using ABR or ASSR, bone conduction assessment that would normally provide information about the presence of air-bone gaps in audiometric testing may be limited in infants. As a result, the use of acoustic immittance testing to infer the function of the middle ear is a particularly important component of the diagnostic assessment process for infants. Decisions about whether or not to proceed with amplification or medical management of middle ear dysfunctions are important distinctions to be able to make. Acoustic immittance assessment allows for quantification of the dynamics of the middle ear system to support those distinctions. The acoustic immittance measures that are discussed in this section are the most commonly used in the diagnosis of hearing loss in children, including tympanometry, wideband reflectance, and acoustic stapedial reflexes.

### *Tympanometry*

Tympanometry quantifies the pressure and mobility of the tympanic membrane to characterize the status of the middle ear system. The tympanometer probe includes a transducer that produces a pure-tone at a specific frequency, usually 226 Hz or 1000 Hz, and a pressure pump that is used to vary the pressure in the ear canal. Tympanometry is based on the idea that the intensity of the probe tone will be lowest when the greatest amount of sound is being absorbed by the tympanic membrane. As the pressure is varied in the ear canal, the sound level of the probe tone is measured with a microphone to determine how much sound is being absorbed into the middle ear as a function of the pressure in the ear canal. A normal middle ear will absorb the most sound at ambient pressure, leading to characteristic peak admittance in a normal tympanogram around 0 daPa, known as a Type A tympanogram (Figure 2–3A). In cases where there is no visible peak admittance due to fluid or other obstruction of the tympanic membrane, a flat or Type B tympanogram will be observed (Figure 2–3B). If the eustachian tube that connects the nasopharynx at the back of the upper throat is not functioning adequately to equalize the pressure behind the tympanic membrane, the peak admittance may occur at negative pressure values, known as a Type C tympanogram (Figure 2–3C). This classification scheme can be useful in identifying middle ear dysfunction as part of the diagnostic process when a 226 Hz probe tone is being used.

The 226 Hz probe tone used in standard tympanometry is popular because of its sensitivity to middle ear fluid, which significantly disrupts the transmission of sound at low frequencies due to mass effects on the tympanic membrane.

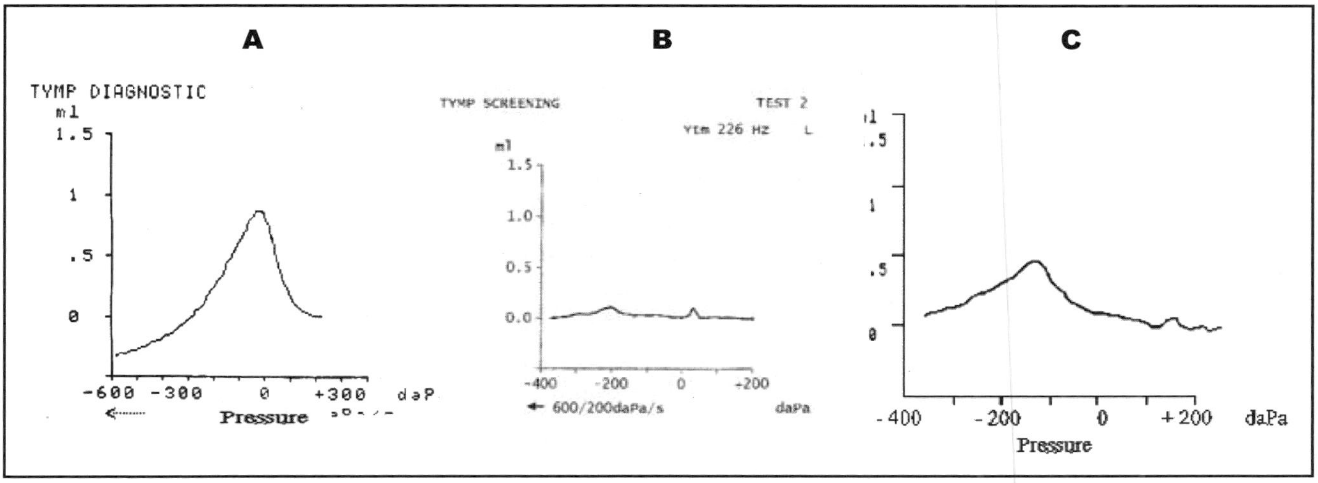


**FIGURE 2–3.** Three primary tympanogram classifications for a 226 Hz probe tone. Type A (Panel A) is consistent with normal middle ear function. Type B (Panel B) is consistent with middle ear dysfunction, such as the presence of middle ear fluid. Type C suggests the presence of negative middle ear pressure.

Despite its popularity, there are some significant limitations to the 226 Hz probe tone related to the dynamics of the middle ear in infants and stiffness-related pathologies of the middle ear that should be considered. Changes in the middle ear system that changes the stiffness of the middle ear system, such as ossicular discontinuity (reduced stiffness) or otosclerosis (increased stiffness), are more likely to cause changes in the high-frequency transmission of sound through the middle ear and may not be apparent if the 226 Hz probe tone is used. Most stiffness-related problems are rare during infancy and early childhood, but are worth considering for older children.

A larger concern with the 226 Hz probe tone for infants is related to the physical characteristics of the infant ear canal. In older children and adults, the outer one-third of the ear canal is soft and cartilaginous, while the inner two-thirds of the ear canal is inside the temporal bone and much harder. The impedance and power transmission characteristics of the middle ear in infants are different than adults in the low frequencies. Therefore, there are occasions where tympanometry conducted with a 226 Hz probe tone in an infant will appear to be normal, and yet the child has middle ear dysfunction. This false negative result occurs because the softer infant ear canal absorbs the sound from the 226 Hz probe tone, even if the middle ear cannot. This issue is a significant problem up to at least 6 months of age. The solutions that have been proposed to this problem are to either use a probe tone with a higher frequency, such as 1000 Hz, or to assess the function of the middle ear at multiple frequencies using wideband reflectance.

The use of 1000 Hz tympanometry has higher sensitivity for middle ear dysfunction in infants who are less than 6 months of age than 226 Hz tympanometry (Alaerts, Luts, & Wouters, 2007; Kei et al., 2003; Sanford et al., 2009). Clinical guidelines have been developed to suggest that 1000 Hz tympanometry should be used in infants under 6 months of age, with 226 Hz tympanometry being used after 6 months of age. The clinical use of 1000 Hz tympanometry has led to some confusion related to classification. Unlike 226 Hz tympanograms, which yield the predictable A/B/C types for classification, 1000 Hz tympanograms can present with a wide range of odd shapes that are more challenging to classify (Figure 2–4). However, a useful classification scheme was developed and presented in a paper by Baldwin (2006). This classification method was validated on a large number of infants with the presence of an air-bone gap on an ABR as the gold standard comparison for diagnosis of conductive hearing loss. The classification scheme requires that the audiologist draw a horizontal line from the negative tail of the tympanogram to the positive tail of the tympanogram (Figure 2–5). If there is a clear peak above the line, the tympanogram is classified as consistent with normal middle ear function. If there is no peak above the line or the tympanogram moves across the line multiple times, the tympanogram is classified as abnormal and consistent with middle ear dysfunction. This classification scheme has excellent sensitivity and specificity, as well as being simple to implement clinically.

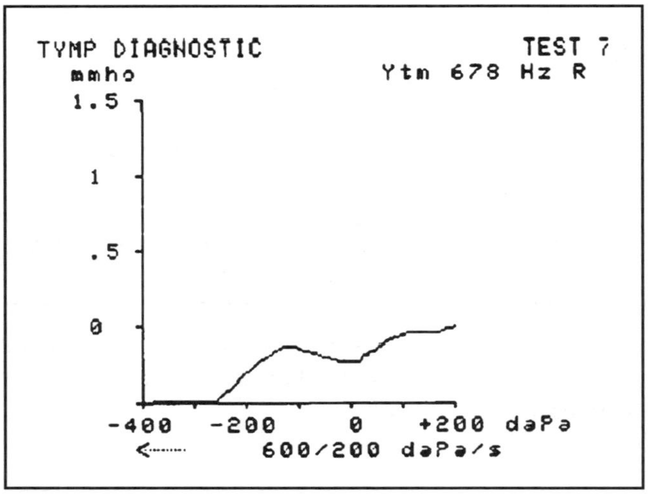


**FIGURE 2–4.** An example of a 1000 Hz tympanogram obtained from an infant. The irregular shape of the tympanogram can make it difficult to classify the type using traditional tympanometric classification schemes.

### *Wideband Reflectance*

A more recent development in the assessment of middle ear function is wideband reflectance. Reflectance is based on the same principles of sound absorption as tympanometry, but has a few advantages. First, as the name of the test indicates, wideband reflectance assesses the function of the middle ear over a wide range of frequencies, typically from 200 to 10,000 Hz. This is accomplished by using a brief click stimulus that has broad energy across a range of frequencies. Wideband

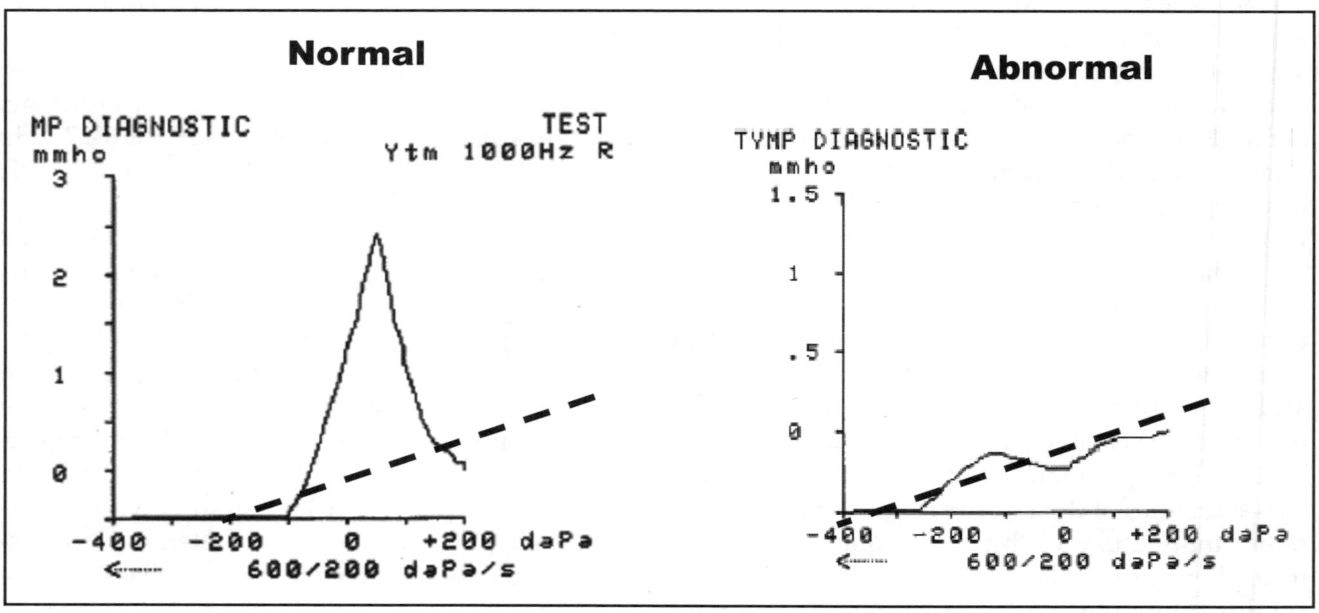


**FIGURE 2–5.** The classification scheme proposed by Baldwin et al. (2006) for high-frequency tympanograms. A line is drawn between the tails of the tympanogram. If there is a peak above the line (left example), the tympanogram is classified as normal. If there is no peak or the tympanogram is below the line, the tympanogram is classified as abnormal.

reflectance can also be conducted at ambient pressure without pressurizing the ear canal, or with a range of pressurization, like single-frequency tympanometry. Because wideband reflectance assesses a broad frequency range of the middle ear system, it offers the potential for greater sensitivity for detecting middle ear problems that might alter the transmission of low (mass) or higher (stiffness) frequencies through the middle ear.

Despite these advantages, the data on the diagnostic value of wideband reflectance is still in its infancy. The limited test performance data that have been published for infants suggests that wideband reflectance performs similarly to tympanometry for predicting which infants might fail newborn hearing screening due to middle ear dysfunction (Sanford et al., 2009). Normative values for children with normal middle ear function have been published for infants (Hunter, Feeney, Miller, Jeng, & Bohning, 2010). One of the challenges in the adoption of wideband reflectance as a clinical test has been that audiologists have been trained and are comfortable with tympanometry, but have had limited training and exposure to wideband reflectance. This issue is somewhat trivial in the sense that wideband reflectance provides nearly identical information to tympanometry, except at multiple frequencies rather than a single frequency. A potentially larger concern with the clinical adoption of wideband reflectance is the fact that the normative ranges for normal middle ear function and middle ear dysfunction in infants show significant variability and areas of overlap, limiting any advantages in test performance that wideband reflectance might have over tympanometry. Researchers continue to work on classification schemes for wideband reflectance that will improve sensitivity and specificity. Eventually, wideband reflectance is likely to be used in place of single-frequency tympanometry to assess middle ear function as part of the diagnostic test battery.

### *Acoustic Stapedial Reflexes*

When loud sounds are presented in the ear canal, the stapedius muscle that is attached to the neck of the stapes contracts, leading to changes in the dynamics of the ossicular chain that can be measured using a tympanometer. The contraction can be measured in individuals with normal hearing and normal facial nerve function (because that is the cranial nerve that provides motor innervation for the stapedius), whether the stimulus is presented to the ipsilateral or contralateral ear. The acoustic reflex has been used to assess the integrity of the auditory pathways from the middle ear, through the cochlea, and the auditory and facial nerves. Contralateral reflexes also rely on decussating pathways at the superior olivary complex in the brainstem. Thus, if acoustic reflexes are present at expected levels, inferences about the function of large portions of the auditory system can be made. If acoustic reflexes are absent, there are a large number of potential sites of lesion in the auditory system that could be affected. Much attention has been given to the sensitivity of acoustic reflexes to retrocochlear hearing problems in adults (e.g., Olsen, Noffsinger, & Kurdziel, 1975).

In pediatrics, acoustic reflexes have unique considerations that are slightly different than when the test is used with adults. As with tympanometry, the use of a 1000 Hz probe tone is recommended for assessing acoustic reflexes in infants who are less than 6 months. Normative data for 1000 Hz acoustic reflexes in infants are available from work published by Keefe, Fitzpatrick, Liu, Sanford, and Gorga (2010). Because acoustic reflexes are measured at the same pressure as the admittance peak from the tympanogram, tympanometry should be measured first to ensure that there is a peak admittance. In the case of Type C tympanograms with significant negative middle ear pressure (<−150 daPa), acoustic reflexes may be absent, even if the negative pressure can be maintained, because of increased stiffness of the tympanic membrane. In the case of Type B tympanograms or other abnormal patterns, it is not advisable to attempt to measure acoustic reflexes, as they would almost certainly be absent, or at least be unable to be measured. Caution must also be taken when setting a maximum presentation level for acoustic reflexes in infants. The stimulus levels for acoustic reflexes are calibrated in a 2-$cm^3$ coupler, which is considerably larger than the average infant ear canal. The level of the stimulus may be 12 to 18 dB higher in the infant ear canal than the calibrated value in the 2-$cm^3$ coupler. For this reason, a maximum stimulus level of 95 dB SPL is recommended for testing infants and young children.

Because acoustic reflexes rely on contraction of the stapedius muscle and stiffening of the ossicular chain, they can be disrupted by the presence of even slight conductive hearing loss. For this reason, acoustic reflexes can be helpful in detecting the presence of conductive hearing loss, particularly when the tympanogram appears to be normal. This can be useful information in cases where young children cannot provide sufficient test data to allow for bone conduction assessment. Children with sensorineural hearing loss up to a moderate degree typically have present acoustic reflexes, whereas the presence of acoustic reflexes can diminish as the degree of hearing loss reaches severe or profound. While acoustic reflexes cannot be used to predict absolute thresholds, they can provide corroborating evidence for the observed degree of hearing loss on other assessments, including ABR. For example, if a child with profound hearing loss had measurable acoustic reflexes, that would raise suspicion that potentially the estimation of the degree of hearing loss might not be accurate.

The other important application of acoustic reflexes is in the diagnosis of auditory neuropathy spectrum disorder (ANSD). As discussed in the section on newborn hearing screening, children with ANSD have normal outer hair cell function, but disrupted auditory function in the neural system. The disrupted neural activity in children with ANSD also disrupts the transmission of neural energy required to elicit acoustic reflexes. In a 2005 study by Charles Berlin and colleagues, none of the children with ANSD had acoustic reflexes that were present at expected intensity levels. While the ABR is the gold standard test for the diagnosis of ANSD, absent acoustic reflexes are a diagnostic finding that would be expected in nearly all cases of ANSD and, therefore, are considered a supportive supplemental indicator. Children with less than moderate degrees of sensorineural hearing loss who have absent acoustic reflexes despite having normal middle ear function could be considered candidates to receive a diagnostic evaluation with an ABR to rule out the presence of ANSD.

### *Conclusions on Immittance*

The ability to quantify the dynamics of the middle ear system provides important information as part of the diagnostic process for children. Children with persistent middle ear dysfunction who do not pass their hearing screening or have measurable hearing loss on diagnostic assessments should be referred to their primary care doctor or an otolaryngologist for medical management. The presence of middle ear dysfunction in children can complicate the diagnostic process of identifying the type of hearing loss and delay the provision of amplification. Early management of middle ear problems can help to ensure that children receive accurate diagnosis and prompt amplification if needed.

## Diagnostic Applications of Otoacoustic Emissions

The same otoacoustic emissions (OAEs) that are used in universal newborn hearing screening programs can also be used in the diagnostic process to help differentiate the site of lesion of hearing loss in the auditory system. The main differences between screening and diagnostic versions of OAEs are worth delineating. Screening OAEs only give an overall result of "Pass," which is consistent with normal cochlear outer hair cells function, and "Refer," which means the test cannot rule out the presence of significant hearing loss. Diagnostic otoacoustic emissions provide more specific information about the sound level of the emission relative to the noise floor at the specific frequencies being tested. For diagnostic emissions, a larger range of frequencies is typically tested than in screening applications, although diagnostic OAEs are still reflective of the function of the cochlea at mid to high frequencies, generally from 1500 Hz to 8000 Hz at most. This section of the chapter discusses the different approaches to measuring OAEs and how these techniques are used as part of the diagnostic process for children with hearing loss.

### *Methods of Generating OAEs*

The discovery of OAEs was completely serendipitous. As described by Kemp (1986), scientists were taking sound measurements in ear canals using sensitive microphones and discovered that there were sounds present in the ear canal whose origins could not be pinpointed in the environment. This led scientists to document the discovery of spontaneous OAEs, which are OAEs that can be measured without specific acoustic stimulation to the ear. While there was some interest in using spontaneous OAEs for evaluation of cochlear function, a rather significant number of infants with normal hearing, around 35%, did not have measurable spontaneous otoacoustic emissions (Burns, Arehart, & Campbell, 1992). To have over a third of normal hearing infants fail the screening measure was not acceptable in terms of levels of sensitivity, which led scientists to consider other methods of generation. For clinical purposes, there are two types of OAE generation that have gained acceptance and have reasonable test performance data to support their application in assessing cochlear function across the lifespan. Those methods are distortion-product OAE (DPOAE) and transient-evoked OAE (TEOAE).

With DPOAEs, two pure-tone sounds are simultaneously presented to the ear canal at specific frequencies. Because the elicitation of DPOAEs requires simultaneous presentation of two pure-tones, the probe for measuring DPOAEs has two receivers for producing the stimuli and one microphone for measuring the response (Figure 2–6). The relationship between the frequencies of the two pure-tones, known as f1 and f2, elicits an OAE at a third specific frequency, known as the cubic distortion product. There are several harmonic distortion products that occur when two pure-tone sounds are introduced to the ear canal, but the cubic distortion product is robust and consistently measurable in individuals with normal hearing. The cubic distortion product occurs at a frequency that is two times f1, minus f2 (sometimes noted as 2f1–f2). For example, if f1 = 3000 Hz and f2 = 4000 Hz, the cubic distortion product will occur at 2000 Hz (2 × 3000 = 6000 − 4000 = 2000 Hz). An f1 to f2 ratio of 1.22 has been found to yield consistent DPOAE responses. The DPOAE response is correlated with behavioral thresholds at the f2 frequency. Different combinations of f1 and f2 are used to generate specific cubic distortion frequencies to assess a wide range of cochlear function. An intensity difference where f1 is presented at 65 dB SPL and f2 is presented at 55 dB SPL tends to generate the most consistent DPOAE responses from ears with normal cochlear function (Gorga et al., 1997). An example of a DPOAE response is shown in Figure 2–7.

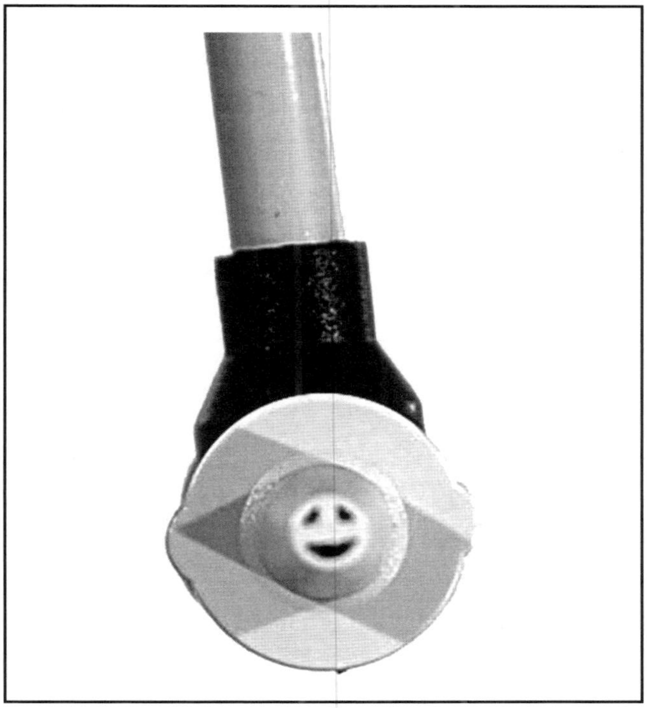

**FIGURE 2–6.** A probe used to measure Otoacoustic Emissions (OAEs). The three openings in the tip are the receivers where sound is produced and the microphone where the response is recorded. Because this probe has two receivers, it can be used to measure either Distortion Product (DP) or Transient Evoked (TE) OAEs.

For TEOAEs, the stimulus is a single broadband click, which has energy that covers a wide range of frequencies because of its brief duration. Instead of attempting to stimulate the cochlea in a frequency specific manner using pure-tone sounds, TEOAEs occur as the result of broadband stimulation, which generates a broadband response from the cochlea. The response is recorded in brief intervals between broadband click stimuli. Because the TEOAE uses a single stimulus, the TEOAE probe requires only a single receiver and a single microphone. The TEOAE response must be higher than the noise floor at specific frequencies in order to be reflective of normal hearing. Criteria for the signal-to-noise ratio for TEOAEs for diagnostic protocols has been +4 or +6 dB SNR in previous

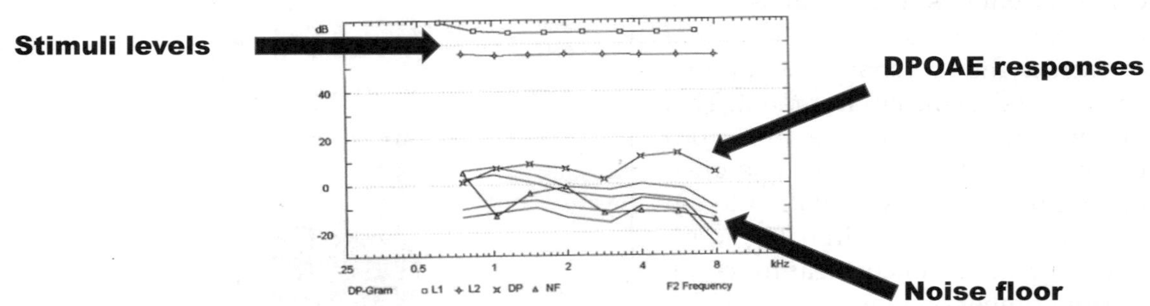


Left: 6-Jul-4: -: 750_8000.lst:

| L1(dB) | L2(dB) | F1(Hz) | F2(Hz) | GM(Hz) | DP(dB) | NF(dB) | DP-NF(dB) |
|---|---|---|---|---|---|---|---|
| 65.0 | 55.2 | 6656 | 7969 | 7283 | 5.2 | -15.3 | 20.5 |
| 64.8 | 55.1 | 4688 | 5625 | 5135 | 13.3 | -12.0 | 25.3 |
| 64.8 | 55.2 | 3328 | 3984 | 3641 | 11.9 | -11.4 | 23.3 |
| 65.1 | 55.5 | 2344 | 2813 | 2567 | 2.2 | -12.4 | 14.6 |
| 64.9 | 55.7 | 1641 | 1969 | 1797 | 6.9 | -1.3 | 8.2 |
| 64.9 | 55.4 | 1172 | 1406 | 1284 | 8.8 | -4.0 | 12.8 |
| 65.8 | 55.0 | 844 | 1031 | 933 | 7.2 | -13.3 | 20.5 |
| 69.4 | 56.0 | 609 | 750 | 676 | 1.0 | 5.0 | -4.0 |

SNR by frequency

**FIGURE 2–7.** Distortion product otoacoustic emissions (DPOAEs) measured on a child. Note the stimulus levels of 65 dB/55 dB SPL and the DPOAE responses (X symbols connected with a line) and noise floor (triangles connected with a line). The signal-to-noise ratio (SNR) at each frequency is highlighted in the box around the column labeled DP-NF.

studies (Hussain, Gorga, Neely, Keefe, & Peters, 1998; Prieve et al., 1993). An example of a TEOAE response is shown in Figure 2–8.

In order to measure either TEOAE or DPOAE, stimuli are presented to the ear numerous times. The responses to each stimulus are averaged over time based on the idea that averaging the responses can reduce the level of the noise across trials and increase the salience of the OAE response, which should be consistently measured across trials. Some clinical OAE systems use different averaging rules that will stop averaging when a specific signal-to-noise ratio criterion or noise level criterion is reached. A minimum of 20 stimuli per frequency for DPOAEs or 20 stimuli total for TEOAEs is preferable. This means that OAEs using either elicitation method can be completed in about 60 to 90 seconds per ear in a cooperative child. The presence of background noise in the test environment or noise from the child will increase the time needed to measure OAEs. Because most sources of noise tend to be lower in frequency, DPOAEs are particularly susceptible to background noise because the cubic distortion product occurs at frequencies slightly lower than the stimuli. The test performance for both TEOAE and DPOAE responses is poor at frequencies less than 1500 Hz, due primarily to the presence of physiological noise from breathing and circulation. Thus, most clinical OAE protocols will not include frequencies below 1500 Hz. As a result, OAEs cannot be used to measure cochlear function at lower frequencies.

The clinical interpretation of OAEs has been enhanced by the development of normative data from ears with normal hearing and ears with significant cochlear hearing losses for DPOAEs (Gorga et al., 1997) and TEOAEs (Hussain et al., 1998). Regardless of the elicitation paradigm, there are ears with sensorineural hearing loss that produce OAE responses, and ears with normal hearing that fail to produce responses. To put this another way, the distributions of OAE responses from ears with normal hearing and ears with hearing loss overlap to some degree. The implication of this overlap is that there is no OAE criterion that will perfectly separate ears with normal hearing from ears with hearing loss. Diagnostically, this means that OAEs are seldom used in isolation of other test methods, including immit-

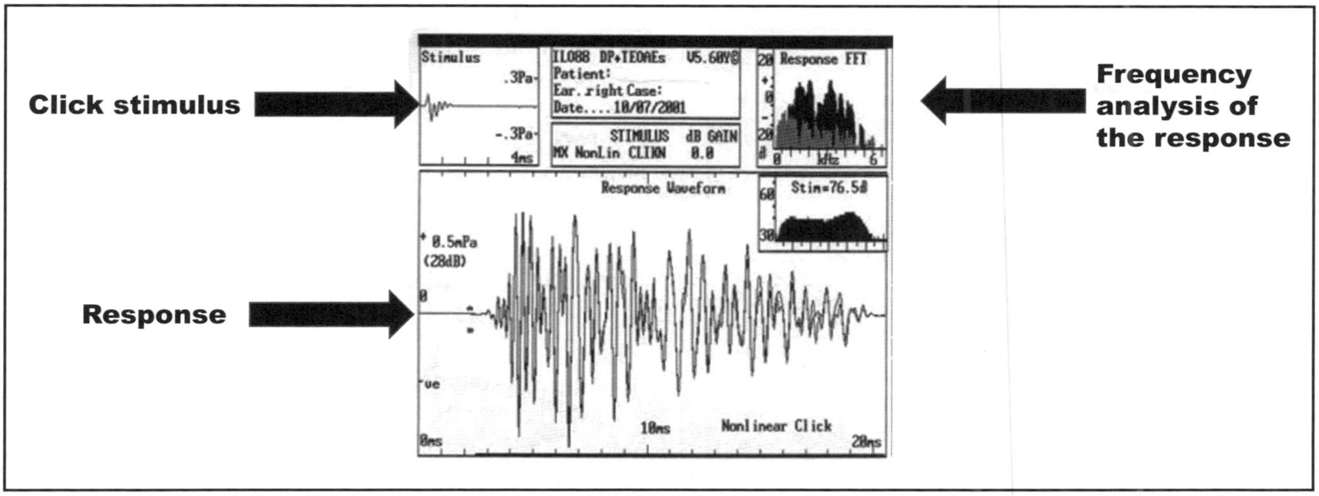


**FIGURE 2–8.** Transient evoked otoacoustic emissions (TEOAEs) measured on a child. Note the click stimulus and broadband response measured in the ear canal. In the upper right corner of the display, a Fast Fourier Transform (FFT) of the TEOAE response is estimated to determine the signal-to-noise ratio as a function of frequency. The black peaks are the TEOAE response and the smaller gray peaks are the noise floor of the averaged response.

tance and auditory brainstem response. Despite these limitations, the clinical normative data from Gorga and colleagues (1997) have been used to develop a clinical form (Figure 2–9) that can be used to plot the level of DPOAE responses on a chart to determine if the responses are consistent with normal hearing, consistent with hearing loss, or in an area of uncertainty, which is the overlap between the DPOAE response distributions for ears with normal hearing and ears with hearing loss. For diagnostic purposes, frequencies where the DPOAE is present in the normal range are likely to be associated with normal hearing or no more than mild hearing loss. Frequencies where DPOAE responses are either in the area of uncertainty or in the range of ears with hearing loss are considered to be abnormal and indicate a need for further evaluation. While similar data are available for TEOAE responses from a later paper by Hussain and colleagues (1998), a clinical form has not been developed, although a clinician with enough ingenuity could easily develop their own form based on the data from that paper.

As noted in the previous section about the use of automated OAEs for newborn hearing screening, OAEs are typically absent in ears with significant middle ear dysfunction. The need for the stimulus and the response to travel through the middle ear means that even mild middle ear dysfunction may disrupt OAEs. This can include middle ear fluid related to otitis media or even negative middle ear pressure from eustachian tube dysfunction (Owens, McCoy, Lonsbury-Martin, & Martin, 1993; Topolska, Hassman, & Baczek, 2000). Therefore, the absence of OAEs in ear with middle ear dysfunction should be considered a nonspecific diagnostic finding in that the presence of cochlear dysfunction cannot be ruled out by OAEs when the status of the middle ear is abnormal. The evidence regarding the effect of tympanostomy tubes on OAE responses has been inconclusive, but several studies have suggested no significant effect (Tas et al., 2004; Topolska et al., 2000), whereas an earlier study indicated a reduction in OAE amplitude in ears with tympanostomy tubes compared to control ears with no tubes (Owens et al., 1993). Collectively, these studies suggest that OAE responses would generally be expected in ears with patent tympanostomy tubes and that absence of OAEs in those cases would be justification for further testing to rule out hearing loss.

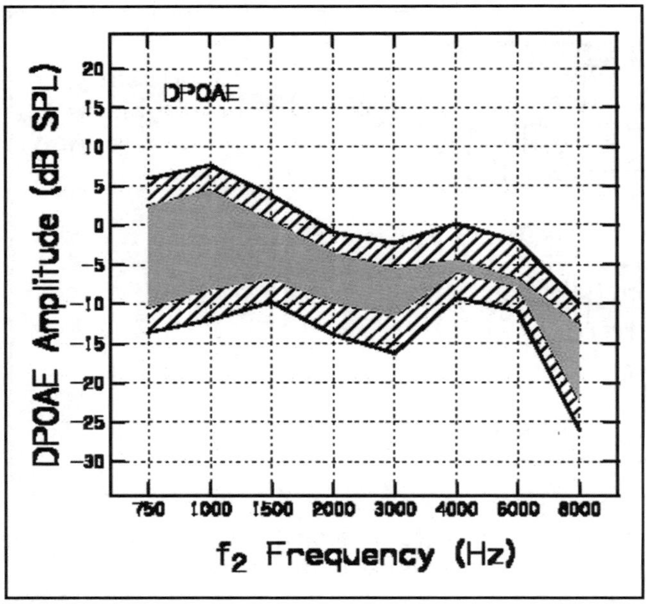


**FIGURE 2–9.** A clinical form for interpreting DPOAE responses. To be plotted on the form, the DPOAE level must be at least 6 dB above the noise floor. Responses that fall above the shaded and hatched area are consistent with normal cochlear function. Responses that fall below the hatched and shaded area are consistent with abnormal cochlear function. Responses that fall within the hatched area occur in the area of overlap between distributions of OAEs from normal ear and ears with hearing loss and indicated that further assessment is needed to determine auditory function.

There are also several specific applications for diagnostic OAEs that clinicians may encounter. In cases of ANSD, OAEs are often present in combination with an absent or grossly abnormal auditory brainstem response. As is discussed in the following section about auditory brainstem response, an absent ABR is typically consistent with profound hearing loss, but in ANSD, the lack of auditory nerve function means that the ABR is rendered an invalid measure of hearing sensitivity. Because ANSD often leaves the cochlear outer hair cells functional, present OAEs are one diagnostic indicator of ANSD when coupled with the absent or abnormal ABR. Another diagnostic application of OAEs is for monitoring ototoxicity from medications or chemotherapeutic agents. Changes in OAE responses have been noted to precede changes in the behavioral audiogram, which means that OAEs may be a useful monitoring tool for adjusting medications during treatment, if possible (Hotz, Harris, & Probst, 1994; Stavroulaki, Apostolopoulos, Segas, Tsakanikos, & Adamopoulos, 2001).

## Auditory Brainstem Response

Up to this point in the diagnostic process, we have discussed measures that assess the function of the middle ear system (immittance) and the cochlea (otoacoustic emissions). These assessments are vital component to the diagnostic audiological process in children, but the key information about the degree and configuration of hearing loss that is needed to diagnose hearing loss and prescribe amplification comes from the auditory brainstem response. As noted in the section about the use of the auditory brainstem response in newborn hearing screening, the ABR represents the response of the auditory nerve and auditory brainstem to sound. In addition to being a useful screening measure for newborn hearing screening, the ABR has the additional benefit of being highly correlated with the behavioral audiogram (Gorga et al., 2006; McCreery et al., 2014). The thresholds responses from ABR assessments in infants can be used to prescribe amplification.

### *ABR Measurement*

A comprehensive discussion of ABR measurement techniques is beyond the scope of a chapter related to diagnostic assessment of hearing for the purposes of fitting hearing aids for children, but interested readers are encouraged to see comprehensive reviews of the topic in books by Hall (2015) and Picton (2010). The use of ABR assessment in infants and young children requires specific training and experience in administering the test and interpreting responses. The potential to misdiagnose the presence or degree of hearing loss can lead to no amplification in cases where it is needed or overamplification in cases where the ABR responses are not interpreted appropriately. For these reasons, ABR assessment on infants and children should only be completed by audiologists with the necessary skills and experience using ABR with infants and children.

A characteristic ABR response to a broadband click is shown in Figure 2–10. At high levels, the three most prominent features of the ABR waveform are visible in individuals with normal hearing. Wave I is thought to correspond with the distal VIIIth nerve, Wave III is thought to correspond with the caudal brainstem, and Wave V is thought to correspond with higher brainstem pathways. As the stimulus level decreases, Waves I and III become less apparent, leaving only Wave V. The level of presence or absence of Wave V is considered to have excellent correspondence with behavioral audiometric thresholds in previous studies (Gorga et al., 2006; McCreery et al., 2014; Vander Werff, Prieve, & Georgantas, 2009). The lowest intensity level where Wave V is observed is considered to be the ABR threshold for a given frequency.

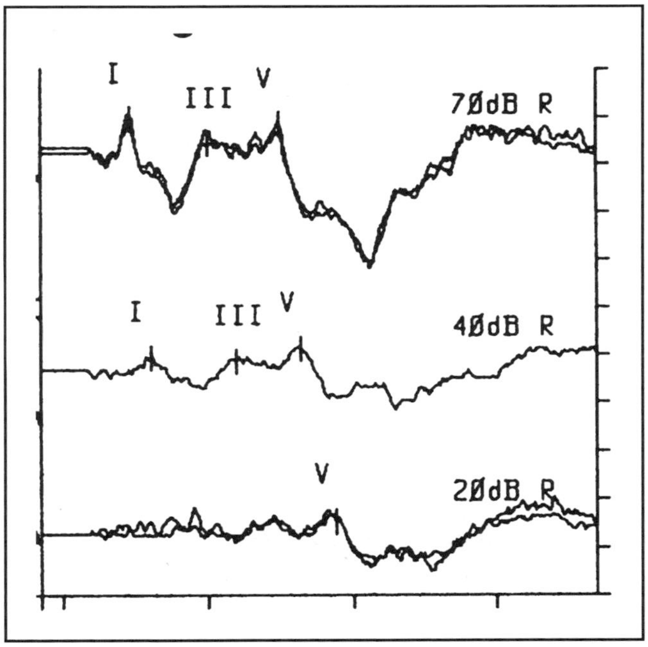


**FIGURE 2–10.** An auditory brainstem response (ABR) for a click stimulus at 70 dB (*top*), 40 dB (*middle*) and 20 dB (*bottom*) nHL for an infant with normal hearing. At high levels, Waves I, III, and V are prominent, but only Wave V is evident as the stimulus level decreases. The latency of Wave V increases as the stimulus level decreases.

**Electrode Montage.** The ABR response can be recorded using multiple arrangements of electrodes placed on the head. The electrode montage used at Boys Town National Research Hospital (BTNRH) is shown in Figure 2–11. One electrode is placed on the high forehead and one electrode is placed on each mastoid process. The mastoid electrode that is ipsilateral to the ear being tested is used as the reference, while the contralateral mastoid electrode is used as the ground. This electrode montage can be used with any ABR equipment that allows electrode switching in the software so that the electrode inputs do not have to be switched each time the tester switches between ears. This electrode montage minimizes the number of electrodes that are required for testing compared to montages that require a separate ground electrode. Placing electrodes on the mastoid process also provides a larger surface to apply the electrodes compared with montages that place the reference electrodes on the ear lobes, which can be quite small in infants. One disadvantage of mastoid placement is the fact that recordings may be contaminated by postauricular muscle artifact in cases where the child's head is moving, although this is typically not an issue since most

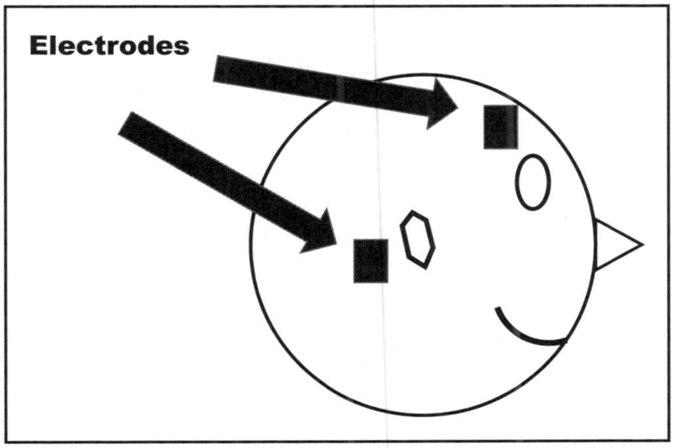


**FIGURE 2–11.** The electrode montage for auditory brainstem response measures used at Boys Town National Research Hospital.

ABR assessment in children is done in natural sleep or with sedation.

**State of Arousal.** Threshold ABR responses are best observed while the child is in a state of sleep. A sleeping child not only has limited self-generated noise, but also reduced movement to minimize the likelihood of muscle artifact during assessment. Some ABR equipment manufacturers have developed specialized signal processing systems that are purported to allow threshold ABR assessment in infants and children while they are awake. However, independent research validating these claims have only been reported in screening ABR applications (Wiegers, Bielefeld, & Whitelaw, 2015), and have not been validated for estimation of thresholds in infants with hearing loss. In general, infants under 3 months of age can be tested in a state of natural sleep, because infants in this age range often sleep around 16 hours per day (Galland, Taylor, Elder, & Herbison, 2012). Scheduling the appointment around a regular nap time or shortly after the baby eats can help maximize the likelihood of extended natural sleep. Between 3 to 6 months of age, daytime sleep becomes much less consistent and more variable, which can make natural sleep more difficult. Because the alternative to natural sleep is to use some form of sedation to induce sleep, most parents of infants in the 3- to 6-month age range are highly motivated to attempt a natural sleep ABR and will often comply with instructions to feed the baby prior to the assessment to help induce sleep. This challenge highlights the need to perform diagnostic assessment following a Refer result on newborn hearing screening within the first few months of life, so that the use of sedation can be minimized. For children who cannot be tested in a state of natural sleep, sedation or anesthesia can be used to induce sleep for ABR assessment. A wide range of anesthetic agents are available, and individual protocols are often dictated by anesthesiologists or physicians at the medical facility where the testing is conducted.

**ABR Stimuli.** In order to obtain sufficient information to describe the degree and configuration of hearing loss which will determine the need for amplification, ear- and frequency-specific thresholds are required. Broadband click stimuli produce an ABR with clear morphology that is easy to interpret. A click threshold generally has a high degree of correspondence with behavioral pure-tone audiometry at 2000 and 4000 Hz, but may underestimate thresholds in cases where the configuration of hearing loss is sloping (see case examples in Gorga et al., 2006). For this reason, tone-burst stimuli that correspond with audiometric test frequencies are the preferred stimuli for ABR assessment. Blackman windowing functions are applied to tone-bursts to maintain frequency specificity, while minimizing the occurrence of energetic side-lobes that occur with brief stimuli. Figure 2–12 shows the ABR stimulus characteristics for tone bursts used at BTNRH. The frequency range of these stimuli is designed to reflect a range of important audiometric frequencies for diagnosis of hearing loss and initiation of amplification. The stimulus presentation rates for tone bursts are

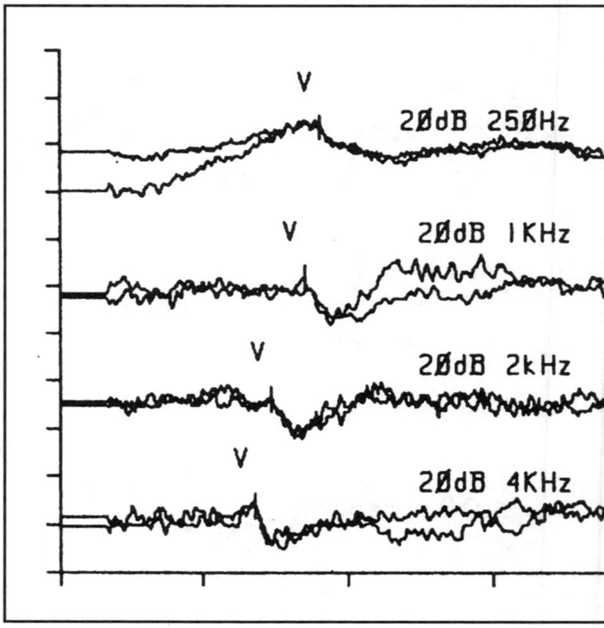


**FIGURE 2–12.** Auditory brainstem response (ABR) recordings from an infant with normal hearing. Each pair of recordings represents ABR responses at a different frequency (*from top*) 250 Hz, 1000 Hz, 2000 Hz, and 4000 Hz at 20 dB nHL. For the same level, the Wave V latency increases as the stimulus frequency decreases, reflecting the tonotopic organization of the basilar membrane in the cochlea.

designed to maximize the collection of information while eliciting high-quality ABR responses.

**Strategies for Maximizing Threshold ABR Assessment.** The goal of threshold ABR assessment in children is to gather the largest number of ear- and frequency-specific thresholds in the shortest amount of time, as the child could wake up during a natural sleep test and the total duration of sedation may be limited. This means that the number of thresholds that can be measured during an ABR is often less than might be available from behavioral audiometric testing. For example, McCreery and colleagues (2014) found that the average number of ABR thresholds obtained was 2.4 for natural sleep and 3.4 for ABR assessments under sedation. Thus, it is important to use strategies to maximize the efficiency of ABR testing to gather the most information possible that would allow an accurate diagnose and permit the fitting of amplification if the child has hearing loss.

At each level that is tested, a minimum of 1000 stimulus presentations should be collected, with threshold responses sometimes requiring around 2,000 presentations. Each threshold response should be replicated to ensure that the waveform morphology is consistent and repeatable. Unlike pure-tone audiometry, which has a specific bracketing procedure based on the Hughson-Westlake method (Carhart & Jerger, 1959), audiologists will use increased step-sizes of 10 dB or more between levels based on the responses that are recorded to minimize the amount of time spent searching for thresholds. For example, a 60 dB nHL starting level is often recommended. If a clear Wave V response is visible at 60 dB nHL, the audiologist may decide to drop the level to 20 dB nHL, which is the lowest intensity level that is tested and is consistent with normal hearing. If no response is visible at 60 dB nHL, the audiologist may wish to increase the level of the stimulus up to 90 dB nHL to elicit a clear response. This method of large changes in presentation level will help ensure that information can be obtained rapidly while the child sleeps.

The minimum amount of information that should be used to fit hearing aids based on an ABR is a high-frequency and low-frequency threshold in each ear. To that end, the ABR protocol at BTNRH starts with a 2000 Hz tone burst in each ear, followed by a 250 Hz tone burst in each ear. If the child wakes up after these two frequencies are obtained in each ear, there would be sufficient information to determine the presence of hearing loss and initiate amplification. The frequencies obtained after this point will depend on the results at 250 Hz and 2000 Hz. In some cases, it may be of interest to evaluate 4000 Hz thresholds to get a higher frequency if the thresholds at 250 Hz and 2000 Hz are similar. In other cases where there is a large discrepancy between 250 Hz and 2000 Hz, 1000 Hz tone bursts may be of greater interest.

There are also helpful cross-checks that can be available to audiologists during ABR threshold assessment that can help to increase confidence that the responses being measured are present and that the thresholds are valid estimates of behavioral threshold. Near threshold, it can be difficult to determine if Wave V is present or absent. Two attributes of ABR responses can help clinicians to gain confidence in their interpretation of ABR. First, the Wave V latency should increase as the stimulus level decreases. This characteristic, known as the latency-intensity function, is an important cross-check, since a feature of the waveform that does not increase in latency as intensity increases is not characteristic of an ABR response. Additionally, thresholds at the same intensity level can be compared across frequency, as in Figure 2–12. Because of the tonotopic organization of the cochlea, where high-frequency sounds are encoded at the basal end and low-frequency sounds are encoded apically, low-frequency stimuli will elicit a longer Wave V ABR latency than high-frequency stimuli due to longer travel time on the basilar membrane. This yields a characteristic frequency-intensity function where the latencies of Wave V get longer as the frequency of the stimulus increases. A 20 dB nHL threshold at different frequencies should follow the same characteristic increases in latency as frequency decreases.

**ABR Correction Factors.** Once ABR thresholds are obtained, there are several methods for converting the ABR thresholds from dB nHL, which is a reference to a specific sound pressure level, to dB eHL, which represents an estimated behavioral threshold. ABR thresholds are measured with short-duration tone-burst stimuli, whereas the behavioral thresholds that are predicted from the ABR are measured with longer duration pure-tone stimuli. Because of differences in temporal integration, thresholds are higher (poorer) for shorter-duration sounds than for pure-tones. Therefore, different methods have been developed to account for the differences in threshold that generally involve incorporating a correction factor to convert ABR thresholds to a behavioral threshold. One method is to measure the ABR in dB nHL and subtract a correction factor from the ABR threshold to estimate the behavioral threshold (Bagatto, Scollie, Hyde, & Seewald, 2010). The correction factors are developed by measuring ABR thresholds on a large group of individuals who are known to have normal hearing from the behavioral audiogram. The average difference between the ABR threshold and the behavioral threshold for each frequency becomes the correction factor that is used for ABR. Another method (Gorga et al., 2006) directly measures the behavioral thresholds of a group of individual with normal hearing to ABR stimuli. The calibration table in the ABR system is set so that the level of the average threshold for listeners with normal hearing is equivalent to 0 dB nHL. This negates the need for an additional correction factor and simplifies reporting of thresholds, so that individuals who are fitting hearing aids based on the ABR can treat the ABR thresholds as already equivalent to the audiogram. Both methods yield similar results and have published data to support them. Audiologists should include details in the reported ABR results to indicate which method was used and whether the reported thresholds have already been equated to the audiogram to avoid errors in threshold estimation.

Despite the widespread use of these approaches for attempting to equate behavioral thresholds and ABR thresholds, recent studies have suggested that attempting to account for differences in temporal integration may lead to errors in threshold estimation, particularly for children with severe or profound hearing loss. A retrospective review of ABR results from infants and children by McCreery and colleagues (2014) found that while the application of a correction factor improved the prediction of behavioral thresholds for children with normal hearing or mild hearing loss, subtracting a correction factor from the ABR threshold led to larger errors in thresholds for children with severe or profound hearing loss. The explanation for these errors is related to the fact that hearing loss reduces the amount of temporal integration and the difference in thresholds between short- and long-duration sounds. In fact, individuals with severe to profound hearing loss show very little temporal integration, so adding a correction factor to account for temporal integration reduces the accuracy of ABR estimates of behavioral thresholds. The study introduced an alternative method where the amount of the correction factor is reduced as the degree of hearing loss increases, leading to more accurate predictions of behavioral thresholds across the entire range of degrees of hearing loss.

**ABR in Auditory Neuropathy Spectrum Disorder.** As noted in the previous section of this chapter on OAEs, children with ANSD often have absent or grossly abnormal ABR responses, along with OAEs that are consistent with normal hearing. In addition to an absent or abnormal ABR response, the cochlear microphonic response might also be present in the early part of the ABR, around the same latency as Wave I. Figure 2–13 shows a picture of the cochlear microphonic obtained from an ABR of a child with ANSD. The cochlear microphonic represents the electrical activity of the cochlear outer hair cells, so it is often considered the electrical analog of otoacoustic emissions. The cochlear microphonic can be distinguished from Wave I of the ABR because the cochlear microphonic maintains the same polarity as the stimulus being used to elicit the ABR. Cochlear microphonic will reverse direction if the polarity of the click stimulus is changed between rarefaction and condensation. Wave I will not reverse with stimulus polarity. The cochlear microphonic must also be distinguished from stimulus artifact, which also can occur early in the ABR response and also reverses polarity since it is an electrical artifact from the transducer. To delineate the cochlear microphonic from stimulus artifact, a control run with the ABR stimulus on, but the insert earphone tubing clamped or removed from the transducer can be used. If the early response

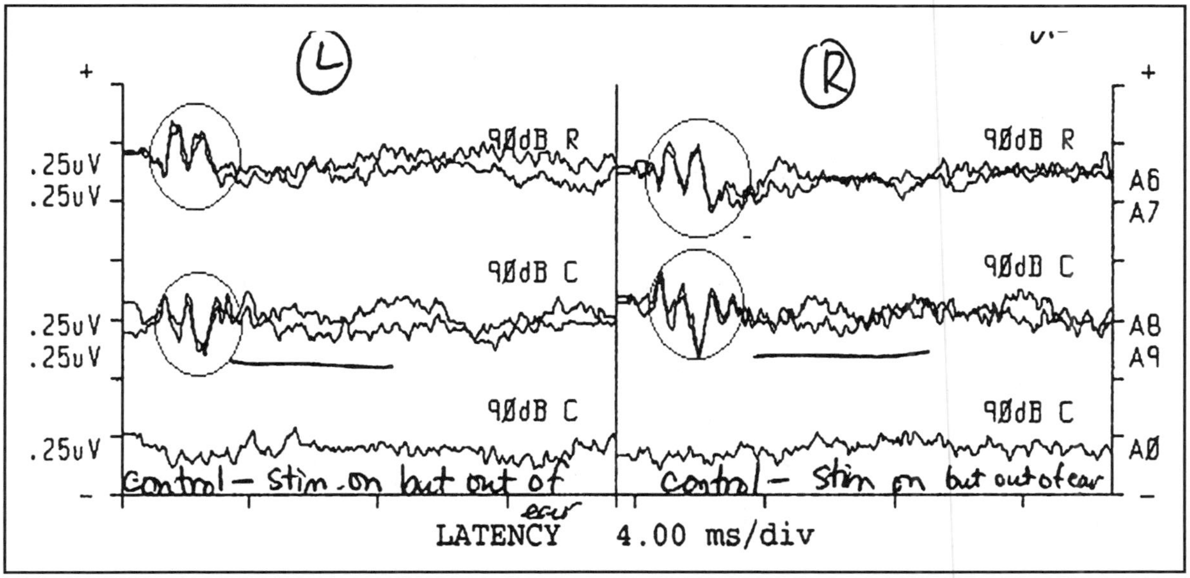


**FIGURE 2–13.** Auditory brainstem response (ABR) recordings to click stimuli from an infant with auditory neuropathy spectrum disorder. Responses in the left panel are from the left ear, and response in the right pane are for the right ear. The stimulus level for all recordings is 90 dB nHL. The top set of recordings in each panel are for rarefaction stimulus polarity, the middle recordings are for condensation polarity, and the bottom recording is a control condition with the stimulus on, but the insert earphone disconnected from the ear. The cochlear microphonic response is circled in each of the recordings and reverses when the stimulus polarity changes from rarefaction to condensation. The absence of cochlear microphonic in the control condition indicates that the early response is not stimulus artifact from the transducer, but a response from the auditory system.

persists without the acoustic stimulation to the ear, but with the transducer on, then the response is electrical stimulus artifact, since no sound is being delivered to the ear. If the early response goes away when the acoustic stimulus is not presented to the ear, but the earphone is on, then the response is the cochlear microphonic. Figure 2–13 shows ABR tracings with rarefaction and condensation, as well as a controlled trial without stimulation to the ear.

Although some children with ANSD will have a measurable Wave V in the ABR at high-intensity levels, the presences of the cochlear microphonic and OAEs and an absent ABR should be an indicator that the level of Wave V is unlikely to correspond to the behavioral threshold, like it does in children with other types of hearing loss. Research suggests that children with ANSD have a wide range of behavioral thresholds, from normal to profound, despite having an absent ABR (Rance, 2005). Other research has shown that the presence of Wave V in individuals with ANSD is not useful in predicting the amount of auditory function that the person might have (Sininger & Oba, 2001). Therefore, ABR responses in individuals with ANSD should not be used to proceed with amplification. Instead, behavioral estimates of threshold must be obtained before the initiation of amplification, which often leads to significant delays in the confirmation of the degree of hearing loss and provision of hearing aids (Walker, McCreery, Spratford, & Roush, 2016). Scientists are working on developing methods using cortical evoked responses that may offer greater promise in estimating thresholds in infants with ANSD (Lightfoot & Kennedy, 2006). Until those tests become clinically available, the ability to provide amplification to children with ANSD will be delayed until behavioral thresholds can be estimated.

**Summary of ABR Threshold Assessment.** The ABR is a cornerstone of pediatric assessment for children who are unable to participate in behavioral assessment, including infants and children with significant developmental disabilities. The ABR provides valid and reliable estimates of behavioral threshold that can be used to provide amplification. Although the amount of threshold information provided by ABR is often more limited than a traditional behavioral audiometric assessment, it is a vital tool that allows the early provision of amplification to children. Additional tools are needed in order to estimate behavioral thresholds in individuals with ANSD.

### Auditory Steady-State Response

An evoked potential that is similar to an ABR response is the auditory steady-state response, or ASSR. The ASSR is recorded using a similar electrode montage that would be used for recording ABR, but instead of relying on brief tone-burst stimuli, the ASSR can use longer duration pure-tone stimuli to elicit a response. The pure-tones used to record ASSR are amplitude and/or frequency modulated at specific rates from 75 to 100 Hz. There are specific nerve fibers in the brainstem that preserve this modulation. The electrical response of the brainstem can be recorded and analyzed for those specific modulation frequencies using a Fast Fourier Transform. The level where the modulation can be measured in the brainstem is used to estimate the behavioral threshold. For a complete review of ASSR detail and recording techniques, see Chapter 10 in Picton (2010).

Data suggest that the ASSR has similar predictive capacity as ABR for estimating the behavioral audiogram in infants with normal hearing and infants with hearing loss (Cone-Wesson, Dowell, Tomlin, Rance, & Ming, 2002; Rance et al., 2005). Additionally, because the ASSR uses stimuli that have a similar duration as the pure-tones used to measure the behavioral audiogram, those stimuli are easier to calibrate and do not have the need for correction factors related to temporal integration like ABR stimuli do. The detection of ASSR is also done automatically, using statistical detection algorithms. This minimizes the need to visually inspect waveforms and identify peaks, as is needed with ABR, so it has been suggested that ASSR might be an easier tool for individuals with limited experience than ABR (Picton et al., 2001).

However, ASSR is not without its limitations. Because different modulation rates can be used for different frequencies and different ears, it was theoretically possible to test up to eight frequencies simultaneously in some early iterations of ASSR (Picton et al., 2001). This appeared to save considerable time compared to ABR responses. However, when this approach was validated in infants, the use of multiple, simultaneous modulation frequencies led to a reduction in the response amplitudes and overestimation of thresholds in infants (Van Maanen & Stapells, 2010). When single ASSR frequencies were tested individually, the advantage in test time over ABR was minimal. Additionally, because ASSR detection is automated and no waveforms are visible, ANSD and associated cochlear microphonic cannot be easily detected. For these reasons, the ASSR has not gained widespread clinical use in the United States at the time of this writing, as it offers similar sensitivity and specificity as ABR, but with limitations for detecting ANSD.

### Behavioral Assessment Techniques with Children

The ABR is the primary method of diagnosing hearing loss in infants and providing early amplification because infants are not able to provide reliable behavioral responses to sound in the first few months of life. However, much of the later information obtained during the amplification process for children are gathered using developmentally appropriate behavioral techniques. Starting at a developmental age of 6 months, different methods of behavioral assessment can be used to supplement findings from electrophysiological tests or diagnose hearing loss in children who have never been tested or passed newborn hearing screening, but have concerns for hearing. The process of obtaining unconditioned responses to sound using behavioral observation will be discussed. Three approaches to measuring thresholds, visual reinforcement auditory, conditioned play audiometry, and conventional audiometry are also highlighted.

**Chronological Age vs. Developmental Age.** An important consideration for behavioral audiological assessment is using developmentally appropriate techniques. A child's chronological age simply refers to how old the child is relative to his or her birthday, whereas the developmental age is an approximation of the child's age based on their developmental skills and abilities. Children need to have developed the physical, cognitive, and behavioral skills to participate in specific types of audiological assessment. Audiologists must be able to quickly assess the child's developmental skills and adapt the assessment techniques to the child's developmental age. Testing a child based on their chronological age can often lead to limited ability to collect test data, as children may not be able to reliably perform the task if the approach is too advanced and may become bored with the task if the approach is not sufficiently advanced or varied. In the case of premature infants, chronological age may be adjusted to account for the child's gestational age, but developmental abilities in premature infants will vary considerably. Therefore, the assessment method used should be based on the child's developmental abilities, rather than chronological or adjusted gestational estimates alone. The success of behavioral audiometric assessment in infants and young children is contingent upon the audiologist's ability to select the appropriate task for behavioral assessment.

**Behavior Observation.** Behavior observation in the context of hearing assessment refers to any unconditioned response to sound. Unconditioned responses can include cessation of sucking, eye widening, gaze shift, startle responses, or head turns. In most cases, behavior observation is used to determine whether a child has awareness of sound, which is typically performed before children reach a developmental age of 6 months. Northern and Downs (2002) describe many of the techniques used to elicit rudimentary responses to sound from infants including rattles and noisemakers, as well as speech and pure-tone sounds presented through the audiometer. The terms behavioral observation audiometry and behavioral response observation have also been used to describe the technique of eliciting unconditioned responses. The term behavior observation audiometry is avoided in this text to avoid conflating this unconditioned approach with other types of behavioral hearing assessment that require a conditioned response from the infant.

Behavior observation can be useful in making dichotomous judgments about whether or not a child has awareness of sound, but is less useful in estimating the child's behavioral thresholds. Unconditioned responses have the disadvantage of being suprathreshold responses, meaning that the level of the sound has to be above the threshold in order to elicit a response. Although some clinicians will use calibrated signals through the audiometer for behavioral observation, many of the sounds used in behavioral observation are generated with noisemakers that are uncalibrated and produce sound with a wide frequency range of energy, limiting the frequency-specificity of the assessment. In most cases, the sounds used for behavioral observation are also delivered in the sound field and cannot be used to determine which ear might be hearing the sound. For these reasons, behavior observation does not meet the requirements of being ear- or frequency-specific and does not have a strong predictive relationship with the child's threshold. As a result, the use of behavior observation in the diagnostic process should be limited to situations where supplemental information about the child's hearing is needed. Behavior observation cannot be used to prescribe amplification.

**Visual Reinforcement Audiometry.** Once infants reach a developmental age of 6 months, several developmental milestones permit the assessment of hearing using visual reinforcement audiometry (VRA). Infants who are able to sit up without assistance and turn their heads can be conditioned to respond to sound in a VRA paradigm. Generally, the infant is placed on a parent or caregiver's lap (Figure 2–14). The parents are often provided with headphones that produce masking noise so that they do not react to sounds that their child might be hearing through headphones or the speakers. The child's attention is drawn forward using a test assistant with toys or a centering toy, which can be a static, lighted picture that can

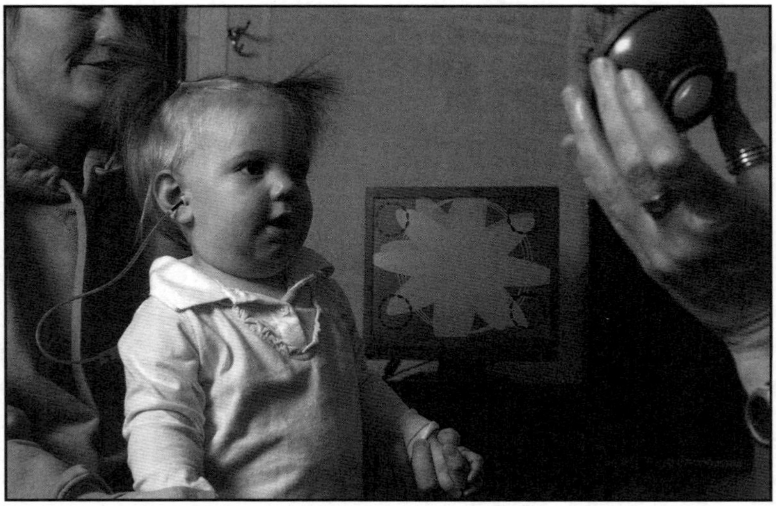

**FIGURE 2–14.** A child seated on her parent's lap for visual reinforcement audiometry assessment.

draw a child's attention forward without being so interesting that the child will not participate in conditioning. Speech, pure-tones, or warble tones are delivered via insert earphones, speakers, or a bone oscillator, at medium to loud intensity levels (generally starting around 60 dB HL). At first, the sounds are paired with a visual reinforcement toy that is located inside of a smoked glass box that is only visible when the toy is illuminated. Viewing screens showing short videos can also be used to provide visual reinforcement, with results comparable to mechanical reinforcers (Schmida, Peterson, & Tharpe, 2003). Once the child consistently responds on several consecutive trials to the paired stimulus and visual reinforcement, the visual reinforcement becomes contingent on the child turning in response to the sound being presented. Behavioral thresholds can be estimated using speech, but also pure-tones or warble tones to estimate frequency-specific thresholds for amplification. If insert earphones are used, the data gathered during VRA also satisfy the ear-specific requirements for initiating amplification.

The prime developmental age range for VRA is between 9 to 18 months. During this age range, the number of potential responses prior to the child habituating to the task reaches a maximum (Widen et al., 2000). The number of responses can be maximized by having multiple toys or videos for the child to respond to. On average, the number of responses that can be obtained using VRA is typically around 18 to 24 (Schmida et al., 2003), so the number of thresholds that can be estimated depends on how efficiently the audiologist can search for thresholds since each threshold requires multiple responses at the same intensity level. Much like ABR, a productive VRA test session will yield two to three thresholds per ear. Ongoing testing is needed to collect enough threshold information for a full audiogram. Starting around 18 months developmental age, children begin to lose interest in the VRA paradigm and the number of responses that can be reliably obtained in a single session begins to decline. By 24 to 30 months developmental age, children may not condition to visual reinforcement consistently at all. Unfortunately, children around 2 years of age also lack the executive function skills to perform the next behavioral audiometric assessment method for children, conditioned play audiometry (CPA). This leads to a period of time between 2 to 3 years of age where the amount of audiological information that can be obtained may be very limited. Despite these limitations, attempts to gather audiological threshold data in this age range are essential to monitoring hearing status and maintaining an appropriate hearing aid fitting. In some cases where audiological information has not been reliably obtained for a year, audiologists may recommend an ABR under sedation to estimate threshold. However, sedation should be avoided whenever possible, and the best strategy for minimizing the need for sedation is consistent behavioral assessment attempts.

**Conditioned Play Audiometry.** When children reach the age of around 24 to 30 months developmental age, an alternative audiological assessment paradigm, CPA, can be used instead of VRA. For CPA assessment, the child generally sits on the parent's lap or by themselves at a small table. A play partner is usually available to help the child play the game and prevent false positive responses. Parents can also be trained to be a play partner during CPA if another option is not available. In some cases, the audiologist runs the audiometer from the patient side of the booth, while also serving as the play partner. Like VRA, a stimulus is paired with a response, but in the case of CPA, the response is performed an action with a toy or part of a game each time a sound is presented. A child may be conditioned to place a peg in a board, drop a block in a bucket, or place rings on a stand in response to the stimulus. Computerized games have also been developed as a way to vary the task and maintain a child's interest during the assessment. As with VRA, CPA can be used to obtain ear- and frequency-specific thresholds for amplification. The number of responses that can be obtained during CPA is also typically greater than what can be obtained during VRA. For a child with a developmental age of 3 to 4 years, an entire audiogram can be obtained in a single test session with a cooperative child. One key to maintaining the child's interest during CPA assessment is to recognize the need to switch the game or task during the assessment before the child habituates to the task. CPA is a viable option to use with children all the way up to the age where they can complete a hearing assessment using conventional techniques that would be used with adults. Often, children may be able to perform conventional audiometry, but may still prefer to play games in a CPA paradigm up until adolescence. Once children reach a developmental age of 5 years, the child may be able to participate in CPA without a play partner or parent to help them with the task.

**Conventional Audiometry.** Starting around the developmental age of 5 years, children can be tested using the same audiometric approaches that are often used with adults. As noted in the previous section, some children may prefer CPA for many years, even if they are capable of completing a conventional audiometric assessment, because it is more fun. Some children will eventually prefer conventional audiometry and good pediatric audiologists will often leave the decision about the method of assessment up to the child once they are old enough to decide. Conventional audiometric techniques rely on the child to press a button or raise their hand when the stimulus is presented. This task can be more efficient than VRA or CPA in terms of both time and the number of responses that can be obtained but may not be sufficiently interesting to engage the child's attention.

## CONCLUSIONS

The first step in the amplification process is to obtain accurate assessment information about the child's type, degree, and configuration of hearing loss. Multiple assessments, including immittance, OAEs, and either ABR or behavioral assessment are needed to make an accurate diagnosis, rule out the presence of temporary conditions like middle ear fluid that can affect hearing, and gather sufficient information to permit the prescription of amplification if that is needed. Comprehensive information about a child's hearing is rarely obtained in a single test session. Instead, thresholds are estimated across multiple test sessions, which are completed more frequently than with older children and adults. Information is often combined across test sessions and the test sessions can occur as frequently as every 3 to 6 months in cases where information is lacking. With ongoing audiological assessment, clinicians can ensure that amplification can be adjusted to meet the child's hearing needs if they change, and also consider the need to move to a cochlear implant if the child's hearing progresses beyond the point where hearing aids are likely to be helpful.

## REFERENCES


American Academy of Pediatrics, & Joint Committee on Infant Hearing. (2007). Year 2007 position statement: Principles and guidelines for early hearing detection and intervention programs. *Pediatrics, 120*(4), 898.

Alaerts, J., Luts, H., & Wouters, J. (2007). Evaluation of middle ear function in young children: Clinical guidelines for the use of 226- and 1,000-Hz tympanometry. *Otology and Neurotology, 28*(6), 727–732.

Bagatto, M., Scollie, S. D., Hyde, M., & Seewald, R. (2010). Protocol for the provision of amplification within the Ontario infant hearing program. *International Journal of Audiology, 49*(sup1), S70–S79.

Baldwin, M. (2006). Choice of probe tone and classification of trace patterns in tympanometry undertaken in early infancy. *International Journal of Audiology, 45*(7), 417–427.

Berg, A. L., Prieve, B. A., Serpanos, Y. C., & Wheaton, M. A. (2011). Hearing screening in a well-infant nursery: Profile of automated ABR-fail/OAE-pass. *Pediatrics, 127*(2), 269–275.

Berlin, C. I., Hood, L. J., Morlet, T., Wilensky, D., Brashears, S., John, P. S., . . . Thibodeaux, M. (2005). The battery principle re-visited physiologically, with special attention to auditory neuropathy and cued speech. *SIG 9 Perspectives on Hearing and Hearing Disorders in Childhood, 15*(1), 5–9.

Bess, F. H., & Paradise, J. L. (1994). Universal screening for infant hearing impairment: not simple, not risk-free, not necessarily beneficial, and not presently justified. *Pediatrics, 93*(2), 330–334.

Burns, E. M., Arehart, K. H., & Campbell, S. L. (1992). Prevalence of spontaneous otoacoustic emissions in neonates. *Journal of the Acoustical Society of America, 91*(3), 1571–1575.

Carhart, R., & Jerger, J. (1959). Preferred method for clinical determination of pure-tone thresholds. *Journal of Speech and Hearing Disorders, 24*, 330–345.

Cone-Wesson, B., Dowell, R. C., Tomlin, D., Rance, G., & Ming, W. J. (2002). The auditory steady-state response: comparisons with the auditory brainstem response. *Journal of the American Academy of Audiology, 13*(4), 173–187.

Galland, B. C., Taylor, B. J., Elder, D. E., & Herbison, P. (2012). Normal sleep patterns in infants and children: A systematic review of observational studies. *Sleep Medicine Reviews, 16*(3), 213–222.

Gorga, M. P., Johnson, T. A., Kaminski, J. K., Beauchaine, K. L., Garner, C. A., & Neely, S. T. (2006). Using a combination of click-and toneburst-evoked auditory brainstem response measurements to estimate pure-tone thresholds. *Ear and Hearing, 27*(1), 60–74.

Gorga, M. P., Neely, S. T., Dorn, P. A., & Konrad-Martin, D. (2002). The use of distortion product otoacoustic emission suppression as an estimate of response growth. *Journal of the Acoustical Society of America, 111*(1), 271–284.

Gorga, M. P., Neely, S. T., Ohlrich, B., Hoover, B., Redner, J., & Peters, J. (1997). From laboratory to clinic: A large-scale study of distortion product otoacoustic emissions in ears with normal hearing and ears with hearing loss. *Ear and Hearing, 18*(6), 440–455.

Hall, J.W. (2015). *eHandbook of auditory evoked responses: Principles, procedures and protocols*. St. Augustine, FL: Pearson.

Hotz, M. A., Harris, F. P., & Probst, R. (1994). Otoacoustic emissions: An approach for monitoring aminoglycoside-induced ototoxicity. *Laryngoscope, 104*(9), 1130–1134.

Hunter, L. L., Feeney, M. P., Miller, J. A. L., Jeng, P. S., & Bohning, S. (2010). Wideband reflectance in newborns: Normative regions and relationship to hearing screening results. *Ear and Hearing, 31*(5), 599–610.

Hussain, D. M., Gorga, M. P., Neely, S. T., Keefe, D. H., & Peters, J. (1998). Transient evoked otoacoustic emissions in patients with normal hearing and in patients with hearing loss. *Ear and Hearing, 19*(6), 434–449.

Jerger, J. F., & Hayes, D. (1976). The cross-check principle in pediatric audiometry. *Archives of Otolaryngology, 102*(10), 614–620.

Keefe, D. H., Fitzpatrick, D., Liu, Y. W., Sanford, C. A., & Gorga, M. P. (2010). Wideband acoustic-reflex test in a test battery to predict middle-ear dysfunction. *Hearing Research, 263*(1), 52–65.

Kei, J., Allison-Levick, J., Dockray, J., Harrys, R., Kirkegard, C., Wong, J., . . . Tudehope, D. (2003). High-frequency (1000 Hz) tympanometry in normal neonates. *Journal of the American Academy of Audiology, 14*(1), 20–28.

Kemp, D. T. (1986). Otoacoustic emissions, traveling waves and cochlear mechanisms. *Hearing Research, 22*(1), 95–104.

Lightfoot, G., & Kennedy, V. (2006). Cortical electric response audiometry hearing threshold estimation: Accuracy, speed, and the effects of stimulus presentation features. *Ear and Hearing, 27*(5), 443–456.

McCreery, R. W., Kaminski, J., Beauchaine, K., Lenzen, N., Simms, K., & Gorga, M. P. (2014). The impact of degree of hearing loss on auditory brainstem response predictions of behavioral thresholds. *Ear and Hearing, 36*(3), 309–319.

Northern, J. L., & Downs, M. P. (2002). *Hearing in children*. Baltimore, MD: Lippincott, Williams & Wilkins.

Olsen, W. O., Noffsinger, D., & Kurdziel, S. (1975). Acoustic reflex and reflex decay: Occurrence in patients with cochlear and eighth nerve lesions. *Archives of Otolaryngology, 101*(10), 622–625.

Owens, J. J., McCoy, M. J., Lonsbury-Martin, B. L., & Martin, G. K. (1993). Otoacoustic emissions in children with normal ears, middle ear dysfunction, and ventilating tubes. *Otology and Neurotology, 14*(1), 34–40.

Paradise, J. L., Rockette, H. E., Colborn, D. K., Bernard, B. S., Smith, C. G., Kurs-Lasky, M., & Janosky, J. E. (1997). Otitis media in 2253 Pittsburgh-area infants: Prevalence and risk factors during the first two years of life. *Pediatrics, 99*(3), 318–333.

Picton, T.W., Dimitrijevic, A., van Roon, P., John, M.S., Reed, M., & Finkelstein, H. (2001) *Possible roles for the ASSR in fitting hearing aids*. Proceedings of the Sound Foundations through Early Amplification Conference. Phonak AG, Chicago, IL.

Picton, T. W. (2010). *Human auditory evoked potentials*. San Diego, CA: Plural.

Pittman, A. L., & Stelmachowicz, P. G. (2003). Hearing loss in children and adults: Audiometric configuration, asymmetry, and progression. *Ear and Hearing, 24*(3), 198–205.

Prieve, B. A., Gorga, M. P., Schmidt, A., Neely, S., Peters, J., Schultes, L., & Jesteadt, W. (1993). Analysis of transient-evoked otoacoustic emissions in normal-hearing and hearing-impaired ears. *Journal of the Acoustical Society of America, 93*(6), 3308–3319.

Rance, G. (2005). Auditory neuropathy/dys-synchrony and its perceptual consequences. *Trends in Amplification, 9*(1), 1–43.

Rance, G., Roper, R., Symons, L., Moody, L. J., Poulis, C., Dourlay, M., & Kelly, T. (2005). Hearing threshold estimation in infants using auditory steady-state responses. *Journal of the American Academy of Audiology, 16*(5), 291–300.

Rogers, D. J., Boseley, M. E., Adams, M. T., Makowski, R. L., & Hohman, M. H. (2010). Prospective comparison of handheld pneumatic otoscopy, binocular microscopy, and tympanometry in identifying middle ear effusions in children. *International Journal of Pediatric Otorhinolaryngology, 74*(10), 1140–1143.

Sanford, C. A., Keefe, D. H., Liu, Y. W., Fitzpatrick, D., McCreery, R. W., Lewis, D. E., & Gorga, M. P. (2009). Sound-conduction effects on distortion-product otoacoustic emission screening outcomes in newborn infants: Test performance of wideband acoustic transfer functions and 1-kHz tympanometry. *Ear and Hearing, 30*(6), 635–652.

Schmida, M. J., Peterson, H. J., & Tharpe, A. M. (2003). Visual reinforcement audiometry using digital video disc and conventional reinforcers. *American Journal of Audiology, 12*(1), 35–40.

Sininger, Y., & Oba, S. (2001). Patients with auditory neuropathy: who are they and what can they hear. In Y. Sininger & A. Starr (Eds.), *Auditory neuropathy: A new perspective on hearing disorders* (pp. 15–35). San Diego, CA: Singular.

Stavroulaki, P., Apostolopoulos, N., Segas, J., Tsakanikos, M., & Adamopoulos, G. (2001). Evoked otoacoustic emissions—an approach for monitoring cisplatin-induced ototoxicity in children. *International Journal of Pediatric Otorhinolaryngology, 59*(1), 47–57.

Tas, A., Yagiz, R., Uzun, C., Adali, M. K., Koten, M., Tas, M., & Karasalihoglu, A. R. (2004). Effect of middle ear effusion on distortion product otoacoustic emission. *International Journal of Pediatric Otorhinolaryngology, 68*(4), 437–440.

Toner, J. G., & Mains, B. (1990). Pneumatic otoscopy and tympanometry in the detection of middle ear effusion. *Clinical Otolaryngology and Allied Sciences, 15*(2), 121–123.

Topolska, M. M., Hassman, E., & Baczek, M. (2000). The effects of chronic otitis media with effusion on the measurement of distortion products of otoacoustic emissions: Presurgical and postsurgical examination. *Clinical Otolaryngology and Allied Sciences, 25*(4), 315–320.

Van Maanen, A., & Stapells, D. R. (2010). Multiple-ASSR thresholds in infants and young children with hearing loss. *Journal of the American Academy of Audiology, 21*(8), 535–545.

Vander Werff, K. R., Prieve, B. A., & Georgantas, L. M. (2009). Infant air and bone conduction tone-burst auditory brainstem responses for classification of hearing loss and the relationship to behavioral thresholds. *Ear and Hearing, 30*(3), 350–368.

Walker, E. A., McCreery, R. W., Spratford, M., & Roush, P. A. (2016). Children with ANSD fitted with hearing aids applying the AAA Pediatric Amplification Guideline: Current practice and outcomes. *Journal of the American Academy of Audiology, 27*(3), 204–218.

Werner, L. A., Levi, E. C., & Keefe, D. H. (2010). Ear-canal wideband acoustic transfer functions of adults and two-to nine-month-old infants. *Ear and Hearing, 31*(5), 587–598.

Widen, J. E., Folsom, R. C., Cone-Wesson, B., Carty, L., Dunnell, J. J., Koebsell, K., . . . Gorga, M. P. (2000). Identification of neonatal hearing impairment: Hearing status at 8 to 12 months corrected age using a visual reinforcement audiometry protocol. *Ear and Hearing, 21*(5), 471–487.

Wiegers, J. S., Bielefeld, E. C., & Whitelaw, G. M. (2015). Utility of the Vivosonic Integrity™ auditory brainstem response system as a hearing screening device for difficult-to-test children. *International Journal of Audiology, 54*(4), 282–288.

# 3

# Hearing Aid Candidacy and Feature Selection for Children

*Ryan W. McCreery and Elizabeth A. Walker*

## INTRODUCTION

Once a diagnosis of hearing loss has been confirmed, audiologists must next make decisions about whether or not amplification can help to improve the child's access to the acoustic cues needed to support speech and language development. The process of determining candidacy for amplification for children differs from the process that is typically considered for adults with hearing loss. The goal of providing children who have hearing loss with cumulative auditory experience can only be met if the device and features selected can provide sufficient audibility for speech, as well as comfortable listening across a wide range of environments. If hearing aids are determined to be appropriate for a specific child, the specific features of the hearing aid should be selected with the listening needs of children in mind. Features that are selected during the amplification process include the physical characteristics of the hearing aid and the earmold, as well as decisions about activation of signal processing strategies that may enhance speech understanding and comfort when wearing the hearing aids. Whenever possible, specific research evidence, based on children with hearing loss, should be used to make decisions regarding hearing aid features. Some types of hearing aids or signal processing features may be activated only at a specific age or when specific developmental milestones have been achieved. Thus, the process of device and feature selection for children is not a one-time event, but part of an on-going process of reassessment of the child's listening needs. Many hearing aid signal processing strategies were developed based on the needs of adults and were not optimized or validated for children. Published evidence on the efficacy and effectiveness of hearing aid signal processing strategies for children has begun to emerge, but remains limited. In the current chapter, we highlight the evidence-based framework of promoting cumulative auditory experience to guide the selection process with hearing aids and signal processing strategies for children.

## HEARING AID CANDIDACY FOR CHILDREN

As noted in Chapter 1, children have unique listening needs compared to adults and are fitted with hearing aids to achieve different objectives. The goal of fitting hearing aids for adults is to minimize the effects of hearing loss by providing amplification that improves audibility, but does not cause loudness discomfort. Adults have fully developed linguistic and cognitive abilities in most cases, which has two main implications for hearing aid candidacy. Knowledge of language and the ability to store and process incoming auditory information are helpful skills for listening under degraded conditions. Therefore, adults may not require hearing aids until hearing loss has become moderate in the high frequencies or mild across a wide frequency range. Additionally, once adults seek help for their hearing loss, hearing aids may only be needed to partially restore audibility of the speech signal to minimize the negative effects of hearing loss. Adults can often recognize continuous discourse accurately with less than half of the speech spectrum audible to them (Sherbecoe & Studebaker, 2002). Thus, adults can function with greater degrees of hearing loss and less audibility than infants and children.

When hearing loss occurs during infancy or childhood, it disrupts the developmental process of speech and language, which requires sensory experience to drive it. The main objective of providing hearing aids to infants and young children is to provide access to these acoustic cues across a wide range of listening environments. The implications for hearing aid candidacy are that infants and children may be fit with hearing aids even when the hearing loss is mild or limited to high frequencies, whereas an adult with the same audiogram might not be considered a hearing aid candidate. Furthermore, when children are fit with hearing aids, the amount of amplification provided is typically greater than what would be provided for an adult with the same audiogram because audibility is needed to promote auditory access (Scollie et al., 2005). The prescription of amplification is discussed in greater detail in Chapter 4. Modern prescriptive approaches for hearing aids prescribe more gain for children than for adults, due to the perceptual evidence that children may need higher sensation levels and greater audibility than adults for speech recognition (Stelmachowicz, Pittman, Hoover, Lewis, & Moeller, 2004b) and word learning (Pittman, 2008; Stelmachowicz, Pittman, Hoover, & Lewis, 2004a).

Because nearly any degree or configuration of permanent hearing loss can affect the development of communication, a child with almost any degree or configuration or permanent hearing loss is likely to be considered a candidate for a hearing aid. Candidacy decisions for amplification for children should be made to err on the side of providing amplification when the benefit may be minimal, rather than waiting for developmental evidence that the hearing loss has had an impact. Once present, developmental deficits may be difficult to ameliorate in the long run and should be avoided through aggressive provision of amplification that occurs as soon after the confirmation of hearing loss as possible. In cases where the potential benefits of amplification may be questionable, families should be given the option to use loaner hearing aids on a trial basis to determine whether benefits can be observed. If amplification is only initiated after a child with hearing loss exhibits significant developmental concerns, those deficits can be difficult to overcome. A comprehensive battery of developmentally appropriate audiological outcome measures, including aided speech recognition assessment and auditory development questionnaires, should be used to assess potential benefits over time, and this is discussed in Chapter 6. The development of key communication and cognitive abilities is too crucial to the child's well-being and quality of life to take a less proactive approach to hearing aid candidacy. Special considerations for hearing aid candidacy, including minimal hearing loss, auditory neuropathy spectrum disorder, and unilateral hearing loss are discussed in greater detail in Chapter 9.

## HEARING AID SELECTION FOR CHILDREN

Hearing aids have a wide range of available features and attributes that must be considered when selecting a hearing aid for children. Once it is determined that a child is a candidate for a hearing aid, the audiologist must select a hearing aid that meets the child's current and future needs, up to the 5-year life span of most of hearing aids. Whereas adults may select devices based on cosmetic or sound quality criteria, the ability to adapt to changes in a child's hearing, as well as durability and connectivity of the hearing device, are among the key criteria for selection for children. There are a wide range of child-specific considerations that may influence decisions about the child's hearing aids. This is discussed in the following sections.

### Hearing Aid Style

Hearing aids are available in a wide range of sizes and styles from behind-the-ear (BTE) hearing aids to tiny completely-in-the-canal (CIC) custom hearing aids (Figure 3–1).

Adults may select CIC or small BTE hearing aids because the devices are discrete and cosmetically appealing. It may seem logical to conclude that smaller devices are also preferable for children who are smaller in size. However, there are a number of other factors that will influence the selection of the hearing aid style for children. Custom hearing aids, including in-the-ear (ITE) and CIC hearing aids, contain all of the circuitry and hardware in a hard shell that is fabricated from the mold of the patient's ear. These custom devices should be avoided with children under 12 years for a number of reasons. The ear canals of infants and children undergo rapid growth during the first few years of life and steady increases in the size of the ear canal in adolescence (Keefe & Levi, 1996). Because the custom shell of ITE and CIC hearing aids cannot be easily adapted to this growth, frequent refabrication of the shell would be needed to maintain a consistent coupling to the child's ear as it grows. Frequent refabrication is expensive. The time period in which the shells are being refabricated would also result in extended

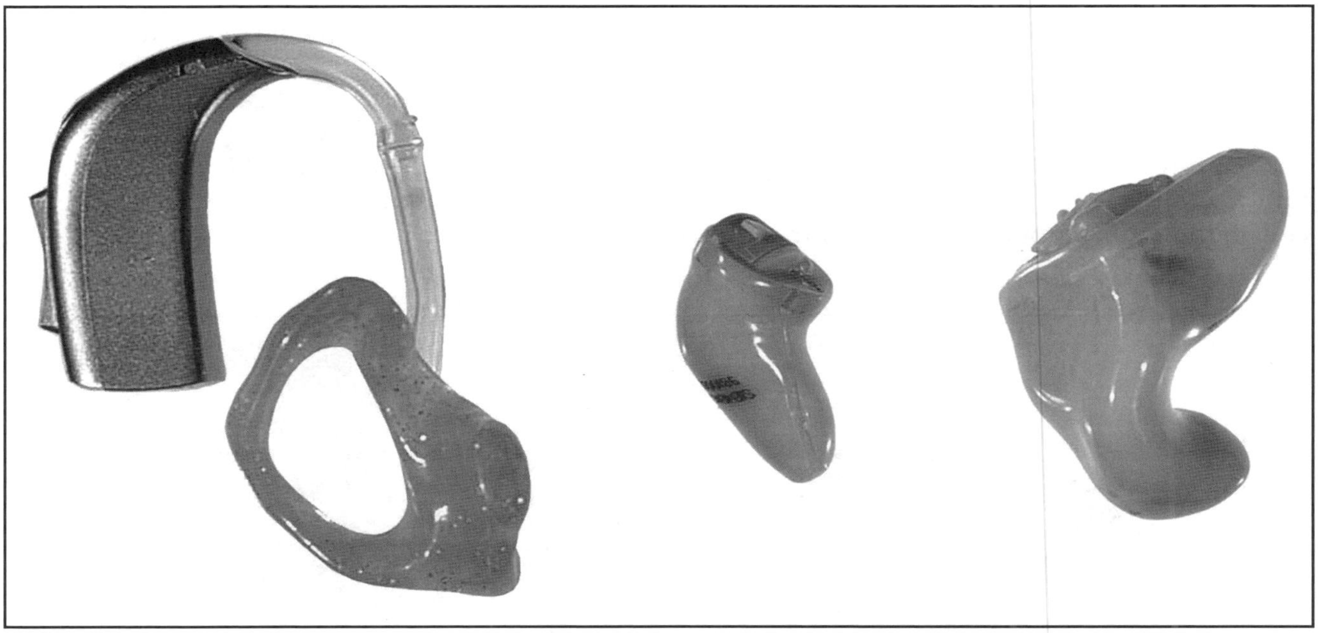

**FIGURE 3–1.** Different hearing aid styles (*from left*) behind-the-ear with earmold (BTE), in-the-ear (ITE) custom device, and in-the-canal (ITC) custom device.

duration of no amplification for the child. The potential fitting range of ITE and CIC hearing aids is generally much more limited than BTE devices, which means that the devices cannot provide adequate gain over the plausible range of hearing losses that a child might develop if their hearing loss progresses. Custom ITE and CIC hearing aids have shorter lifespans, and are less durable than BTE hearing aids. They often have a smaller battery that needs to be replaced more frequently. The ability to connect ITE and CIC hearing aids to hearing assistance technologies is also limited or may require additional accessories.

The advantages of BTE hearing aids make them the preferred style of hearing aid for infants and children. Unlike the custom shell that comprises the ITE or CIC hearing aid, BTE hearing aids are coupled to an earmold (Figure 3–2).

Earmolds can be easily modified or remade as the child's ear canal grows and develops. Earmolds are also typically constructed of a soft material, such as vinyl or silicone, which may be more comfortable for children than an acrylic shell. Another advantage of BTE hearing aids is that they are more durable, require fewer repairs, and have a longer lifespan than ITE or CIC hearing aids, which can reduce the costs of amplification over the child's lifetime. The connectivity of BTE devices to hearing assistance technologies, such as remote-microphone frequency or digital modulation systems, is also easier than with custom devices, as BTE hearing aids often have multiple options for connectivity, including telecoil, Bluetooth, or other wireless transmission options. The larger size of BTE device also allows for a larger battery, which increases the length of the battery life and reduces the number of hearing aid batteries that must be purchased and disposed of. The fitting range of BTE hearing aids often covers the entire range of degrees of loss that would be fit with hearing aids from mild up to severe, which means that if the child's hearing loss progresses, an entirely new hearing aid may not be needed. Finally, tamper-resistant features, including a locking battery door to minimize the likelihood that batteries will be ingested by the child, are available on nearly all models of BTE hearing aids that would be appropriate for infants and children.

There are a wide range of color options for BTE hearing aids, from colors that match the child's skin or hair color, to bright, primary colors such as red, pink, blue, and green. Audiologists may wish to discuss color options with parents first, so that the options meet the parents' specifications prior to being presented to children. Children and some parents may prefer devices that are the child's favorite color, not only to give the child choices about the hearing aids that they will wear, but also because bright colors are often easier to find if the hearing aid is misplaced. If the parents or child does not want the hearing aid itself to be a bright color, selecting a bright color for the earmold can be an alternative. Earmolds often need to be changed every few months in infants and several times a year until a child reaches 5 years of age, so parents may find that the commitment to a specific color of earmold to be more acceptable

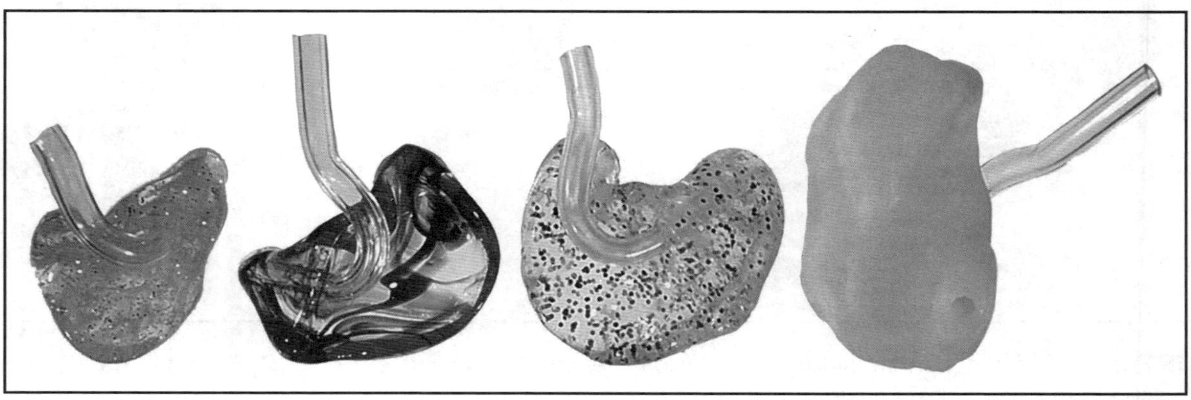

**FIGURE 3–2.** Examples of earmolds for BTE hearing aids.

than committing to 5 years with a specific BTE hearing aid color.

## Level of Technology

Hearing aid manufacturers offer multiple levels of technology with most of their product lines. The different tiers within a specific product are generally categorized based on their features. The most basic models of hearing aids may have more limited signal processing features, while higher levels of technology may offer a greater number of frequency channels or more automatic features, such as adaptive program switching, or other signal processing. Evidence suggests that many outcomes are comparable across levels of hearing aid technology for adults (Cox et al., 2016). At the time of this writing, there is no published evidence to suggest differences in outcomes across levels of hearing aid technology in children. The only proven difference between the different technology levels of hearing aids is the cost, which tends to be significantly higher at each tier of technology. Audibility can be provided with even the most basic levels of technology, which should be the primary motivating factor for children with hearing loss. As is noted later in this chapter, the evidence for the advanced signal processing strategies for children is extremely limited and should not be used to justify the purchase of higher levels of hearing aid technology for children.

## Hearing Aid Coupling

Because BTE hearing aids are the style of choice for infants and children nearly all the way through adolescence, the device must be coupled to the child's ear using an earmold, in most cases. The earmold is made from an impression taken of the child's ear canal. As noted previously, earmolds for children are fabricated using soft materials, such as silicone or vinyl, because they tend to be more comfortable and can be modified by the audiologist if needed.

Earmolds should be replaced when the coupling between the ear and the hearing aid becomes compromised by either the child's ear canal growth or shrinkage of the earmold material over time. Signs that earmolds need to be replaced include the presence of audible whistling or buzzing when the hearing aid is fully inserted into the child's ear (known as acoustic feedback) or when the retention of the device on the child's ear becomes poorer. However, modern feedback suppression algorithms have minimized the occurrence of acoustic feedback in some cases, to the point where acoustic feedback may not be present when the device is out of the child's ear. As the earmold fit becomes less optimal over time, the audibility of speech can change as low-frequency sounds leak out of the ear around the earmold. The best method for assessing earmold fit is through ongoing verification of the child's hearing aid to ensure that prescriptive targets for amplification can be met with the device. If the child's amplification must be increased considerably to compensate for a poor earmold fit, then it may be time to consider replacing the child's earmold, even if feedback and retention are not major concerns. In most cases, earmolds have to be replaced every 3 months for children under 1 year of age due to rapid ear canal growth during the first year of life. After a year, earmolds often need to be replaced every 6 to 12 months for children up to age 5 years, with 12 months or greater earmold life expected for children over 5 years of age. These are only average replacement timelines, and considerable variability is often present across children or within the same child over time because physical growth is not a uniform or linear process. However, earmolds do not need to be automatically replaced on a regular schedule. Rather, replacement should be based on the integrity of the fitting, retention, and the presence of acoustic feedback as noted above. Earmold problems related to cracks or breaks in the tubing can be resolved by replacing the tubing of the earmold, rather than replacing the earmold.

Improvements in feedback suppression algorithms have led to the ability to develop BTE hearing aids that either do not occlude or minimally occlude the ear canal. There are a host of acronyms for these devices, including receiver-in-the-ear (RITE), receiver-in-the-canal (RIC), and open-fit (OF) hearing aids. For the purposes of this discussion, we will describe devices where the receiver of the hearing aid is in the ear canal using the term

RITE, and describe devices with minimal occlusion of the ear canal as OF. Note that RITE devices can vary in the amount of occlusion of the ear canal, ranging from complete to minimal. Thus, the terms RITE and OF refer to different aspects of the hearing aid coupling and should not be viewed as synonymous. Occlusion in hearing aid coupling is an issue that is related to the discussion on venting and acoustic modifications, and this is reviewed in another section. The viability of RITE devices for children will be the focus of this section.

The popularity of RITE devices in adults is driven by the fact that the devices are often small and cosmetically appealing and can be fit with minimal occlusion of the ear canal. Occlusion is an important consideration for many adults with hearing loss because the processes of noise exposure and aging—the most common culprits of noise-induced hearing loss—often result in high-frequency hearing loss with relatively preserved low-frequency thresholds. Occluding the ear canal for an individual with normal low-frequency hearing can result in limited audibility of the unamplified sound through the ear canal, as well as complaints of sound quality for the listener's own voice or chewing. Along with advances in feedback suppression algorithms, RITE devices can be fit with minimal occlusion of the ear canal. This combination of features makes RITE devices an excellent choice for adults with high-frequency sensorineural hearing loss.

The popularity of RITE devices for adults has led to questions about whether or not RITE devices could also be effective for children with hearing loss, particularly children with high-frequency hearing loss and normal low-frequency hearing. Whereas RITE devices may be appropriate for some older children and teenagers, there are several limitations that limit the utility of these devices for infants and younger children. First, the thin wire and loudspeaker of RITE devices are delicate. This can lead to breakdowns related to loudspeaker problems. Although the loudspeaker can be replaced fairly easily, this replacement necessitates additional clinic visits for parents and children, which may be an added burden. An additional limitation is that RITE devices have been developed for a specific population of adults with high-frequency hearing loss related to aging. Thus, some RITE devices provide very limited gain in the low frequencies. This may seem appropriate for children with high-frequency hearing loss; however, children are more likely than adults to have configurations of permanent hearing loss that require low-frequency amplification (Pittman & Stelmachowicz, 2003). Children are also much more likely than adults to experience middle ear dysfunction, which can introduce temporary or permanent changes to low-frequency hearing, as well as the changes in the low frequencies that can occur with perforations of the tympanic membrane or tympanostomy tubes. These factors enhance the need to use devices that can provide flexibility in the amount low-frequency amplification that the child receives. The presence of middle ear dysfunction can also result in drainage or fluid in the ear canal and can compromise the function of the receiver, whereas an earmold can be easily cleaned and disinfected if it comes into contact with drainage from middle ear dysfunction.

Retention is also a major limitation of most RITE devices. Some RITE devices are coupled to the ear with a soft dome or other noncustom piece that fits in the ear canal, whereas other RITE devices must be coupled to the ear with a hard acrylic shell, also known as a micro-earmold (Figure 3–3). Neither of these coupling options are ideal for infants and young children. The limitation of custom shells for ITE and CIC hearing aids similarly applies to RITE devices that are coupled to the ear with a hard micro-earmold; if the micro-earmold needs to be replaced, the child may not be able to use their hearing aid during that process. Even when soft, noncustom domes are available in an appropriate size for the child's ear, these solutions do not provide sufficient retention for most young children, who may be physically active or frequently try to remove their own hearing aids. The coupling options for RITE devices are currently not optimal for infants and young children.

Another limitation of RITE devices for children is that because the devices are small and developed for use by adult listeners who want discrete and cosmetically appealing devices, some RITE devices do not include a broad range of

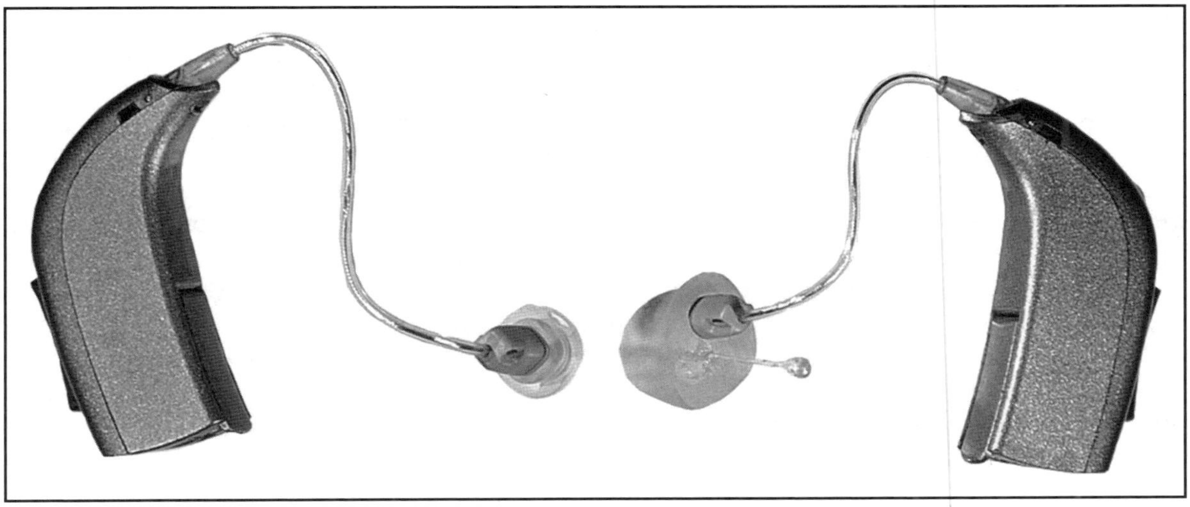

**FIGURE 3–3.** A receiver-in-the-ear (RITE) hearing aid with a noncustom dome coupling (*left*) and a RITE hearing aid with a micro-earmold coupling (*right*). Neither coupling offers an effective solution for infants and young children, though adolescents and teenagers may be able to use these coupling options as they get older.

options for connectivity to hearing assistance technologies, computers, or phones. In manufacturing smaller devices, manufacturers may have to omit components that offer connectivity, such as telecoils, Bluetooth, or other wireless transmitters. As noted in Chapter 7, connectivity is an essential consideration for children who wear hearing aids, and should not be compromised when alterative options are available that offer connectivity, particularly if the objective is to limit the visibility of the device or other cosmetic objectives. Connectivity offers children who wear hearing aids a way to access all of the devices and communication options that are available to children with normal hearing. Some RITE devices have options for connectivity that require an intermediary device to connect to other devices. However, the cost of that intermediary device, as well as the practicality of having a young child wear the accessory should be considered against providing a device with greater connectivity that does not require an additional piece of hardware.

Despite the limitations of RITE devices, there are situations in which the devices may be effective for children. Older adolescents and teenagers may prefer a cosmetically appealing solution; in fact, some may only wear the hearing aid if the appearance can be minimized. As with adults who wear hearing aids, the preference for discrete devices is highly individualized. In some cases, providing a discrete solution may be the only way that the child will use their device. After all, a larger device that the child will not wear will not meet the objectives of promoting consistent auditory access. If an RITE device is selected for an older child, the device should provide enough gain for the child's current hearing loss and have the option to increase the gain if the child's hearing loss becomes poorer over time. Compromising audibility in favor of a cosmetically appealing solution does not meet the objectives of promoting auditory access. Devices should be selected that provide the child with the greatest amount of connectivity that is available. Though retention with RITE devices may not be as limited with older children, as it might be with younger children, a RITE option that offers sufficient retention is still an important requirement. If all of these objectives can be met, some RITE devices may be an appropriate solution for older children, particularly as they begin to independently make choices about the type of amplification they receive.

## Venting, Earmold Acoustics, and Occlusion of the Ear

Another important aspect of the selection process is determining the amount of venting or occlusion of the ear canal that the child will receive. This consideration may be overlooked for several reasons. In the case of infants, the ear canal is very small and may not permit the introduction of a vent. With the advent of digital hearing aids that offer a high level of precision in the control and adjustment of hearing aid output compared to previous generations of analog hearing aids, the acoustic effects of venting and earmold modification has not been as widely discussed or considered in recent years. Occlusion of the ear canal is often minimized in children to improve retention of the hearing aid in the child's ear. As children get older, there is an increasing need to consider the effects of venting and the degree of occlusion provided by the fitting, as well as the acoustic modifications to the signal that can be achieved through the selection of earmold characteristics. Consideration of these effects can offer benefits to the child and increase the potential to provide audibility across a wide range of frequencies.

### *Degree of Occlusion and Venting*

The amount of occlusion of the ear canal that occurs with a fitting and venting have often been considered to be separate considerations. For the purposes of this discussion, they should be considered to represent a continuum from an earmold with no vent that maximally occludes the ear canal to an open fitting, where there is minimal occlusion of the ear canal. Earmolds with increasing sizes of vents form the middle of the continuum. As noted above, most infants start with a fully occluding earmold due to limited ear canal size and the goal of maximizing retention of the device, but as children get older, the amount of venting or degree of occlusion may be varied based on several considerations. Feedback suppression algorithms have been developed so that hearing aids can be fit with minimal occlusion of the ear canal and limited likelihood of feedback. In general, occlusion of the ear canal may not only have undesirable effects on sound quality but also may affect the health of the ear canal, as fungal and bacterial infections can develop in the external ear canal without ventilation (Rosenfeld et al., 2006). For these reasons, audiologists should seek to limit the occlusion of the ear canal to the greatest extent possible as soon as the child's ear canal is sufficiently large enough to permit venting or as soon as retention can be achieved with an open fitting.

An important caveat to this goal is that limiting occlusion should never occur at the expense of audibility. Increasing the size of the vent or providing an open fitting restricts the amount of amplification that can be provided in the low frequencies below 2000 Hz (Studebaker & Zachman, 1970). Small vents or completely occluding earmolds may be needed in order to provide sufficient gain in the low frequencies. Fortunately, most companies that fabricate earmolds have an option for a vent plug that varies in its internal diameter, sometimes known as variable venting or select-a-vent. This can allow for a vent that varies from completely plugged to several millimeters in diameter, so that the size of the vent can be adjusted for increased low-frequency amplification if the need arises. The verification process described in Chapter 4 can be used to assess how much amplification the child needs and will help assist the audiologist in determining how much venting can be achieved without limited audibility.

Another way that earmold venting can affect acoustics is dependent on the orientation of the vent related to the sound bore of the earmold. The sound bore is simply the hole in the earmold where sound is routed from the hearing aid. Vents can either run parallel to the sound bore and have their own opening into the ear canal or can intersect the sound bore. Intersecting sound bores are the most frequently used method used to create a vent when there is insufficient ear canal size to allow for a parallel vent. However, the use of intersecting vents also has the unintended effect of limiting the high-frequency resonance of the sound as it comes through the sound bore (Studebaker & Cox, 1977). In the care of intersecting vents, decisions should be made about whether or not to have a vent and potentially minimize the high-frequency audibility of the signal. Audiologists must make judgment calls on an individual basis to determine whether or not a vent is necessary, but in most cases, the preferred course of action would be to not vent the earmold rather than to provide a vent that intersects the sound bore. If an intersecting vent is present in the earmold, the clinician can retube the earmold so that the earmold tubing extends beyond the intersecting vent or plug the vent to minimize the negative effects on the high-frequency resonance of the earmold.

### Acoustic Modifications From the Earmold

For BTE hearing aids that are coupled to an earmold, the sound is routed from the hearing aid receiver through a tone hook, which couples to the tubing on the earmold. The tubing routes the sound from the hearing aid into the child's ear. The length and diameter of the earmold tubing can affect the acoustic properties of the hearing aid because the tube acts as a transmission line, which will have its own resonant characteristics. An audiologist can use this transmission line to their advantage to help maximize audibility and minimize resonant effects that negatively affect audibility and sound quality. The acoustic effects of earmolds can be categorized as being related to venting, damping, and resonance.

Damping effects occur with the introduction of resistance to the transmission line. A damper is a physical resistor of sound that is introduced into the sound channel, typically in the tone hook or the earmold tubing. The addition of resistance to the sound transmission line most often has the effect of reducing the presence of resonant peaks in the hearing aid output in frequencies between 750 Hz and 2000 Hz, roughly. Damping can be achieved by placing these materials in the tone hook or in the earmold tubing itself, though increasing the distance between the hearing aid and the damper can differentially affect the specific frequencies where the damping occurs. In some early attempts to minimize the resonant peaks in the hearing aid response, lamb's wool was placed in the earmold tubing. As noted above, the high degree of control that most digital hearing aids offer over the frequency response of the hearing aid has minimized the need to use damping to smooth the response of the device. In most cases today, tone hooks have specific dampers that are designed to minimize resonant peaks at specific frequencies, but additional damping is not required. Damping is not as widely used in hearing aids today because of the high degree of control over programming afforded by digital hearing aids.

Resonance effects, on the other hand, still have an important role in the design of earmolds because of the potential to enhance the high-frequency response of the device. Like a musical instrument, increasing the internal diameter of the sound bore can increase the high-frequency output of the hearing aid (Libby, 1991). These effects can be achieved through a specific earmold tubing that increases in internal diameter at the sound bore, known as a Libby horn. The effect can also be achieved by terminating the earmold tubing before the end of the sound bore, creating an increase in the diameter of the sound channel at the end of the sound bore. Any of these modifications increase the high-frequency response of the hearing aid, which can increase the audible bandwidth of the device. Increased audible bandwidth has been associated with better word recognition (Stelmachowicz, Pittman, Hoover, & Lewis, 2001) and word learning rates (Pittman, 2008) in children who wear hearing aids. A horn effect is likely to be a desirable earmold feature for infants and children with hearing loss to increase the audible bandwidth of the hearing aid to the greatest extent possible.

Increasing the internal diameter of the earmold tubing has a positive effect on the high-frequency output of the hearing aid, but decreasing the diameter of the earmold tubing can have the opposite effect on the high-frequency output. This effect of reduced high-frequency output is known as a reverse horn effect. In most cases, reverse horns are not intentionally applied in earmold fittings for children because of the desire to provide the widest possible bandwidth. However, reverse horn effects may occur unintentionally in situations where the earmold tubing becomes compressed at the end of the earmold. The restriction of the earmold tubing is particularly a risk for infants or children with very small ear canals, where the ear canal may become stenotic. Audiologists should work with the company that fabricates their earmolds to avoid reverse horn effects for infants and children. Reverse horn effects can be avoided by using smaller diameter earmold tubing or terminating the earmold canal portion before the point at which the ear canal begins to taper. Reverse horn effects may also be compensated through increasing the high-frequency gain of the hearing aid in the programming software, but the high-frequency output of the hearing aid is likely to be limited, particularly once thresholds reach moderate levels in the high frequencies (Moore, Stone, Füllgrabe, Glasberg, & Puria, 2008).

### Safety Considerations and Tamper-Resistant Features

Another aspect of hearing aid selection for children versus adults is the need to consider child safety when using the device. The U.S. National Poison Control Center estimates that hearing aid batteries are among the most commonly ingested foreign bodies by children and can lead to damage to the digestive system in extreme cases (Thomson & Sharma, 2015). Hearing aids and earmolds are increasingly small and may present a hazard for choking. If a hearing aid has external controls, such as a volume control or program switch, the child may accidentally alter the intensity of the hearing aid or change the program of the device. Fortunately, several hearing aid features can be selected to minimize the likelihood of these undesirable outcomes.

Tamper-resistant features, including a locking battery door, should be considered mandatory features for hearing aids for infants and young children in order to minimize the likelihood of battery ingestion. In most modern digital hearing aids, external controls are becoming increasingly uncommon and those that are on the hearing aid can be disabled in the programming software. Retention devices, which are discussed in greater detail in Chapter 5, can also help to reduce the likelihood that removable parts can be ingested. Once children reach an age where they can manage changing the batteries of their hearing aids, tamper-resistant features may be discontinued. However, other children in the home, such as siblings or friends, may access the child's hearing aids when not worn, and tamper-resistant features should be considered until all children in the home reach an age where battery ingestion risk is minimal, usually by kindergarten. Program switches and volume controls should also be deactivated in the programming software to prevent unintentional changes in the output of the hearing aid or desired program.

### Conclusions Regarding Hearing Aid Device and Feature Selection

Children have unique listening needs that influence clinical decisions about the type of hearing aids and features that are selected. In most cases, BTE hearing aids, with a fitting range that can accommodate changes in the child's hearing over time, are the most effective and durable style of hearing aid for children. The hearing aid coupling is an important consideration because it influences the acoustics of the fitting and can have a direct impact on the ability to make speech audible through the hearing aid. The acoustics of the earmold and venting are two examples where the coupling can be used to affect the acoustic output of the hearing aids in ways that need to be considered for children. Devices with tamper-resistant features also can minimize the likelihood of safety concerns with hearing aids, including accidental battery ingestion. In the next section of the chapter, evidence-based decisions about selection and activation of the signal processing features of hearing aids for children are discussed.

## SELECTION OF HEARING AID SIGNAL PROCESSING FOR CHILDREN

The selection of the physical hearing aid characteristics, including the style and coupling, is an important first step in the hearing aid selection process for children. Once the physical characteristics are determined, audiologists must also consider which hearing aid signal processing features will be selected or activated. In the past, decisions about physical device often included implications for signal processing, as many devices offered a fixed set of signal processing features. With digital hearing aids, nearly all hearing aids include some form of the most common hearing aid signal processing features, including amplitude compression, digital noise reduction, directional microphones, frequency lowering, and feedback suppression algorithms. The complexity of the available signal processing features can vary across different levels of hearing aid technology and manufacturers. Audiologists who fit children with hearing aids must decide which hearing aid signal processing features should be activated for a given child, based on a wide range of factors, including age and degree of hearing loss. Many hearing aid manufacturers offer pediatric feature sets based on the age of the child entered into the programming software. While some of these feature sets are based on research from children, there are often features excluded from a specific age group due to a lack of supportive evidence for activation. However, many of these automated feature sets may include default settings that are not optimized for individual children. Therefore, audiologists should use an individualized, evidence-based rationale for feature activation for children.

The major components of the model of cumulative auditory experience serve as an excellent framework for feature activation, just as they do for physical hearing aid device selection. Hearing aid signal processing features that enhance audibility should be activated for children of all ages. Features such as amplitude compression and frequency lowering can enhance audibility, if appropriately prescribed on an individual basis. Other features may not directly enhance audibility, but may promote consistent use of hearing aids across a range of different listening situations. Digital noise reduction, for example, may reduce the likelihood of loudness discomfort for children in noisy listening situations. While digital noise reduction does not enhance audibility or speech recognition in noise, the ability of the child to comfortably use their device in background noise is important if the goal of consistent hearing aid use is to be achieved. Similarly, feedback suppression algorithms may have no effect on audibility, but can improve the likelihood of consistent hearing aid use by minimizing the occurrence of acoustic feedback, which can annoy parents and children alike. The extent to which the benefits of hearing aid signal processing features can be realized may also be contingent on the child's age. Directional microphones are contingent on the ability of the listener to locate and orient toward the talker of interest, which may not occur developmentally until children reach school age. Developmental considerations are also informative for making decisions about feature activation for children. In the following sections of this chapter, hearing aid signal processing features are presented, along with the activation rationale for children based on the model of cumulative auditory experience and developmental considerations.

## Amplitude Compression

One major sequela of sensorineural hearing loss is a loss of the function of the outer hair cells in the cochlea, which serve as amplifiers to sounds that are received at the basilar membrane (see Moore, 2007, for a review). Damage to the outer hair cells results in elevation of hearing thresholds at soft levels. Outer hair cell damage also results in an abnormal growth of loudness perception once sounds are above threshold, known as recruitment. The functional consequence of the loss of the cochlear amplifier is a more limited dynamic range of hearing. Early generations of hearing aids were linear over the input range of speech, meaning that there was a 1:1 relationship between the input to the hearing aid and the output of the hearing aid. A 5 dB increase in the input resulted in a 5 dB increase in the output (Figure 3–4). At input levels near the listener's upper limit of comfort, linear hearing aids often used compression limiting, which applies extremely high compression ratios (often on the order of 9:1 or 10:1) to prevent the output from saturating the hearing aid amplifier and to prevent distortion. For individuals with abnormal loudness growth related to sensorineural hearing loss, the linear growth of the hearing aid output meant that hearing aid users would often have to alter the volume control of the hearing aid as the sound level in the environment changed. Volume control settings that resulted in audibility for soft sounds were often uncomfortably loud in listening situations with background noise (Leijon, Lindkvist, Ringdahl, & Israelsson,

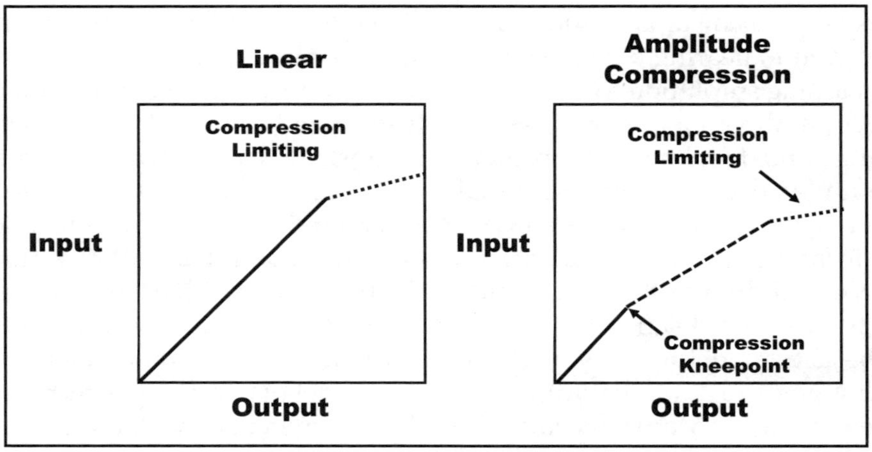


**FIGURE 3–4.** Input-output functions for a hearing aid with a linear frequency response and amplitude compression. In each figure, the solid line represents the linear portion of the input output function. The dotted line in each panel represents compression limited that is applied to high input levels to avoid saturation for both linear and amplitude compression. The dashed line in the right panel represents amplitude compression above the compression kneepoint.

1990). For infants and young children who could not adjust the volume control of their hearing aids, linear hearing aids had to be set to optimize audibility and minimize loudness discomfort, which often resulted in poorer audibility for soft sounds (Marriage, Moore, Stone, & Baer, 2005).

As an alternative to linear amplification with compression only at high input levels, amplitude compression was designed as a signal processing strategy in hearing aids that would better reflect normal hearing processes related to the cochlear amplifier that are compromised with sensorineural hearing loss. Specifically, the output of the hearing aid is compressed above a specific input level, known as the compression threshold or compression knee point. Instead of the 1 dB change in the output with every 1 dB change in the input, a 2 to 3 dB change in the input is needed for a 1 dB change in the output (see Figure 3–4). The 30 dB dynamic range of speech can be compressed into a 10 to 15 dB range, leading to the ability to restore audibility across a wide range of input levels without the increased likelihood of loudness discomfort that occurs with linear amplification. Amplitude compression is known as wide dynamic range compression (WDRC), because it compresses the output of the hearing aid over a wide range of input levels. Amplitude compression also uses compression limiting, like linear amplification, to minimize the likelihood that the hearing aid will exceed the listener's loudness discomfort levels or saturate the hearing aid amplifier.

Multiple studies have examined the benefits of amplitude compression for children with hearing loss. These studies have been summarized in two different evidence-based systematic reviews of the literature (Palmer & Grimes, 2005; McCreery, Venediktov, Coleman, & Leech, 2012a). Outcomes in studies of amplitude compression for children with hearing loss have focused on three specific areas of outcomes: audibility, speech recognition, and self-report measures of hearing aid satisfaction or sound quality. For audibility, Jenstad, Pumford, Seewald, and Cornelisse (2000) reported that WDRC better normalized audibility for environmental sounds and speech than linear amplification. A similar study by Marriage and colleagues (2005) found higher standardized measures of audibility across soft, average, and loud speech input levels for WDRC than for linear amplification. These studies suggest that

WDRC can achieve the goal of improving audibility across a range of input levels, which is easy to predict based on predictions of the output from simulations.

While improvements in audibility with WDRC compared to linear amplification are important, improvements in audibility can occur without concomitant improvements in speech recognition. The improvements in audibility that occur with WDRC would be expected to result in improvements in speech recognition for children compared to linear amplification that have been evaluated across multiple studies using a wide range of different speech stimuli. Another study by Jenstad, Seewald, Cornelisse, and Shantz (1999) found that the improvements in audibility with WDRC compared to linear amplification resulted in better recognition for nonsense words in quiet, but equivalent performance compared to linear amplification for sentences in quiet. Similarly, Gou, Valero, and Marcoux (2002) found advantages in speech recognition for WDRC over linear amplification for monosyllabic and bisyllabic words at input levels equivalent to soft speech (<50 dB SPL), but not for average speech input levels (~65 dB SPL). Marriage and colleagues (2005) found improvements in monosyllabic words in quiet with WDRC compared to linear amplification for monosyllabic words in quiet, but not in background noise. Differences in the benefit from WDRC amplification were also evident among children with severe and profound hearing loss, with children with greater degrees of hearing loss receiving less benefit from WDRC than children with better hearing.

These differences in speech recognition benefit across studies may appear to suggest that the benefit from WDRC is not uniform across studies. While there has been some variability, the overall patterns from these studies fit with predictions based on audibility differences between WDRC and linear amplification and other factors that are known to influence speech recognition in children with hearing loss. Differences in speech recognition with sentences may be more difficult to document than with monosyllabic words or nonsense words, due to the ability of children to use the semantic and syntactic cues in sentences that are not present in shorter stimuli to assist in speech recognition. The largest improvements in audibility for WDRC compared to linear amplification are for soft input levels, which is consistent with the findings that WDRC is often better than linear amplification at soft input levels, but not at average or loud input levels. In fact, many WDRC and linear hearing aids provide similar amounts of audibility for average speech but only vary at higher or lower input levels. Thus, differences in speech recognition for average speech input levels with WDRC may not be predicted to occur. Additionally, children with great degrees of hearing loss may require significant amounts of amplitude compression due to their narrow dynamic range. This may result in limited audibility regardless of whether or not amplitude compression or linear amplification is prescribed. Additionally, some listeners with profound hearing loss may have the peaks of speech compressed by the compression-limiting phase of the amplitude compression algorithm. Therefore, the differences between these processing strategies for listeners with profound hearing loss may be quiet small. This is one reason that cochlear implants are increasingly indicated for children with profound hearing loss instead of hearing aids. All of these aspects of speech recognition benefit with amplitude compression are important considerations when speech recognition is used as a clinical outcomes measure.

The final area of outcome measures for amplitude compression in the literature for children who wear hearing aids is self-reported outcomes of listening satisfaction or loudness discomfort. Because amplitude compression normalizes the dynamic range of hearing, greater listening comfort is expected to occur across different listening situations. Laboratory ratings of loudness discomfort should be reduced for higher input levels compared to linear amplification. Overall, amplitude compression is preferred to linear amplification and does result in more favorable sound quality ratings across a wide range of listening environments (McCreery et al., 2012a). Like speech recognition, there are a few caveats to this general conclusion about listener preference. A child's experience with a specific signal processing strategy might affect their listening preferences. For example, Christensen (1999) found significant differences in preference for WDRC over linear amplification for a group of school-age children, where about half of the children in the study preferred WDRC and the other half preferred linear amplification. There was some speculation that previous signal processing experience in the child's own hearing aid might have affected their preference for one signal processing strategy over another. This is consistent with a comparison of listening preference and loudness ratings, two different prescriptive approaches for children that offer different amounts of amplification for school-age children (Scollie et al., 2010). Children who were fit with one prescriptive approach preferred that prescription over the other consistently. Thus, a child's experience with how they are fit with amplification may influence their preference ratings in ways that are not predictable based on audibility.

Self-report measures may also provide valuable information about amplitude compressions that cannot be gleaned from either audibility or speech recognition data. The Gou et al. (2002) study discussed above found that children's preferences for WDRC over linear amplification were stronger, even in conditions where speech recognition was not significantly better with WDRC. Measures of listener preference and sound quality are often difficult to define in terms of what specific aspects of the signal processing they are sensitive to. This may be part of the reason why measures of listening preference for children with hearing loss may not align with variables such as audibility and speech recognition (e.g., Speech, Spatial, and Qualities questionnaire measures in McCreery et al., 2015). Nonetheless, measures of a child's preference for a specific type of signal processing has strong face validity, in that children who are old enough to express a strong opinion about how their hearing aids sound are also old enough to make decisions about whether or not to wear their hearing aids. Clinicians may wish to incorporate measures of listening preference for children when making changes to signal processing features in the child's hearing aids, including amplitude compression.

Amplitude compression increases audibility, improves speech recognition, and results in either equivalent or preferable sound quality and self-reported comfort in school-age children. The evidence supports the use of amplitude compression for children of all ages as a way to balance audibility and listening comfort across listening situations that vary in sound level. All of the research to date has been conducted with school-age children, but there is little reason to believe that the benefits of amplitude compression related to audibility and speech recognition would not extend to younger children. Unlike other hearing aid signal processing features, audiologists do not have to make decisions about whether to choose linear or amplitude compression, as they had to in the past. Instead, amplitude compression is now the default approach to processing inputs to the hearing aids for children and adults. The amount of amplitude compression varies based on the listener's degree of hearing loss and is specified by the prescriptive formula that is selected for the child. Details about prescription are discussed in the next chapter, but all prescriptive formulae used for children use nonlinear input-output functions that prescribe decreasing gain as the degree of hearing loss increases. The amount of compression varies depending on the prescriptive formula and degree of hearing loss. Most prescriptive formulae also prescribe different amounts of compression for different frequency bands, a reflection of the capability of digital hearing aids with multiple channels that process sounds at different frequencies. Audiologists do not make decisions about whether or not to activate amplitude compression, as is the case with other hearing aid features, but may vary the amount of amplitude compression to meet the specific prescription that they have selected to optimize audibility.

Amplitude compression helps children to meet both the audibility and hearing aid use goals that are associated with increasing cumulative auditory experience. Amplitude compression increases the amount of audibility that can be achieved, particularly for input levels that are equivalent to soft speech. The increased access associated with amplitude compression can increase the cumulative auditory experience for children through their hearing aids. Amplitude compression also limits the amount of loudness discomfort that can occur as the input level to the hearing aid rises, which increases the likelihood that children can wear their hearing aids across a wide range of listening environments or as the sound levels increase or decrease within a specific environment. These are two reasons that amplitude compression is prescribed for children of all ages in modern hearing aid prescriptions.

## Feedback Suppression Algorithms

Acoustic feedback is distortion, typically a buzzing or whistling sound that is generated when amplified sound from the hearing aid is received at the microphone, creating a feedback loop where the sound is amplified repeatedly. Feedback occurs most frequently at higher frequencies due to the shorter wavelengths and resonant peaks at those frequencies (Figure 3–5). For many years, acoustic feedback was a major concern, particularly for individuals with severe or profound hearing loss who required the most gain from their hearing aids. Infants and children may also be at particular risk for acoustic feedback because their heads and hearing aids may be in close proximity to surfaces that reflect sound back into the hearing aid microphones, such as car seats, parent's bodies, or surfaces when lying down. Early feedback management strategies in hearing aids often worked by limiting the amount of high-frequency gain in the hearing aid through filtering (Maxwell & Zurek, 1995). Gain reduction, or filtering, were not always successful in reducing feedback in the worst cases and also had the negative side effect of reducing high-frequency audibility. However, feedback may limit a person's ability to wear their hearing aid, so some reduction in audibility was acceptable over not being able to wear the hearing aid at all.

Over the last two decades, significant progress has been made in signal processing strategies to minimize the occurrence of acoustic feedback (see Van Waterschoot & Moonen, 2011, for a comprehensive review of feedback control strategies in hearing aids). The advances that have occurred in feedback suppression are one of the main signal processing advances that have permitted the development of open-fit hearing aids. Perhaps most importantly, many feedback suppression algorithms can reduce the occurrence of feedback without compromising gain in the hearing aid or only compromising gain as a last resort, keeping audibility in the high frequencies intact to the greatest possible extent. Many hearing aids employ multiple types of feedback suppression signal processing to address different potential sources of feedback or limitations of one particular approach. Different feedback suppression approaches are described in Box 3–1.

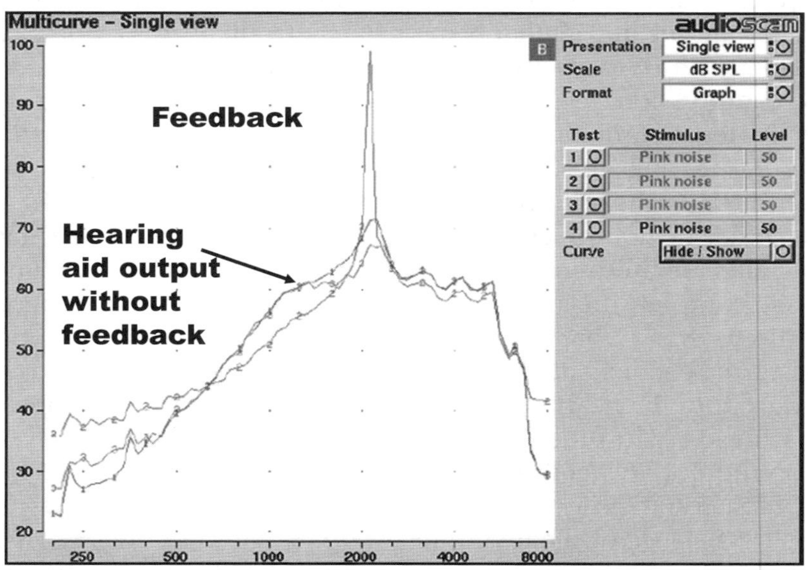


**FIGURE 3–5.** An example of acoustic feedback measured through a hearing aid.

**Box 3–1: Types of Feedback Suppression Algorithms**

- Frequency shifting: The hearing aid shifts the output signal by 5 to 10 Hz so that feedback signals do not align in frequency. Most frequency shifting is inaudible to the listener for speech and music signals. The increase in gain that is available is generally limited to about 6 dB compared to the signal without frequency shifting (Vila, 2005).
- Gain reduction: The output of the hearing aid is reduced in either broadband (Kates, 1991) or narrowband (Maxwell & Zurek, 1995).
- Adaptive filtering: The output of the hearing aid is modified only if feedback is detected at the microphone (Spriet, Proudler, Moonen, & Wouters, 2005).

Much of the research on feedback suppression research to date has either been done using acoustic modeling or with adult hearing aid users (Guo, Jensen, & Jensen, 2013). Those investigations have suggested that most hearing aid feedback-suppression algorithms can achieve significant increases in the maximum stable gain of the hearing aid, which can increase audibility and high-frequency output of the hearing aid, thereby increasing audibility. The way that feedback suppression algorithms function is not dependent on whether the hearing aid is in the ear of an adult or a child. Therefore, the increases in maximum stable gain that have been reported in simulations and in behavioral studies with adults with hearing loss can be expected to translate into similar benefit for infants and children who wear hearing aids.

Like amplitude compression, feedback suppression may be activated automatically or by default in many digital hearing aids. Thus, the audiologist is not required to make decisions in some cases about whether or not to activate the feature in the hearing aids for children. However, the audiologist must complete verification of the hearing aid (as discussed in Chapter 4) after feedback suppression has been activated, so that any changes in the output of the hearing aid will be quantified in that process. In older children who can report on sound quality, feedback suppression may occasionally result in signal processing artifacts, such as persistence of tonal stimuli that occur in the environment or a sound echo. In those cases, most hearing aid manufacturers offer settings within their programming software to alter the feedback suppression algorithms in order to minimize the artifacts that can influence sound quality.

Feedback suppression also manages to support both audibility and hearing aid use aspects of promoting cumulative auditory experience in children who wear hearing aids. By increasing the maximum stable gain that is available in the hearing aid, feedback suppression can permit greater high-frequency output and audibility than devices without feedback suppression. This can increase the child's access to high-frequency sounds and overall audibility for speech. Feedback suppression also increases the likelihood that infants and children can consistently wear their hearing aids. While feedback may not be audible to the child, parents often have reported feedback as a challenge to establishing hearing aid use in infants and young children (Sjoblad, Harrison, Roush, & McWilliam, 2001). Minimizing feedback can also extend the life of earmolds, as long as problems with maintaining sufficient gain and retention with the earmold are not encountered. In these ways, feedback suppression is recommended for children of all ages in order to increase audibility and consistent hearing aid use, as long as audibility can be verified and sound quality is not reduced.

## Frequency Lowering

Feedback suppression and increasing hearing aid receiver bandwidth have both increased the ability to make high frequencies audible in recent years.

As noted previously, high-frequency sounds are particularly important for children with hearing loss in terms of speech recognition (Stelmachowicz et al., 2004b), word learning (Pittman, 2008), and phonological development (Koehlinger, Van Horne, Oleson, McCreery, & Moeller, 2015). However, the audible bandwidth of hearing aids remains limited in many cases by the child's degree of high-frequency hearing loss, the bandwidth of the hearing aid receiver, or a combination of these two factors (Kimlinger, McCreery, & Lewis, 2015). As an alternative approach for making high-frequency sounds audible for listeners where the signal cannot be made audible through conventional means, frequency lowering signal processing has been introduced by nearly all major hearing aid manufacturers. While there are differences in how manufacturers implement frequency lowering, the general purpose is to move high-frequency sounds in the input to lower frequencies in the output. The premise is that audibility may be easier to achieve at lower frequencies, where the child's degree of hearing loss and the ability of the hearing aid receiver to provide amplification may be less restricted than at higher frequencies.

Currently, two of the most common methods for frequency lowering are frequency compression and frequency transposition. Frequency compression reduces the bandwidth of the input to the hearing aid by a specified compression ratio above a specified start frequency. Phonak's Sound Recover is one example of frequency compression that has been extensively studied in previous research. Frequency transposition extracts a high-frequency band and moves it to a lower frequency band. The lowered band is often processed in the same frequency channel as the speech signal that was originally in the destination band. Widex's Audibility Extender algorithm uses frequency transposition. Some methods combine frequency compression and transposition, such as Oticon's Speech Rescue algorithm, where three high-frequency source bands are combined, compressed and transposed to a lower-frequency destination band. In each case, the goal of the frequency lowering signal processing is to increase the audibility of high-frequency sounds.

Research on the benefits of frequency lowering for children has been limited mainly to one form of frequency lowering, nonlinear frequency compression (Phonak Sound Recover). An evidence-based systematic review found that the literature on the effects of frequency lowering on audibility, speech recognition, and speech and language outcomes showed mixed results for both frequency compression and frequency transposition (McCreery, Venediktov, Coleman, & Leech, 2012c). Since that systematic review was published, additional evidence has been published to support the use of nonlinear frequency compression with children. If appropriately prescribed (as discussed in the next chapter), frequency lowering can improve audibility and speech recognition in children with hearing loss (McCreery et al., 2014) without major sacrifices in sound quality for speech or music (Brennan et al., 2014). Two longitudinal studies have demonstrated that nonlinear frequency compression can achieve speech and language outcomes equivalent to conventional processing (Bentler, Walker, McCreery, Arenas, & Roush, 2014), including a randomized controlled trial where children were randomly assigned to either nonlinear frequency compression or conventional amplification (Ching et al., 2013). Collectively, these studies suggest that nonlinear frequency compression can lead to improvements in audibility, speech recognition and maintain speech and language outcomes when used in children.

Several manufacturers of frequency lowering signal processing algorithms have the feature activated by default in the hearing aid fitting software. Audiologists must determine whether a specific child needs frequency lowering based on how much of the high frequencies are audible to the listener, known as audible bandwidth. The process for determining the audible bandwidth for a given listener will be described in Chapter 4. If the audible bandwidth with conventional processing is less than 6000 Hz, the use of frequency lowering to restore high-frequency audibility should be considered. This rationale is based on evidence that children may need bandwidth up to 9 kHz to identify /s/ sounds when spoken by a child or female talker (Stelmachowicz et al., 2004b), as well as studies that show improvements for /s/ detection when frequency lowering is applied (Glista et al., 2009). The amount of frequency lowering that is prescribed for a given child should be the weakest setting that brings the /s/ phoneme into audibility, using methods described by Scollie et al. (2016). This is more fully described in Chapter 4. This approach provides access to the highest frequencies that are needed to detect the /s/ phoneme, while minimizing the amount of distortion that is present in the signal. Frequency lowering settings that increase distortion without adding audibility have been shown to negatively affect both speech perception (Souza, Arehart, Kates, Croghan, & Gehani, 2013) and sound quality (Parsa, Scollie, Glista, & Seelisch, 2013).

Frequency lowering has potential positive and negative implications for promoting cumulative auditory experience for children who wear hearing aids. Increasing high-frequency audibility, including access to phonemes like /s/ that are not consistently audible through hearing aids, is a potentially positive aspect of frequency lowering that can promote auditory access for children with hearing loss. As noted above, improvements in speech recognition can be achieved with frequency lowering without sacrificing sound quality (Brennan et al., 2014). However, clinicians should only activate frequency lowering for children if there is evidence that the processor can improve high-frequency audibility for a given child. Applying frequency lowering with minimal benefits for audibility can lead to distortion, which may result in less hearing aid use or even rejection of hearing aids due to poor sound quality. It should also be emphasized that frequency lowering is an example of a processing strategy that is continually improved over time. It is in the clinicians' best interest to stay current with developments and improvements of these signal processing strategies.

## Signal Processing Strategies to Minimize Background Noise

Background noise is a serious problem for children with hearing loss in terms of limiting speech recognition (McCreery et al., 2015) and comfort (Crukley & Scollie, 2012). Many digital hearing aids offer noise reduction signal processing strategies to minimize the negative perceptual consequences of background noise. Two specific signal processing strategies have been developed in hearing aids to reduce the effects of background noise: digital noise reduction and directional microphones. A systematic review of these noise management algorithms for children suggests that despite children's susceptibility to background noise, that there is limited evidence to support the implementation of either strategy routinely in children (McCreery, Venediktov, Coleman, & Leech, 2012b). Clinicians must make decisions about the activation of digital noise reduction and directional microphones based on the listening needs of the child and the limited evidence in the research. Each of these features will be discussed separately in the sections that follow to provide a rationale for activation of these features for children who wear hearing aids.

### *Digital Noise Reduction*

Digital noise reduction refers to signal processing strategies that are designed to limit the perceptibility of background noise by reducing the gain of the hearing aid when background noise is present. Because digital noise reduction algorithms function by reducing gain, there is typically a reduction in audibility. The goal of most digital noise reduction algorithms is to reduce gain as little as possible, with the goal of improving listening comfort in background noise. Note that by reducing gain and audibility, improvements in speech recognition in noise with digital noise reduction are not anticipated to occur with digital noise reduction. Although some digital noise reduction algorithms function in a frequency-specific manner where gain is reduced in specific channels of the hearing aid where noise dominates the input, the spectra of speech and noise are overlapping (Kates, 2008). Noise reduction algorithms work using a variety of signal processing strategies to determine if the input to the hearing aid is speech or noise. A review of digital noise reduction studies with adults who wear hearing aids supports these expectations based on the behavior of noise reduction algorithms: speech recognition is often unchanged, while listeners rate listening in noise to be preferable with digital noise reduction (Bentler & Chiou, 2006). As a result, digital noise reduction is routinely recommended for improving listening comfort in noise for adults who wear hearing aids.

Unfortunately, the evidence from adults cannot be extrapolated down to the pediatric population. Children require more audibility than adults to maintain speech recognition, so it is possible that gain reductions that occur with digital noise reduction might affect children in ways that would not be predictable from data obtained from adults. Several studies with school-age children have been conducted to test this prediction in children. Stelmachowicz and colleagues (2010) measured speech recognition for a group of 5- to 10-year-old children with mild to moderate hearing loss using nonsense syllables, monosyllabic words, and sentences in noise for conditions with and without digital noise reduction. The results found no improvement or degradation in speech recognition for children in the study with digital noise reduction activated. Significant individual variability in the pattern of benefit from digital noise reduction was observed, though none of the participants showed consistent patterns of performance across all three types of stimuli. A study by Pittman (2011a) found a similar null effect for digital noise reduction on speech recognition in children with hearing loss, but a separate study from the same author (Pittman, 2011b) found that older children (>10 years) had faster word learning rates in noise with digital noise reduction activated than without the feature. These studies suggest that gain reductions that may occur with digital noise reduction are unlikely to negatively affect speech recognition in noise for children and enhance word learning in older children.

Few studies have examined the effects of digital noise reduction on listening comfort in children with hearing loss. A study by Gustafson, McCreery, Hoover, Kopun, and Stelmachowicz (2014) asked children with normal hearing to rate the clarity of speech in noise that had been processed with or without digital noise reduction. Generally, children had higher ratings of clarity for speech in noise processed with digital noise reduction than without digital noise reduction for two different manufacturers' digital noise reduction algorithms. This study suggests that children can experience the same improvements in sound quality that have been reported in studies with adults using digital noise reduction. However, the results should be interpreted with caution because children with normal hearing were the sample for the study and would not be expected to use hearing aids or related digital noise reduction strategies.

Collectively, the evidence suggests that the pattern of speech recognition results for school-age children with hearing loss with digital noise reduction is similar to studies with adults with no improvement or decrement in understanding with the feature activated. This suggests that digital noise reduction may be an effective signal processing feature for school-age children. The evidence from infants and preschool children is too limited at the present time to recommend digital noise reduction in those cases. Audiologists must also determine the amount of digital noise reduction that they would like to prescribe. Different hearing aid manufacturers' digital noise reduction algorithms are likely to vary based on the amount of noise reduction that occurs, the amount of time over which the reduction in gain occurs, and the frequencies where gain is reduced (Hoetink, Körössy, & Dreschler, 2009). Each digital noise reduction algorithm may also have different settings that affect the amount of noise reduction that occurs (Figure 3–6). The most conservative amount of noise reduction that can achieve improved listening comfort in background noise is preferred for children to minimize the impact on audibility. If digital noise reduction can be prescribed in a way that improves listening comfort without sacrificing speech recognition in noise, the feature provides a way of potentially increasing the number of environments where a child can comfortably use their hearing aids. This supports the hearing aid use goal of the model of cumulative auditory experience for children who wear hearing aids.

### *Directional Microphones*

Another hearing aid feature that has been designed to minimize the negative consequences of background noise is directional microphones. Directional microphones use differences in spatial cues, either between two ports on a single microphone or multiple different microphones,

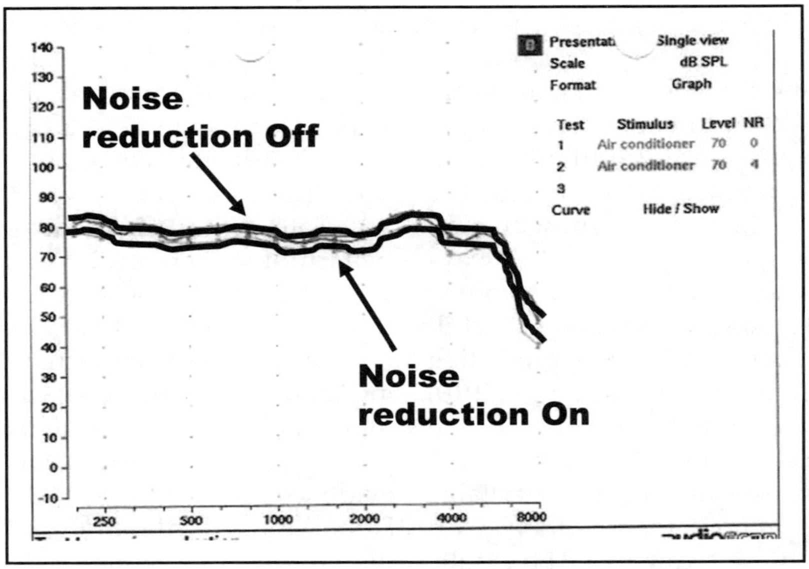


**FIGURE 3–6.** Hearing aid output as a function of frequency for digital noise reduction off compared to digital noise reduction on for a steady-state air conditioner noise.

to determine the spatial location of sound relative to the listener and differentially amplify the signal based on the direction of the sound. Most directional microphones have a response pattern that maintains amplification from the front of the device and reduces amplification from the sides or behind the listener (Figure 3–7). Some directional microphones have a fixed directivity pattern, which does not change. More recently, directional microphones that automatically adapt to the listening environment have been introduced, known as adaptive directional microphones. Directional microphones can be adaptive in terms of activation, where the hearing aid automatically switches from an omnidirectional to a directional response when noise is detected in the environment. Directional microphones can also be adaptive in the directional response as well, shifting the sensitivity of the directional pattern based on the location of the noise in the environment relative to the listener. To date, there have been few studies even in adults to assess adaptive directional systems.

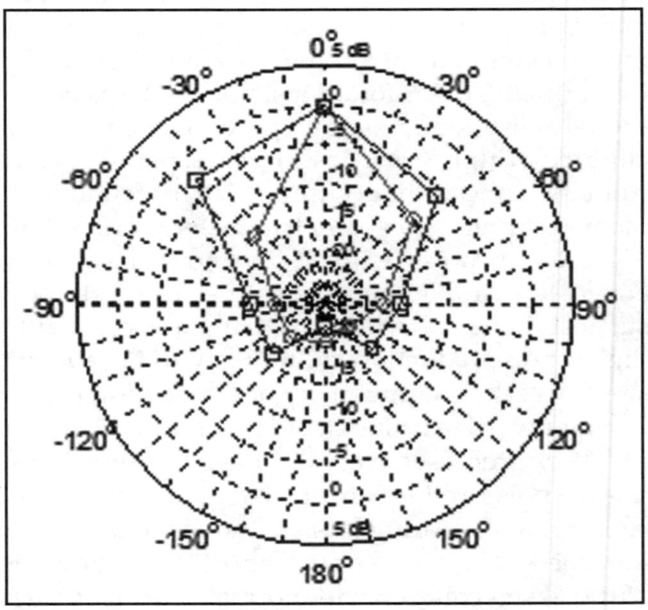


**FIGURE 3–7.** A polar plot for a directional microphone on two different hearing aids at 2000 Hz. Note that the hearing aid polar plot with the squares has a broader response than the hearing aid polar plot with the circles at this frequency.

Fixed directional microphones have been studied in school-age children. Ricketts, Galster, and Tharpe (2007) examined the directional benefit that would be encountered in various classroom listening situations, including having the teacher in front, teacher to the side or behind the listener, or listening to another student to the side or behind the listener. In general, the findings reflected the acoustics of directional microphones and previous studies with directional microphones with adults who wear hearing aids. For situations where the talker was in front of the listener and the noise was behind the listener, the benefit of directional microphones for speech recognition was positive compared to a microphone setting where the hearing aids are equally responsive to sounds from all directions, known as omnidirectional. This finding is predictable based on the fact that directional microphones are maximally responsive to sounds arriving from the front of the listener. Similarly, when the noise was diffuse or in front of the listener and the talker of interest was to the side or behind the listener, the directional benefit was null or even slightly negative compared to an omnidirectional setting. The authors concluded that the benefit of directional microphones in these realistic listening situations was dependent on the ability of the child to orient toward the target talker. A follow-up study from the same group of researchers (Ricketts & Galster, 2008) determined that school-age children with hearing loss do orient toward talkers appropriately, though the students in that classroom observation study were not wearing directional microphones during as part of the study. For school-age children who can direct their visual attention toward a talker, directional microphones appear to provide benefit in some listening situations with background noise.

Like most other hearing aid signal processing strategies, research with infants and young children with directional microphones has not been conducted. One study evaluated looking behavior in infants and preschoolers with hearing loss to attempt to predict what the directional benefits might be for this younger age group. Ching and colleagues (2009) used real-world observations and listening diaries completed by parents to determine what proportion of the time infants and young children were looking at the talker of interest in different listening configurations that are common to this age range. Listening situations included one-on-one play with a parent, playing alone with an adult in the room, a preschool classroom situation, and a playground/recess listening situation. The predicted benefits of directional microphones were when the talker of interest was in front of the child and noise sources were either behind or to the sides of the child. As predicted, the improvements in the signal-to-noise ratio with directional microphones were greatest in one-on-one play with the adult talker in front of the child, whereas the benefits were either negligible or slightly negative for the other listening configurations. The parent diaries suggested that the infants and young children in the study were in those one-on-one listening situations less than half of their day, suggesting that the potential benefits of directional microphones in this age range may be limited. However, the authors concluded that the small potential benefits of directional microphones in those listening situations outweighed the potential for negative outcomes with directional microphones, and recommended that they be provided to infants and young children.

There are several other considerations with directional microphones that could affect audibility and perception in infants and young children. Because directional microphones maintain amplification from the front of the listener, they may reduce opportunities for incidental learning, though this has not been directly evaluated. Importantly, the Ching et al. (2009) study did not measure looking behavior in children with hearing loss while they were wearing directional microphones, so the potential positive or negative effects could not be directly assessed. Because of the limited evidence, some pediatric amplification guidelines have suggested that directional microphones may only be appropriate for school-age children who are old enough to orient toward the talker of interest (American Academy of Audiology, 2013). However, another guideline from Australia Hearing suggests the directional microphones should be provided to children of all ages (King, 2010). This leaves clinicians with inconsistent recommendations about whether or not directional microphones should be provided to infants and young children and limited evidence to support clinical decisions.

The model of cumulative auditory experience may provide some assistance in this decision-making process. Directional microphones can improve the signal-to-noise ratio for sounds that are in front of the listener when the noise is spatially separated and to the side of the listener or behind. Thus, directional microphones can promote enhanced audibility in background noise, assuming that the listener can orient toward the target talker. Directional microphones might also make hearing aids more effective in background noise, which can make them easier to use in noisy situations. Ease of use in noisy situations can promote the consistent use of hearing aids, which is a major part of promoting cumulative auditory experience. However, both of these aspects are contingent on the listener being able to orient their head appropriately toward the talker in a difficult listening environment, which is a developmental process that is still maturing into the school-age years. Until additional evidence regarding the benefits of directional microphones in infants and young children can be provided, the best course of action appears to be limiting the use of directional microphones to school-age children when it is developmentally appropriate.

### Summary of Selection of Advanced Hearing Aid Signal Processing for Children

Hearing aid signal processing strategies have undergone rapid development over the last 20 years with the widespread availability of digital signal processing. Advanced signal processing features that used to be limited to higher end signal processing models are available even in the most basic hearing aids. At the same time, a new generation of infants and young children with hearing loss are being identified and fit with these devices within a few months of birth. These two parallel developments have converged to generate a wide range of questions about what hearing aid features should be used for children with hearing loss, what age should these technologies be activated, and once activated, how the settings of these features should be optimized for children. If there is one main point of this chapter, it should be that there are many more questions along these lines than answers at the present time. Our hope is that by making decisions about activation of advanced hearing aid features from the perspective of how these features may promote or hamper a child's auditory experience, then this theoretical model can be informative for clinical decision making about advanced features until such time as research studies can be completed to provide direct evidence of benefit for children with hearing loss. If background noise is a serious concern for infants and young children, remote-microphone hearing assistance technology may be a valuable addition to hearing aids to minimize the negative perceptual consequences of background noise.

## CONCLUSIONS

Prior to the fitting of hearing aids for children, a number of decisions must be made related to the selection of appropriate devices, coupling, and the signal processing features that will provide the best outcomes. The BTE style of hearing aid remains the most flexible and durable option for children and can be adapted to fit a wide range of degrees and configurations of hearing loss. Basic or entry-level technology can provide adequate audibility and signal processing features for children in most cases. Signal processing strategies, such as amplitude compression and feedback suppression, can be applied with children of all ages, as these features not only promote audibility, but also consistent hearing aid use as well. Frequency-lowering signal processing should be utilized for children with limited audible bandwidth with conventional processing. Digital noise reduction and directional microphones have an emerging evidence base for school-age children, but little to no evidence to support their use in infants or young children at the present time. Additional strategies for managing background noise are highlighted in Chapter 7, focusing on connectivity, and reviewing the hearing assistance technologies that can be used with hearing aids.

## REFERENCES

American Academy of Audiology. (2013). *Clinical practice guidelines: Pediatric amplification.* Reston, VA. Retrieved from http://www.audiology.org/sites/default/files/publications/PediatricAmplificationGuidelines.pdf

Bentler, R., & Chiou, L. K. (2006). Digital noise reduction: An overview. *Trends in Amplification, 10*(2), 67–82.

Bentler, R., Walker, E., McCreery, R., Arenas, R. M., & Roush, P. (2014). Nonlinear frequency compression in hearing aids: Impact on speech and language development. *Ear and Hearing, 35*(4), e143.

Brennan, M. A., McCreery, R., Kopun, J., Hoover, B., Alexander, J., Lewis, D., & Stelmachowicz, P. G. (2014). Paired comparisons of nonlinear frequency compression, extended bandwidth, and restricted bandwidth hearing aid processing for children and adults with hearing loss. *Journal of the American Academy of Audiology, 25*(10), 983–998.

Ching, T. Y., Day, J., Zhang, V., Dillon, H., Van Buynder, P., Seeto, M., . . . Wong, A. (2013). A randomized controlled trial of nonlinear frequency compression versus conventional processing in hearing aids: Speech and language of children at three years of age. *International Journal of Audiology, 52*(Suppl. 2), S46–S54.

Ching, T. Y., O'Brien, A., Dillon, H., Chalupper, J., Hartley, L., Hartley, D., . . . Hain, J. (2009). Directional effects on infants and young children in real life: Implications for amplification. *Journal of Speech, Language, and Hearing Research, 52*(5), 1241–1254.

Christensen, L. A. (1999). A comparison of three hearing aid sound-processing strategies in a multi-memory hearing aid for adolescents. *Seminars in Hearing, 20*, 183–195.

Cox, R. M., Johnson, J. A., & Xu, J. (2016). Impact of hearing aid technology on outcomes in daily life I: The patients' perspective. *Ear and Hearing, 37*(4), e224-e237.

Crukley, J., & Scollie, S. D. (2012). Children's speech recognition and loudness perception with the desired sensation level v5 quiet and noise prescriptions. *American Journal of Audiology, 21*(2), 149–162.

Glista, D., Scollie, S., Bagatto, M., Seewald, R., Parsa, V., & Johnson, A. (2009). Evaluation of nonlinear frequency compression: Clinical outcomes. *International Journal of Audiology, 48*(9), 632–644.

Gou, J., Valero, J., & Marcoux, A. (2002). The effect of nonlinear amplification and low compression threshold on receptive and expressive speech ability in children with severe to profound hearing loss. *Journal of Educational Audiology, 10*, 1–14.

Guo, M., Jensen, S. H., & Jensen, J. (2013). Evaluation of state-of-the-art acoustic feedback cancellation systems for hearing aids. *Journal of the Audio Engineering Society, 61*(3), 125–137.

Gustafson, S., McCreery, R., Hoover, B., Kopun, J. G., & Stelmachowicz, P. (2014). Listening effort and perceived clarity for normal hearing children with the use of digital noise reduction. *Ear and Hearing, 35*(2), 183.

Hoetink, A. E., Körössy, L., & Dreschler, W. A. (2009). Classification of steady state gain reduction produced by amplitude modulation–based noise reduction in digital hearing aids. *International Journal of Audiology, 48*(7), 444–455.

Jenstad, L. M., Pumford, J., Seewald, R. C., & Cornelisse, L. E. (2000). Comparison of linear gain and wide dynamic range compression hearing aid circuits II: Aided loudness measures. *Ear and Hearing, 21*(1), 32–44.

Jenstad, L. M., Seewald, R. C., Cornelisse, L. E., & Shantz, J. (1999). Comparison of linear gain and wide dynamic range compression hearing aid circuits: Aided speech perception measures. *Ear and Hearing, 20*(2), 117–126.

Kates, J. M. (1991). Feedback cancellation in hearing aids: Results from a computer simulation. *IEEE Transactions on Signal Processing, 39*(3), 553–562.

Kates, J. M. (2008). *Digital hearing aids*. San Diego, CA: Plural.

Keefe, D. H., & Levi, E. (1996). Maturation of the middle and external ears: Acoustic power-based responses and reflectance tympanometry. *Ear and Hearing, 17*(5), 361–373.

Kimlinger, C., McCreery, R., & Lewis, D. (2015). High-frequency audibility: The effects of audiometric configuration, stimulus type, and device. *Journal of the American Academy of Audiology, 26*(2), 128–137.

King, A. M. (2010). The national protocol for paediatric amplification in Australia. *International Journal of Audiology, 49*(Suppl. 1), S64–S69.

Koehlinger, K., Van Horne, A. O., Oleson, J., McCreery, R., & Moeller, M. P. (2015). The role of sentence position, allomorph, and morpheme type on accurate use of *s*-related morphemes by children who are hard of hearing. *Journal of Speech, Language, and Hearing Research, 58*(2), 396–409.

Leijon, A., Lindkvist, A., Ringdahl, A., & Israelsson, B. (1990). Preferred hearing aid gain in everyday use after prescriptive fitting. *Ear and Hearing, 11*(4), 299–305.

Libby, E. R. (1991). Measures to verify achievement of desired real-ear gain in adults. *Seminars in Hearing, 12*(1), 42–52.

Marriage, J. E., Moore, B. C., Stone, M. A., & Baer, T. (2005). Effects of three amplification strategies on speech perception by children with severe and profound hearing loss. *Ear and Hearing, 26*(1), 35–47.

Maxwell, J. A., & Zurek, P. M. (1995). Reducing acoustic feedback in hearing aids. *IEEE Transactions on Speech and Audio Processing, 3*(4), 304–313.

McCreery, R. W., Alexander, J., Brennan, M. A., Hoover, B., Kopun, J., & Stelmachowicz, P. G. (2014). The influence of audibility on speech recognition with nonlinear frequency compression for children and adults with hearing loss. *Ear and hearing, 35*(4), 440.

McCreery, R. W., Venediktov, R. A., Coleman, J. J., & Leech, H. M. (2012a). An evidence-based systematic review of amplitude compression in hearing aids for school-age children with hearing loss. *American Journal of Audiology, 21*(2), 269–294.

McCreery, R. W., Venediktov, R. A., Coleman, J. J., & Leech, H. M. (2012b). An evidence-based systematic review of directional microphones and digital noise reduction hearing aids in school-age children with hearing loss. *American Journal of Audiology, 21*(2), 295–312.

McCreery, R. W., Venediktov, R. A., Coleman, J. J., & Leech, H. M. (2012c). An evidence-based systematic review of frequency lowering in hearing aids for school-age children with hearing loss. *American Journal of Audiology, 21*(2), 313–328.

McCreery, R. W., Walker, E. A., Spratford, M., Oleson, J., Bentler, R., Holte, L., & Roush, P. (2015). Speech recognition and parent ratings from auditory development questionnaires in children who are hard of hearing. *Ear and Hearing, 36*, 60S–75S.

Moore, B. C. (2007). *Cochlear hearing loss: Physiological, psychological and technical issues*. Hoboken, NJ: John Wiley & Sons.

Moore, B. C., Stone, M. A., Füllgrabe, C., Glasberg, B. R., & Puria, S. (2008). Spectro-temporal characteristics of speech at high frequencies, and the potential for restoration of audibility to people with mild-to-moderate hearing loss. *Ear and Hearing, 29*(6), 907.

Palmer, C. V., & Grimes, A. M. (2005). Effectiveness of signal processing strategies for the pediatric population: A systematic review of the evidence. *Journal of the American Academy of Audiology, 16*(7), 505–514.

Parsa, V., Scollie, S., Glista, D., & Seelisch, A. (2013). Nonlinear frequency compression effects on sound quality ratings of speech and music. *Trends in Amplification, 17*(1), 54–68.

Pittman, A. L. (2008). Short-term word-learning rate in children with normal hearing and children with hearing loss in limited and extended high-frequency bandwidths. *Journal of Speech, Language, and Hearing Research, 51*(3), 785–797.

Pittman, A. (2011a). Children's performance in complex listening conditions: Effects of hearing loss and digital noise reduction. *Journal of Speech, Language, and Hearing Research, 54*(4), 1224–1239.

Pittman, A. (2011b). Age-related benefits of digital noise reduction for short-term word learning in children with hearing loss. *Journal of Speech, Language, and Hearing Research, 54*(5), 1448–1463.

Pittman, A. L., & Stelmachowicz, P. G. (2003). Hearing loss in children and adults: Audiometric configuration, asymmetry, and progression. *Ear and Hearing, 24*(3), 198.

Ricketts, T. A., & Galster, J. (2008). Head angle and elevation in classroom environments: Implications for amplification. *Journal of Speech, Language, and Hearing Research, 51*(2), 516–525.

Ricketts, T., Galster, J., & Tharpe, A. M. (2007). Directional benefit in simulated classroom environments. *American Journal of Audiology, 16*(2), 130–144.

Rosenfeld, R. M., Brown, L., Cannon, C. R., Dolor, R. J., Ganiats, T. G., Hannley, M., . . . Stinnett, S. S. (2006). Clinical practice guideline: Acute otitis externa. *Otolaryngology-Head and Neck Surgery, 134*(4), S4–S23.

Scollie, S., Ching, T. Y., Seewald, R., Dillon, H., Britton, L., Steinberg, J., & Corcoran, J. (2010). Evaluation of the NAL-NL1 and DSL v4. 1 prescriptions for children: Preference in real world use. *International Journal of Audiology, 49*(Suppl. 1), S49–S63.

Scollie, S., Glista, D., Seto, J., Dunn, A., Schuett, B., Hawkins, M., . . . Parsa, V. (2016). Fitting frequency-lowering signal processing applying the American Academy of Audiology Pediatric Amplification Guideline: Updates and protocols. *Journal of the American Academy of Audiology, 27*(3), 219–236.

Scollie, S., Seewald, R., Cornelisse, L., Moodie, S., Bagatto, M., Laurnagaray, D., . . . Pumford, J. (2005). The desired sensation level multistage input/output algorithm. *Trends in Amplification, 9(4)*, 159–197.

Sherbecoe, R. L., & Studebaker, G. A. (2002). Audibility-index functions for the connected speech test. *Ear and Hearing, 23*(5), 385–398.

Sjoblad, S., Harrison, M., Roush, J., & McWilliam, R. A. (2001). Parents' reactions and recommendations after diagnosis and hearing aid fitting. *American Journal of Audiology, 10*(1), 24–31.

Souza, P. E., Arehart, K. H., Kates, J. M., Croghan, N. B., & Gehani, N. (2013). Exploring the limits of frequency lowering. *Journal of Speech, Language, and Hearing Research, 56*(5), 1349–1363.

Spriet, A., Proudler, I., Moonen, M., & Wouters, J. (2005). Adaptive feedback cancellation in hearing aids with linear prediction of the desired signal. *IEEE Transactions on Signal Processing, 53*(10), 3749–3763.

Studebaker, G. A., & Cox, R. M. (1977). Side branch and parallel vent effects in real ears and in acoustical and electrical models. *Ear and Hearing, 3*(2), 108–117.

Studebaker, G. A., & Zachman, T. A. (1970). Investigation of the acoustics of earmold vents. *Journal of the Acoustical Society of America, 47*(4B), 1107–1115.

Stelmachowicz, P. G., Pittman, A. L., Hoover, B. M., & Lewis, D. E. (2001). Effect of stimulus bandwidth on the perception of/s/in normal-and hearing-impaired children and adults. *Journal of the Acoustical Society of America, 110*(4), 2183–2190.

Stelmachowicz, P. G., Pittman, A. L., Hoover, B. M., & Lewis, D. E. (2004a). Novel-word learning in children with normal hearing and hearing loss. *Ear and Hearing, 25*(1), 47–56.

Stelmachowicz, P. G., Pittman, A. L., Hoover, B. M., Lewis, D. E., & Moeller, M. P. (2004b). The importance of high-frequency audibility in the speech and language development of children with hearing loss. *Archives of Otolaryngology-Head and Neck Surgery, 130*(5), 556–562.

Stelmachowicz, P., Lewis, D., Hoover, B., Nishi, K., McCreery, R., & Woods, W. (2010). Effects of digital noise reduction on speech perception for children with hearing loss. *Ear and Hearing, 31*(3), 345–355.

Thomson, M., & Sharma, S. (2015). The hazards of button battery ingestion. *Archives of Disease in Childhood, 100*(11), 1010–1011.

Van Waterschoot, T., & Moonen, M. (2011). Fifty years of acoustic feedback control: State of the art and future challenges. *Proceedings of the IEEE, 99*(2), 288–327.

Vila, C. (2005, May). *Digital frequency shifting for electroacoustic feedback suppression.* Paper presented at the 118th Audio Engineering Society Convention. Barcelona, Spain (pp. 1–6). New York, NY: Audio Engineering Society.

# 4

# Hearing Aid Verification for Children

*Ryan W. McCreery and Elizabeth A. Walker*

## INTRODUCTION

Electroacoustic verification of hearing aid function is an essential step in the process of providing amplification to children. Measuring the output of the hearing aid, either in the child's ear or in a coupler with an appropriate correction for the child's ear canal acoustics, is one of the most important steps for ensuring that the child will have adequate aided audibility for speech. Recent evidence suggest that despite years of research to support the use of hearing aid verification practices, many clinicians continue to use outdated methods that do not adequately assess audibility for speech (McCreery, Bentler, & Roush, 2013). The methods used to verify hearing aids have a profound influence on the accuracy of the hearing aid fitting, which in turn, affects how much access the child will have to speech and language from their environment. Audiologists have a responsibility to use verification methods that are validated for children. They also have a responsibility to use advanced verification methods to ensure that any advanced signal processing features do not sacrifice audibility. In this chapter, the fundamental concepts that form the basis of hearing aid verification are presented, as well as the clinical processes that provide the most accurate assessment of audibility. Clinical approaches for documenting the impact of advanced signal processing features, including frequency lowering, digital noise reduction, and directional microphones are highlighted. By the end of the chapter, the reader should have an understanding of the reasons and clinical protocols for hearing aid verification with children.

## WHAT IS HEARING AID VERIFICATION?

Hearing aid verification refers to electroacoustic measurements of hearing aid function. Hearing aid verification is completed by measuring the output of the hearing aid in either the listener's ear using a probe microphone, known as real-ear or in situ verification or in a 2-$cm^3$ coupler with a microphone, known as simulated real-ear verification (Figure 4–1).

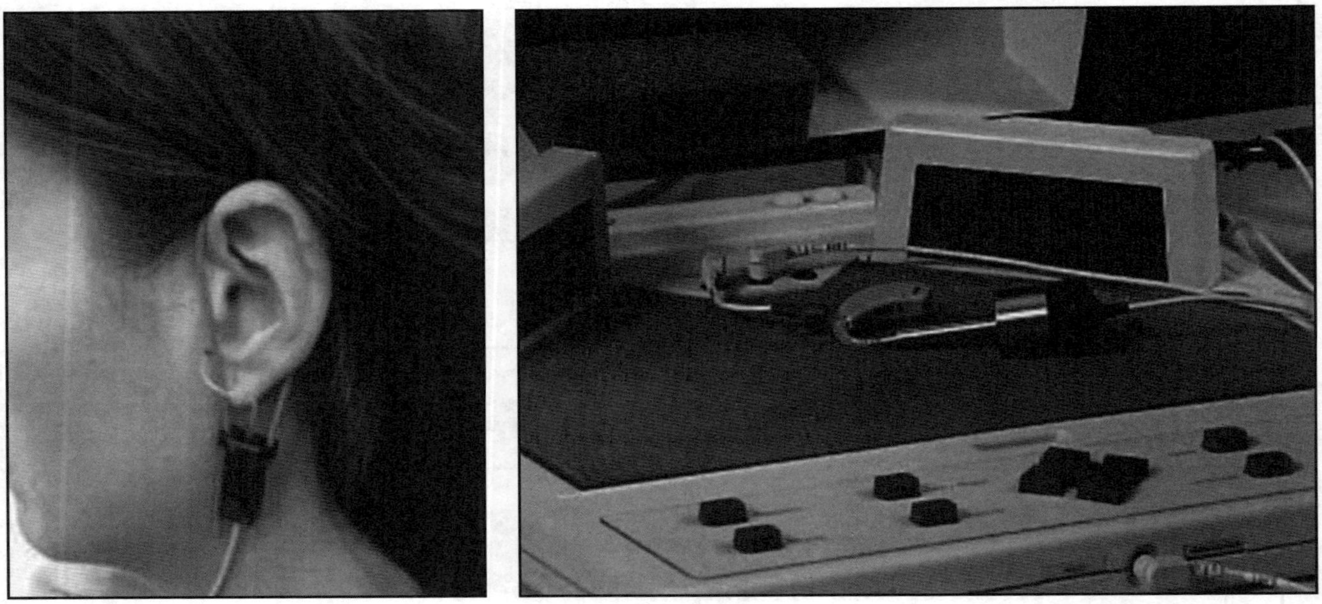

A B

**FIGURE 4–1.** A comparison of real-ear or in situ hearing aid verification (**A**) to simulated real-ear measurements in a 2-cm$^3$ coupler (**B**).

The most valid and frequently used stimulus for hearing aid verification is a calibrated recording of speech. The measurement of the speech signal is averaged to generate a long-term average speech spectrum (LTASS) that characterizes the frequency and intensity range of average speech. The hearing aid measurements of speech obtained during verification are typically compared to the listener's audiometric thresholds to ensure that the output of the hearing aid is sufficient to make speech audible. The graph that plots the intensity of the LTASS against the listener's audiometric thresholds as a function of frequency is known as the SPL-o-gram (Figure 4–2). Mathematical comparisons of the LTASS and the listener's thresholds can be used to estimate audibility for speech.

## REAL-EAR-TO-COUPLER DIFFERENCE (RECD) AND EAR CANAL ACOUSTICS

Verification measurements are objective and do not require a response from the listener, which makes them ideal measures for listeners of any age. Generally, verification during infancy is completed by measuring the child's real-ear-to-coupler difference (RECD) and applying the RECD to hearing aid measurements in the 2-cm$^3$ coupler. The RECD is the difference in dB between the level of a broadband signal recorded in the child's ear canal and the same sound measured in the 2-cm$^3$ coupler. The RECD accounts for the acoustic differences between a coupler that was designed for an adult ear canal used for verification and the child's ear canal. This allows the incorporation of the child's individual ear canal acoustics into the hearing aid verification process without having to take multiple measurements of speech in each of the child's ear canal because many infants and children cannot maintain cooperation across multiple in situ measurements. Once children can maintain sufficient head control in front of a speaker, the verification approach can switch from using an RECD to simulate real-ear to in situ measurements with the probe microphone in the child's ear canal. Many infants can maintain sufficient head control around 6 months developmental age. However, many clinicians continue to use RECD measurements even after the point where children can maintain head control for in

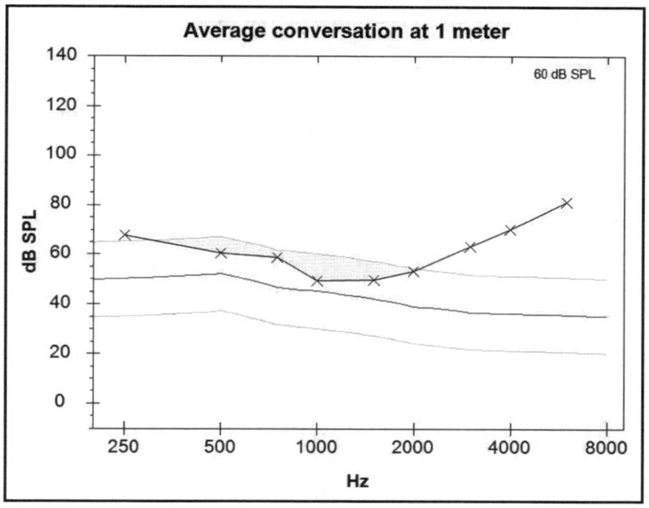


**FIGURE 4–2.** The unamplified long-term average speech spectrum (LTASS) represents the range of frequency and intensity of speech averaged over time. The LTASS is also referred to as the dynamic range of speech. This SPL-o-gram shows the unaided LTASS as a function of frequency for a listener with moderate hearing loss. Portions of the LTASS that fall below the listeners thresholds (*plotted as X symbols for the left ear*) are inaudible.

situ measures, as many infants and toddlers will continue to be limited in their ability to cooperate with multiple in situ measurements through the first few years of life. The transition from RECD to in situ verification should occur as early as the child's cooperation will allow, as in situ measurements more accurately model the variations in ear canal occlusion than simulated hearing aid verification measures with RECD (Bagatto et al., 2005).

In cases where a child cannot cooperate with a measured RECD or in situ measures, age-related average RECD data are available in one-month intervals for children under 5 years of age (Bagatto, Scollie, Seewald, Moodie, & Hoover, 2002). However, age-related average RECD measures should be applied only in cases where an actual measurement of the child's ear cannot be measured. The range of individual RECD values for children who are the same age can be 15 to 20 dB for children with intact tympanic membranes and larger for children with middle ear dysfunction, tympanic membrane perforations or tympanostomy tubes (McCreery et al., 2015). Similarly, children with atypically small ear canals or ear canal stenosis may have RECDs that are substantially higher than the age-related average values. Age-related average RECD result in larger deviations from the prescriptive target than measured RECD or in situ verification methods (McCreery et al., 2013). Even if an RECD can only be measured in one ear, RECD have been found to be symmetrical between ears within 2 to 3 dB as long as there are no obvious structural anomalies that affect one ear and not the other (Munro & Howlin, 2010). In cases where there is a difference between ears, such as tympanic membrane perforation, tympanostomy tube or unilateral defects of the ear canal, the contralateral RECD should not be used nor should an average age-related RECD be applied. The goal of measuring the RECD is to accurately account for individual differences in ear canal acoustics for an individual child in order to accurately predict the amount of amplification that is needed to restore audibility.

An understanding of hearing aid verification requires a review of some basic principles of acoustics. When an earmold is coupled to a hearing aid and placed in the ear canal, the sound level that the hearing aid delivers is determined by two factors: (1) the output of the hearing aid and (2) the volume of the ear canal between the earmold and the tympanic membrane. If the output of the hearing aid is held constant and the volume of the ear canal is varied, the sound level will increase as the volume of the ear canal decreases. In practical terms, this means that the same hearing aid will have a different output depending on the volume of the ear canal in which it is placed. This acoustic fact means that there will be two sources of variability that must be accounted for when fitting a hearing aid for a child. As the ear canal grows, the output of the hearing aid will decrease over time for a given child as the volume of the ear canal increases. Because ear canal size can vary across children of the same age, it also means that even children who are the same age will have a lot of individual variability in their ear canal acoustics due to normal variation in the volume of their ear canals. The implications of these facts are that hearing aid verification must be completed at regular intervals as the child grows and develops to account for differences across children and changes in an individual child's ear canal acoustics over time. The pattern of variability across children and decreasing RECD as children grow older is evident in Figure 4–3.

## The SPL-O-Gram and Hearing Aid Verification

The primary visualization of the hearing aid verification process is based on a plot of the output of the hearing aid known as the SPL-o-gram. The SPL-o-gram has its name because the output of the hearing aid across frequency is plotted in dB Sound Pressure Level (SPL) instead of the dB Hearing Level (HL) convention used for the audiogram. The SPL-o-gram (Figure 4–4) minimally includes the audiometric thresholds converted from HL to SPL. The unamplified or amplified LTASS is plotted along with thresholds to assess audibility. A measure of the hearing aid output to a loud pure-tone sweep, known as the maximum power output (MPO), is also displayed to show the response of the hearing aid to a high input level. The MPO is generally used to assess the level at which the hearing aid might move from a wide dynamic range compression amplitude compression to a compression limiting where the output of the hearing aid is significantly compressed to avoid saturation. The SPL-o-gram not only serves as a good visual tool to assess audibility, but also forms the basis for audibility calculations for the Speech Intelligibility Index (SII; ANSI S3.5-1997).

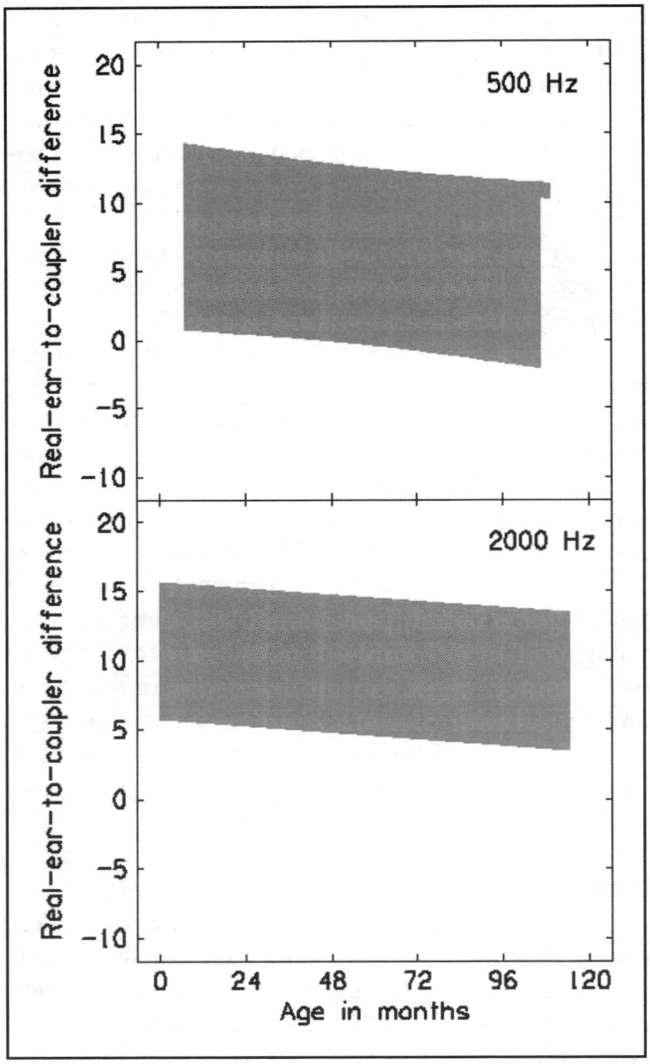


**FIGURE 4–3.** The range of RECD values at 500 Hz (*top panel*) and 2000 Hz (*bottom panel*) for children with normal middle ear status adapted from McCreery et al., 2015.

For the SPL-o-gram, the hearing thresholds from the audiogram are converted to SPL. The formula for converting dB HL thresholds to dB SPL thresholds is:

$$\text{dB SPL threshold} = \text{dB HL} + \text{RETSPL} + \text{RECD}$$

The transducer-specific reference-equivalent threshold for SPL (RETSPL) is added to the HL threshold. A transducer-specific RECD is also applied to account for ear canal acoustics for specific transducers. If the RECD is measured as part of the verification process, the measured RECD will be applied at this stage. If an age-related average RECD is used, the average RECD is applied. The hearing aid output for the SPL-o-gram is either based on either the SPL measurement of the hearing aid output in the ear canal for in situ verification or the simulated real-ear measurement in the 2-cm$^3$ coupler. Coupler measures of hearing aid output are converted to an estimated ear canal SPL with the following formula:

$$\text{dB SPL in the ear canal} = \text{dB SPL hearing aid output in the 2 cm}^3 + \text{MLE} + \text{RECD}$$

The MLE refers to the microphone location effects for behind-the-ear hearing aids, which is an acoustic difference between having a microphone in the ear canal and the hearing aid microphone at the top of the ear. As with the threshold conversion, the RECD that is applied to the hearing aid measurements depends on whether the RECD was measured or average.

The application of the RECD in two different stages of the generation of the SPL-o-gram and estimates of hearing aid output has resulted in multiple questions about how to maximize the accuracy of hearing aid verification for children. A recent article summarizes many of the pertinent clinical issues related to the application of RECD (Moodie et al., 2016a). In most cases, clinicians measure a single RECD as part of the hearing aid verification process and that RECD is applied to both the threshold conversion and the conversion of hearing aid output in the coupler to simulated real-ear measures. However, the RECD for threshold estimation is most often based on the transducer that was used to measure thresholds, typically insert earphones for children. Because RECD has been thought of as part of the hearing aid verification process, most clinicians measure the RECD with the child's earmold (Moodie et al., 2016b). This creates a mismatch between the RECD that is used to measure thresholds and the RECD used to estimate hearing aid output in the coupler. In some clinics, the solution is to measure the child's thresholds using the child's earmold coupled to the insert earphones (Figure 4–5).

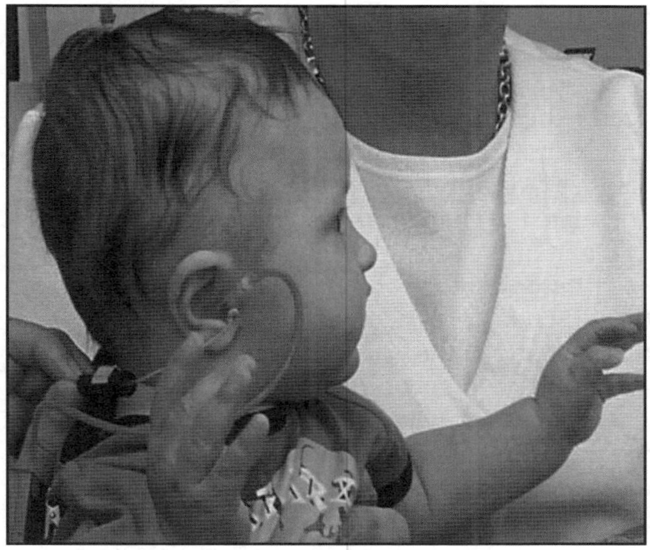

**FIGURE 4–5.** A child with their earmold coupled to insert earphones for hearing assessment.

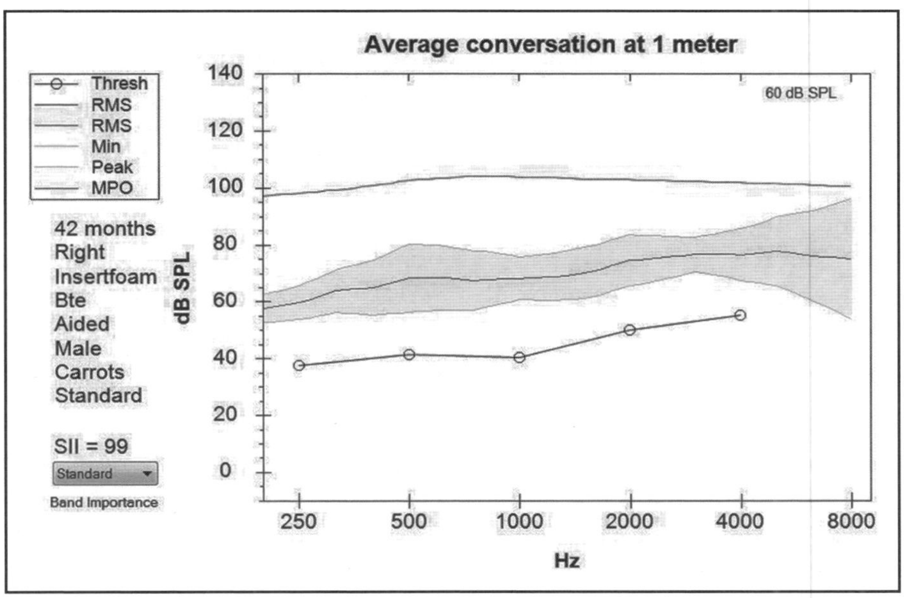


**FIGURE 4–4.** An example SPL-o-gram for a child with mild hearing loss. Note the hearing thresholds in SPL (*plotted as O symbols for the right ear*), amplified LTASS (*shaded area*), and maximum output of the hearing aid plotted as function of frequency.

This approach eliminates the mismatch between the two RECDs because the earmold RECD is used for both threshold and hearing aid measures. Using the earmolds during threshold estimation also has the benefit of increasing the child's acceptance of insert earphones compared to foam insert tips because the child is presumably used to their own earmold (Scollie & Bagatto, 2016). This practice has not received wide clinical acceptance because the earmold may not be available or may need to be replaced at appointments where behavioral assessment is completed. This approach may also lead to apparent changes in thresholds that are related to changes in ear canal acoustics related to the fit of the earmold, though these changes can be differentiated from changes in hearing using the RECD as a benchmark. Acoustic changes in the coupling of the earmold to the child's ear canal should be evident from changes in the RECD.

The alternative approach that has gained greater clinical acceptance is to use an RECD measured with an insert foam tip for both hearing assessment and hearing aid verification. This approach prevents the RECD mismatch problem, but also has been shown to provide reasonably consistent results compared to in situ verification measures (Gustafson, Pittman, & Fanning, 2013). The obvious limitation of this approach is that the effects of earmold acoustics related to horn or damping effects will not be quantified using this method. The child may also not find the insert foam tip to be as comfortable or as acceptable as their own earmold. In either case, the mismatch between the two different RECDs is avoided by maintaining the same coupling for assessment and hearing aid verification.

A third option that has recently become available is to measure two separate RECDs: one for the assessment phase with an insert foam tip, and one for the hearing aid verification phase with the child's earmold. This change was made available by the development of hearing aid verification equipment that allows for the specification and measurement of separate RECDs. While this approach may be the most technically accurate in terms of specifying the contributions of each RECD to the hearing aid verification process, the requirement to measure the RECD using two methods for each ear at each appointment is likely to be a significant limiting factor for clinicians who may face challenges measuring a single RECD for each child with hearing aids that they see in their clinic. The gains in accuracy compared to either the earmold or insert foam tip methods also are likely to be minimal, which may raise questions among even the most particular pediatric audiologists about the benefit of taking separate RECD measurements for assessment and hearing aid verification.

Regardless of the method, the application of the RECD to the hearing thresholds and the hearing aid output allows for an accurate estimation of the SPL in the child's ear canal for the purposes of matching prescriptive targets and calculating audibility for the LTASS. A fitting with a close proximity to prescriptive targets will allow audiologists to provide consistent audibility for children who have a wide range of degrees of hearing loss. The quantification of audibility over time will ensure that the goals related to maintaining auditory access over time in children with hearing loss can be accomplished. In the following sections, the use of the SPL-o-gram to quantify the proximity of the fitting to prescriptive targets and the aided audibility for speech is discussed in greater detail.

## HEARING AID PRESCRIPTION FOR CHILDREN

The process of providing consistent audibility for speech for children who wear hearing aids is dependent on the use of validated pediatric prescriptive methods to determine how much amplification is needed for a given child. Hearing aid prescription refers to a method of estimating the amount of amplification that is needed for a given child, typically based on the child's audiometric thresholds and average data about loudness discomfort levels. Several hearing aid prescriptions have been developed for adults and children. Two prescriptive methods have been validated for children: The National Acoustics Laboratory-Nonlinear formula Version 2 (NAL-NL2; Keidser, Dillon, Flax, Ching, & Brewer, 2011) and the Desired Sensation Level, multistage input/output (DSL m i/o or DSL v.5; Scollie et al., 2005). Both the NAL-NL2 and DSL prescriptive algorithms have separate prescriptive formulae that are specifically designed to be used for children. The NAL-NL2 prescriptive formula is based on a rationale of loudness normalization, whereas the DSL algorithm is designed to restore audibility, with loudness normalization as a secondary goal. This difference between the fundamental goals of each prescription means that NAL-NL2 generally prescribes less amplification than DSL overall. The differences in prescribed gain between NAL-NL2 and DSL increase as the degree of hearing loss increases, due to specific predictions in NAL about decreasing benefits of amplification from distortion as the degree of hearing loss increases (Ching et al., 2010; Ching, Johnson, Seeto, & Macrae, 2013a). In practical terms, some differences between the two algorithms, particularly at higher frequencies, are minimized by the limited high-frequency bandwidth of hearing aids, greater degrees of hearing loss or a combination of those two factors.

Multiple studies have been completed to compare a wide range of outcomes for children fitted with DSL and NAL prescriptions. Earlier versions of both prescriptions (NAL-NL1 and DSL version 4) were compared across a number of different outcomes as part of a cooperative research effort between developers of both algorithms. Children were fitted with either NAL-NL1 or DSL 4 as part of a double-blinded, crossover trial, so that children changed prescriptions halfway through the trial. Small, but statistically significant, differences in speech recognition at input levels equivalent to soft speech (55 dB SPL) were observed with DSL resulting in higher speech recognition scores in quiet (Scollie et al., 2010b). At an 80 dB SPL input level, children reported more favorable loudness ratings for NAL than DSL, but patterns of individual variability in preference were observed among children. Differences in loudness ratings across prescriptions decreased as the children wore their hearing aids. In an analysis of listening preference in real world listening conditions, children who had been fitted with DSL before the trial preferred the DSL prescriptive approach, whereas children who had been fitted with NAL preferred NAL. Most of the differences between prescriptions in speech recognition and listening preference will relatively small for the group of children with moderate to severe hearing loss that were part of the study.

More recently, a follow-up study completed a randomized controlled trial was completed comparing the NAL-NL2 and DSL v5 prescriptions on a wide range of developmental outcomes for infants with hearing loss (Ching, 2013b). Language development outcomes and parent-report measures of auditory development were used to determine if children who were randomly assigned to either NAL or DSL prescriptions exhibited differences in language outcomes at three years of age. The study did not find a difference in language or parent-report outcome measures at three years of age between the NAL and DSL prescriptive approaches, suggesting that the differences between the two approaches are not significant enough to impact developmental outcomes in children with hearing loss who wear hearing aids. Because NAL prescribes hearing aid characteristics that result in less audibility than DSL, this finding might initially seem in contrast to longitudinal research that suggests that children who were fitted with hearing aids that provide less audibility have poorer language growth over time than peers who receive more audibility (Tomblin et al., 2015). However, differences in audibility between prescriptive approaches should be distinguished from differences in audibility related to poor fitting practices and lack of hearing aid verification. Though the NAL and DSL prescriptions place different amounts of importance on the relative balance between loudness and audibility for speech, both prescriptions balance these factors in a systematic way. The results suggest that NAL and DSL are both likely to provide sufficient amplification to support language development in children under most circumstances.

In North America, the DSL prescriptive approach is used exclusively for children (McCreery et al., 2013), despite the fact that there is limited evidence to suggest that DSL provides more favorable outcomes than NAL. The main reason for this clear preference is that DSL emphasizes audibility and that loudness complaints among young children are rare and often managed on an individual basis through fine-tuning of the hearing aid fitting. If a child exhibits significant difficulty with loudness discomfort with DSL when wearing their hearing aids that require major reductions in the output, the use of NAL-NL2 may be a valid option that provides a modest reduction in audibility and may improve loudness discomfort for high input levels. The use of prescriptive approaches is important for providing consistent amplification for children with hearing loss, but should not be viewed as a mandate in cases where the child expresses concerns about loudness discomfort or refuses to wear the hearing aids in specific listening situations with high noise levels. Research suggests that some loudness discomfort related to amplification will lessen over time with experience using the hearing aids (Scollie et al., 2010b). Reductions in amplification for children to address complaints of sound quality should be done cautiously with the goal of maintaining audibility of speech to the greatest extent possible.

The comparative studies of DSL and NAL raise interesting questions about the use of one prescriptive approach for all listening situations. In one comparative study (Scollie et al., 2010a), it was generally reported that children preferred to use DSL when listening in quiet or to low-level speech, and that children preferred NAL when listening to louder sounds or in background noise. This finding suggests that a single hearing aid frequency response may not be appropriate for all listening conditions and led the scientists who developed DSL to implement versions of the DSL m i/o formula for noise, known as DSL-Child Noise or DSL-Adult Noise (Scollie et al., 2005). The Noise versions of the DSL prescription are designed to maintain speech audibility, while reducing loudness discomfort in situations with background noise by reducing amplification in a way that effectively targets the frequency regions that are likely to be dominated by noise and have minimal speech importance. A comparison of the DSL-Child and DSL-Child Noise prescriptions reveals that the most significant differences between prescriptions are at high levels and lower frequencies (Figure 4–6).

Recent evidence suggests that the DSL-Noise prescription achieves the dual goals of maintaining speech recognition, while reducing loudness discomfort in noise. Crukley and Scollie (2012) compared the DSL-Child and DSL-Child Noise prescriptions for a group of school-age children with hearing loss. Speech recognition in quiet at low input levels was slightly poorer in quiet with the DSL-Child Noise prescription compared to the standard DSL-Child prescription, but speech recognition in noise was equivalent between the two versions of the prescription. Loudness ratings were more favorable at high input levels (80 dB SPL) with DSL-Child Noise. This pattern of findings is similar to the differences between NAL and DSL reported in the earlier comparative study of these algorithms (Scollie et al., 2010a). Changes in audibility that reduce performance at low input levels may provide benefits in noisy listening situations for discomfort.

A potential solution to this paradox could be to provide children with multiple programs that have different frequency responses for difference listening situations (quiet or noise). This option raises questions about whether children would be able to change the program in their hearing aid in response to different listening situations. Another potential option would be to offer some form of noise management signal processing, such as digital noise reduction, which would automatically engage when the hearing aid detects that the listener is in noise, either based on the level or modulation spectrum of the stimulus (Scollie et al., 2016). The use of noise management may be preferable over having dedicated programs that the child may have to switch, as infants and young children may not be able to switch their hearing aids as the environment changes, and some older children may be unable to do so. One study of adult hearing aid use in real world listening situations suggested that adults stay in the same hearing aid program about 80% of the time, which raises questions about whether or not even adults can make changes to their hearing aids in response to changes in the listening environment (Banerjee, 2011). At the time of this writing, the DSL-Child Noise prescription is not widely used by clinical audiologists for children, but could be incorporated into pediatric hearing aid fittings for older children who can provide feedback about their listening environments and desire greater comfort when listening in background noise.

The hearing aid prescription is an important first step in providing amplification for infants

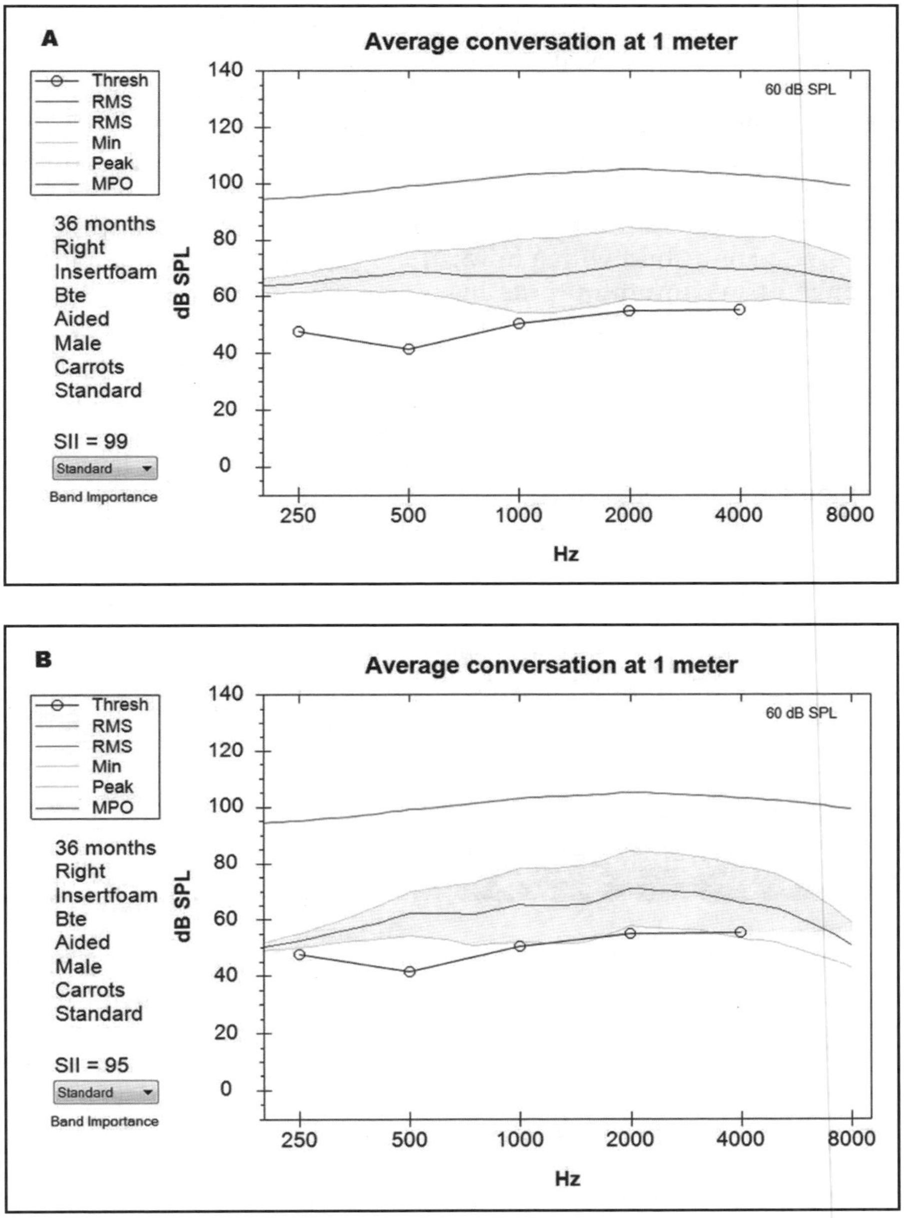


**FIGURE 4–6.** A comparison of the DSL–Child (**A**) and DSL–Child Noise (**B**) prescriptive algorithms for the same audiogram.

and children because it provides a standardized method of determining how much amplification is needed to make speech audible. Many hearing aid manufacturers have implemented both NAL-NL2 and DSL m i/o in their proprietary programming software as an aid to clinicians. However, the existence of the hearing aid prescription in manufacturers' programming software does not obviate the need for electroacoustic verification. A study by Seewald, Mills, Bagatto, Scollie, and Moodie (2008) attempted to determine the accuracy of manufacturer implementation of the DSL prescriptive approach by electroacoustically assessing hearing aids that were programmed by selecting the DSL prescriptive in the manufacturer's software. The results were generated for nine audiograms for a hypothetical 6-month-old infant for five different manufacturers. The accuracy of the manufacturers' implementations of the DSL prescription varied considerably in terms of both the amount of aided audibility and the maximum output of the hearing aid. The range of the maximum output for the same audiogram was greater than 30 dB in some cases. For a child with a mild hearing loss, the range of maximum outputs in one example was between 102 dB SPL peak and 133 dB SPL peak. The range of audibility provided by the manufacturers' implementations for the same audiogram was 10 to 20%. The pattern of the errors was also not predictable with some manufacturers' implementations of DSL providing too little amplification and others providing too much. The main implication of this study is that while selecting a manufacturer implementation of DSL in the programming software may minimize the amount of programming that needs to be done to match prescriptive targets, electroacoustic verification is still required.

## VERIFYING AUDIBILITY

The process of verifying hearing aids generally occurs in one of two ways: either the hearing aid is measured in the child's ear canal, known as in situ verification, or the child's RECD is measured and subsequent measurements of the hearing aid are taken in the coupler, known as simulated real-ear measures. In cases where an individually measured RECD cannot be measured due to limited cooperation from the child or other factors, an age-related average RECD can be used in place of a measured RECD, keeping in mind the limitations that doing so places on the accuracy of the resulting fitting. In most cases, a speech signal is played either through a speaker in front of the child (in situ) or from a speaker inside the test box in front of the hearing aid (simulated real-ear measurements). The following sections will discuss considerations for how electroacoustic verification can be accomplished for either in situ or simulated real-ear measurements for children so that the audibility of speech can be verified.

### Verification Stimuli

The specific stimulus used for verification ideally should have the spectral and temporal characteristics of speech, as well as modulation spectrum and fundamental frequency of speech. This ensures that the hearing aid is processing the input to the hearing aid in the same way that it would be when the person wearing the device is listening to speech. The most direct way to achieve this goal is to use a calibrated passage of speech spoken by a male, female, or child talker as a verification stimulus. Some have argued that passages of speech that are in a particular language may not be suitable for judgments of sound quality from patients who do not speak that language. As a result, there are also international standard stimuli available, such as the International Speech Test Stimulus (ISTS; Holube, Fredelake, Vlaming, & Kollmeier, 2010). The ISTS is based on multiple samples of a female talker speaking different languages, which are purposefully unintelligible due to the mixing of brief segments from each language. The resulting stimulus has temporal and spectral characteristics of speech, but can be used with a patient who speaks any language. The same stimulus should be used whenever possible to promote comparability between verification measures over time and across different settings. Clinicians may wish to use recordings of women and children to better assess the impact of the hearing aid fitting for talkers with higher-frequency speech spectra in specific cases.

### Stimulus Levels

Generally, the response to the hearing aid is measured for speech at three input levels that correspond to soft, average, and loud speech. The actual levels that are recommended for each of these input levels varies between clinics with some clinics measuring soft/average/loud as 50/60/70 dB SPL, and others at 55/65/75 dB SPL. In practice the specific levels that are tested are less important than assessing the hearing aid's response to speech and resulting audibility for a broad range of input levels. The prescriptive algorithm will provide prescriptive targets at each frequency for each specific input level that is assessed to guide the clinician in setting the hearing aid. An example of an SPL-o-gram with hearing aid verification completed at soft, average, and loud speech levels is shown in Figure 4–7.

However, there are some considerations that might influence the clinician's choice about which set of levels to choose. Some clinicians may choose the higher 55/65/75 dB SPL levels because recordings at 50 dB can be susceptible to room noise for in situ verification in some rooms where hearing aids are fitted. Using higher levels can avoid contamination of the recording, though this is not a major issue for simulated real-ear measurements conducted in the test box, as most verification test boxes are sound-treated. The available normative range for aided audibility from Bagatto et al. (2016) includes fitting ranges for both 55 dB and 65 dB SPL, which can be useful for determining whether or not a hearing aid fitting has provided an adequate amount of audibility, as described in the following section on fitting outcomes. Another key consideration is the level(s) where aided speech recognition is likely to be completed during the outcomes validation phase of the hearing aid fitting process. Having aided audibility values from verification that are the same levels as aided speech recognition assessment can be valuable for determining whether or not a child's aided speech recognition is adequate for the amount of aided audibility that they have. Audiologists must consider these factors when determining what combination of stimulus levels to assess during hearing aid verification.

## Assessing Maximum Output

In addition to verifying that a speech signal is audible through the hearing aid, the maximum

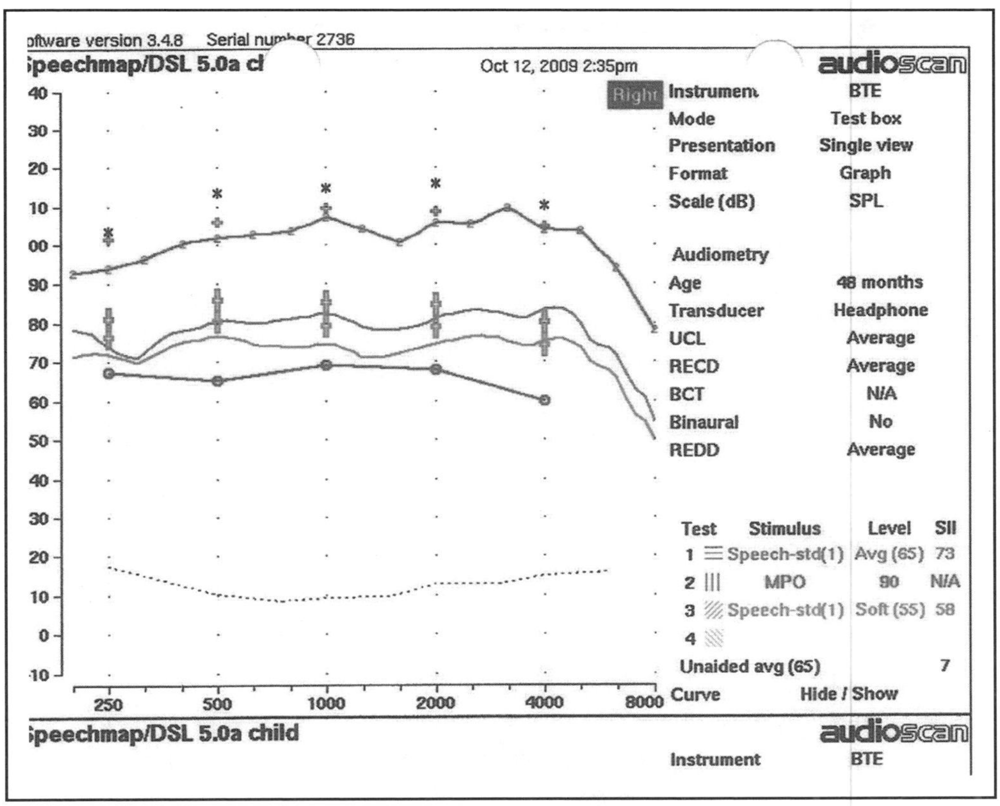


**FIGURE 4–7.** An SPL-o-gram showing the aided verification measures of soft (55 dB SPL) and average (65 dB SPL) speech input levels for a child with mild to moderate hearing loss. The aided SII values increase as the input level increases.

output of the hearing aid is also measured during the verification process. Known as the maximum power output (MPO) or real ear saturation response (RESR), a narrowband sweep of discrete pure-tones is presented to the hearing aid at a high input level, usually around 85 dB or 90 dB SPL. The goal of using the narrowband signal is to attempt to drive the hearing aid into saturation to estimate the maximum level of the hearing aid at each frequency. Prescriptive formulae provide specific targets for MPO (Figure 4–8) and the goal of the fitting is to maintain the MPO at that level. However, the MPO should not be set too conservatively, as limiting the maximum output of the hearing aid may reduce the peaks of speech and negatively affect speech recognition in noise (Kuk, Peeters, Lau, & Korhonen, 2011). Recent evidence suggests that the likelihood of causing damage to a child's hearing through amplification is low as long as the output of the hearing aid can be verified and matched to prescriptive targets (McCreery et al., 2016). Many hearing aid verification systems also have conservative safety mechanisms that limit the output of the hearing aid in the child's ear during in situ measurements to a prespecified safety limit.

Although the MPO is generally safe to measure in the child's ear using in situ verification procedures, the swept pure-tone signals used for the MPO may be unfamiliar to the child, in addition to being loud or sounding like an alarm. As a result, some children may become frightening or startled if the MPO is measured in their ear canal. One solution for this problem is to measure the MPO of the hearing aid in the coupler using simulated real-ear measurements with an RECD. Another potential solution is to familiarize the child with the MPO sweep prior to taking the measurement

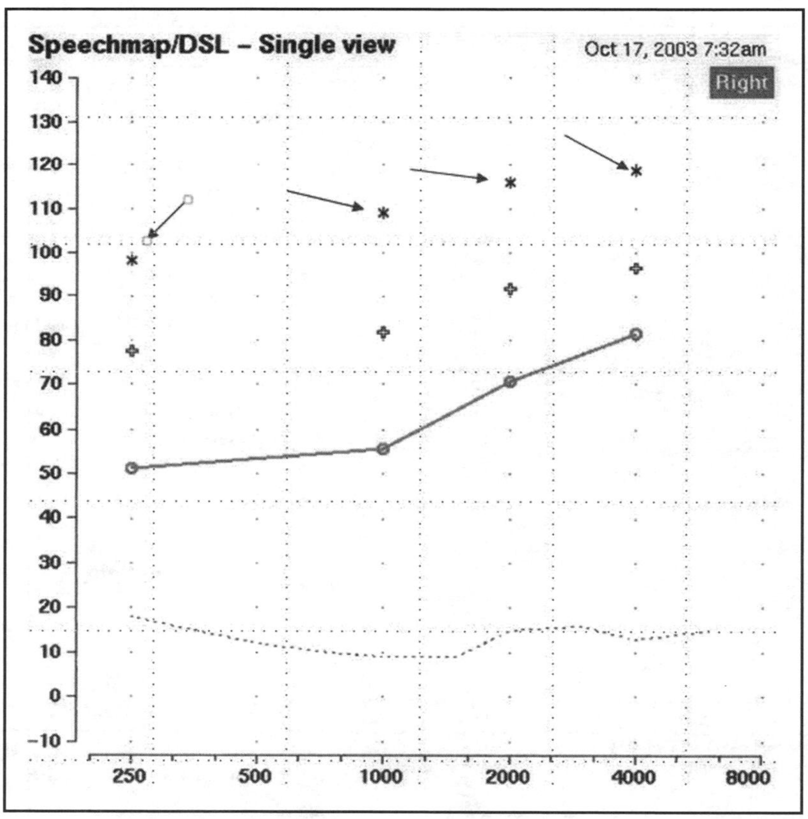


**FIGURE 4–8.** Targets for maximum power output (MPO) are represented by the star symbols at each frequency for a child with moderate hearing loss (*pointed to by arrows*).

of the hearing aid in their ear canal. Experienced audiologists can often recognize whether or not children will be willing to complete in situ measures of MPO and plan accordingly.

Because hearing aids are designed to process speech inputs, some manufacturers have settings in the programming software that can be used to disable advanced signal processing features, such as feedback suppression, during the verification process. These advanced signal-processing features may alter the MPO measurement and lead to inaccurate estimates in some cases. If the manufacturer recommends changing the settings for the hearing aid during verification for MPO, it is advisable to use those settings only for MPO measurements, and complete measurements of the hearing aid with speech with any and all advanced features activated. The goal of this approach is to determine how those features might interact with speech in ways that can be quantified through the verification process. The verification mode in many manufacturers' hearing aid programming software can be activated just for the MPO portion of the verification process to prevent interactions with the pure-tone sweep.

## Measuring Aided Audibility

One of the key components of the cumulative auditory experience model is that speech must be made audible across a range of listening situations. Estimating aided audibility for speech is the primary goal of hearing aid verification and is treated like a key outcome measure that is documented at each hearing aid verification appointment throughout the child's life. Consequently, audiologists may question the amount of audibility that is needed to promote optimal speech and language development in children with hearing loss. Restoring full audibility for speech, with an aided SII value of 1 or 100 would obviously be an ideal goal. The ability to restore full audibility in children with hearing loss, unfortunately, is limited by several factors. While the bandwidth of hearing aids has certainly increased over the past decade, the hearing aid acts as a bandpass filter for speech, generally amplifying speech information from around 100 to 6000 Hz for most degrees of hearing loss (Kimlinger, McCreery, & Lewis, 2015). This bandwidth captures the vast majority of speech information, but does exclude some important speech cues in the high frequencies, particularly for female and child talkers. This means that even a child with mild hearing loss may be unlikely to achieve full restoration of audibility with amplification, though many children with mild hearing loss can achieve audibility in the 0.9 to 1 SII range. As noted in the discussion of amplitude compression in Chapter 3, the dynamic range of hearing narrows with sensorineural hearing loss, which can also limit the ability to fully restore audibility with hearing aids. The unamplified range of speech has an assumed dynamic range of approximately 30 dB, with an asymmetrical distribution around the mean of peaks, which are approximately 12 dB above the average and valleys, which are 18 dB less than the average. The dynamic range of the LTASS can be reduced to 10 to 15 dB with amplitude compression. Even with amplitude compression characteristics that allow prescriptive targets to be matched across a range of input levels, the lowest levels of the LTASS may not be made audible by hearing aids, due in part to the asymmetrical distribution of energy skewed toward the valleys. The ability to map the dynamic range of the LTASS onto the individual patient's dynamic range becomes more difficult as the degree of hearing loss increases and the dynamic range becomes narrower. The degree to which aided audibility can be restored decreases as the degree of hearing loss increases. The implications that this relationship has for decisions about cochlear implantation is discussed in Chapter 8.

The interaction between the amount of audibility that can be achieved with a hearing aid and the child's degree of hearing loss means that there is no single SII value criterion that can be defined as adequate for all children who wear hearing aids. In past years, the lack of an SII criterion for children with hearing loss had limited the applicability of the aided SII as an outcome of the verification process because there was little agreement about what amount of audibility constituted an adequate fitting. There is still some uncertainty around this question, but recent research evidence has substantially clarified the anticipated range of SII values that can be expected for children who wear hearing aids, and the fact that children who are fit to prescriptive targets have adequate audibility to experience growth in language ability that exceeds the expected rate of growth for peers with normal hearing (Tomblin et al., 2015). The normative range for the SII for children fitted to DSL was first published by Bagatto et al. (2011) as part of the University of Western Ontario Pediatric Amplification (PedAmp) Protocol. The normative range was based on a large sample of children who had been fitted in reasonable proximity to DSL targets. It covers a range of hearing losses from mild to severe. Data for children with severe-to-profound hearing losses (pure-tone average >70 dB HL) have been limited by the fact that many of the children with greater degrees of hearing loss in North America receive cochlear implants. Further refinement of the normative SII range was published by Bagatto and colleagues in 2016 and is shown in Figure 4–9. The SII value for average speech is plotted against the child's pure-tone average from the audiogram at 500 Hz, 1000 Hz, 2000 Hz, and 4000 Hz. Values that fall between the dashed lines are considered to be consistent with previously published data for children who wear hearing aids. Children who have aided SII values below the normative range for their degree of hearing loss should have amplification adjusted to attempt to increase their aided audibility for speech.

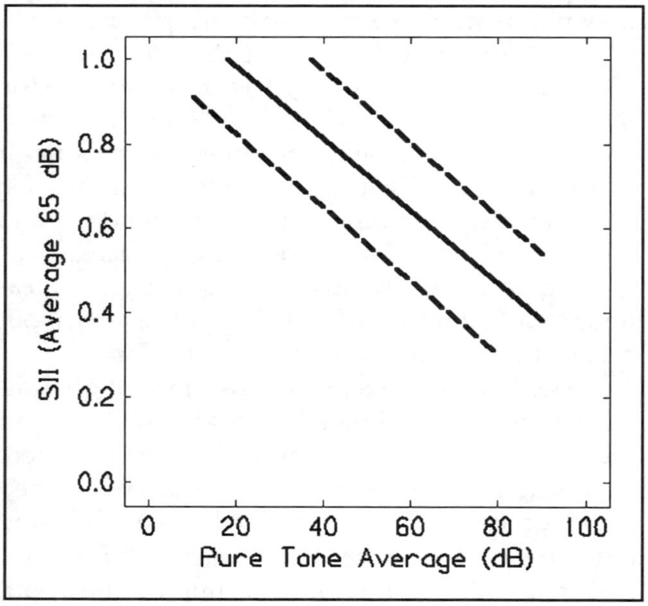


**FIGURE 4–9.** The normative range for the Speech Intelligibility Index (SII) for average speech (65 dB SPL), adapted from data from Bagatto et al., 2010. The SII value measured during hearing aid verification is plotted in correspondence with the child's pure-tone average (500 Hz, 1000 Hz, 2000 Hz, and 4000 Hz). Values that fall within the dashed lines are considered acceptable.

The normative range for the SII is a useful reference for clinicians who want to provide consistent amounts of aided audibility for children with a range of degrees of hearing loss. It is evident from the normative range for the SII that the ability to make speech audible decreases rapidly as the child's degree of hearing loss increases. As noted in the previous paragraph, there is emerging evidence to suggest that having an aided SII within the normative range places a child with hearing loss at an advantage over a peer with a comparable degree of hearing loss who is below that range. However, this fact should be carefully distinguished from statements about providing optimal audibility for a child who wears hearing aids. The normative range simply reflects the expected SII values for children who were fitted to DSL prescriptive targets, but does not provide evidence that some greater amount of audibility might not be more optimal. Despite the previously cited evidence supporting the importance of audibility in predicting language growth in children (Tomblin et al., 2015), children who wear hearing aids also continue to show persistent areas of vulnerability in their communication development, including areas related to morphosyntactic development (Koehlinger, Van Horne, Oleson, McCreery, & Moeller, 2015). Therefore, it remains unclear if the current levels of aided audibility provided by DSL are optimal for children with hearing loss. Audiologists recognize this fact and often have questions about whether or not there is evidence to support providing even greater aided audibility for speech than is prescribed by DSL. At the present time, there is no available evidence in the literature to suggest that further increases in audibility beyond what is provided by DSL or NAL prescription would confer additional benefits for language development beyond those that are being documented. Further increases in audibility may impose specific costs related to the ability to wear the hearing aid comfortably in noisy or reverberant listening conditions. It is also unclear whether an alternative prescriptive approach that provided additional audibility would be able to overcome the previously discussed limitations of the dynamic range and bandwidth of hearing aids. At the present time, the normative range for the SII is the best tool that audiologists have at their disposal for documenting audibility in children with hearing loss.

## Hearing Aid Fitting Accuracy

Another important outcome of the verification process that can be documented to ensure consistent audibility is the proximity of the hearing aid fitting to the prescriptive target. A recent study of hearing aid fitting outcomes for the Outcomes of Children with Hearing Loss study suggested that nearly half of children fitted with hearing aids had unacceptably large deviations from prescriptive targets in at least one of their ears. These deviations from prescriptive target were a significant impediment to their aided audibility (McCreery et al., 2015). One positive interpretation of these results is that the proximity of the hearing aid fitting to the prescriptive targets is an aspect of the hearing aid fitting process that the audiologist has a direct influence on. There are several strategies that can be used to quantify the accuracy of the fitting relative to prescriptive targets.

As described by McCreery, Bentler, and Roush (2013), one strategy is to calculate the root-mean-square (also known as the geometric mean) of the deviations of the fitting from prescriptive targets at 500 Hz, 1000 Hz, 2000 Hz, and 4000 Hz. The resulting estimate of the fitting proximity to prescriptive targets is known as the RMS error. The RMS error has several advantages over a traditional arithmetic mean for estimating fitting error. One of the greatest advantages is the fact that the RMS error treats both positive and negative differences from prescriptive targets as errors, and does not allow them to offset each other. The process of taking the RMS error removes the positive or negative signs from the deviations, meaning that it is potentially a better estimate of fitting error than an arithmetic mean, where positive and negative differences can counteract each other. Clinicians should still pay close attention to the direction of the errors when fitting. The RMS error approach has also been validated in the sense that children with less than 5 dB RMS error for their fittings typically fall within the normative SII range that was highlighted in the previous section.

Although the arithmetic involved with calculating the RMS error is relatively straightforward, busy audiologists may want a simpler method for estimating the fitting error that does not require any calculations. The most basic method of ensuring a close proximity to prescriptive targets without calculating the RMS error is to ensure that the average of the LTASS is in close proximity to DSL targets across the entire range of speech. This can easily be achieved by ensuring the line that represents the average of the LTASS intersects the prescriptive targets at each frequency or by examining the numeric output of the hearing aid verification equipment in tabular form. In most cases, clinicians will not need to calculate the RMS error to minimize the error in the fitting process, but clinicians may find the RMS error to be a useful outcome measure for documenting the quality of their clinical pediatric amplification program, as well as troubleshooting why fitting errors are likely to occur. Examples of estimating the proximity of the fitting to prescriptive targets are shown in Figure 4–10.

A number of different situations, including poor hearing aid bandwidth, sloping audiometric configuration, or severe or profound degree of hearing loss at specific frequencies, may limit the ability to approximate the prescriptive target at key frequencies. As these situations are expected and unresolvable with current technology, those reasons should be documented to ensure that the reason for the lack of correspondence with prescriptive targets can be fully understood. The use of RMS error may also be problematic in cases where frequency lowering signal processing is being used. Some frequency lowering processors function as low-pass filters, particularly at 2000 Hz and 4000 Hz, which may limit the ability of the clinician to match prescriptive targets at those frequencies. Because the low-pass filtering is related to the signal processor, which is hopefully increasing the overall audibility of high-frequency

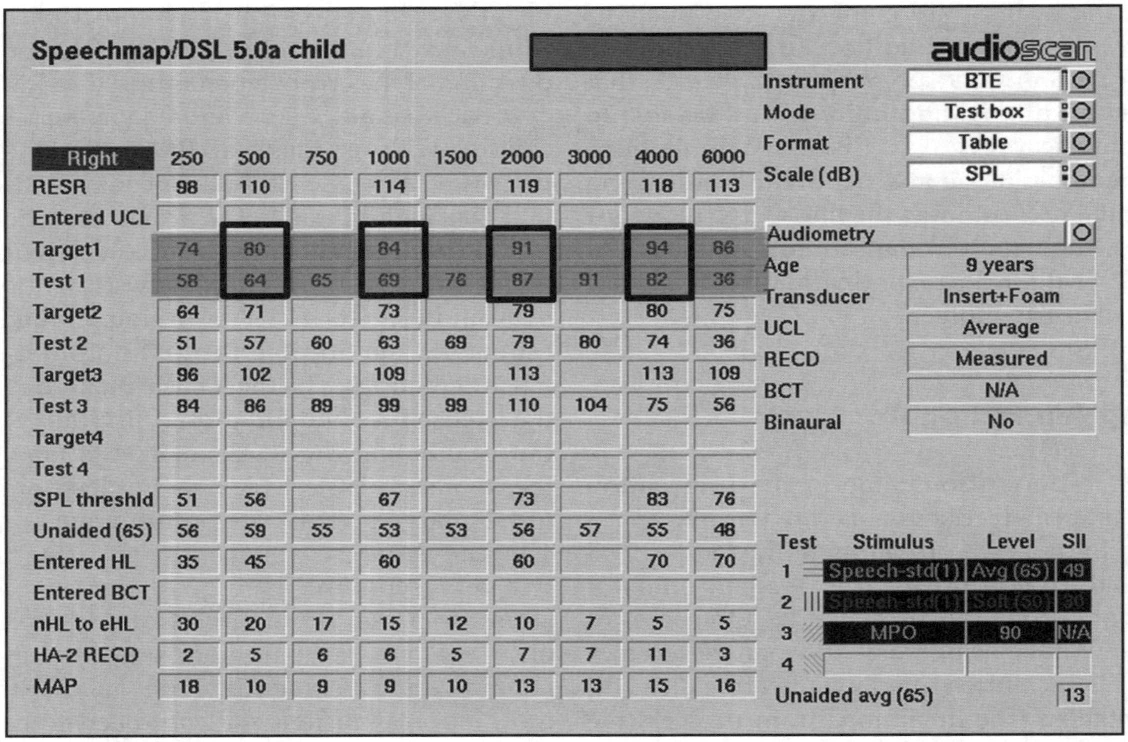


**FIGURE 4–10.** Estimating the proximity of the electroacoustic verification for hearing aids is most easily accomplished by comparing the numerical output of the hearing aid verification measurements compared to targets either visually or in tabular form.

speech, the RMS error calculation should exclude frequencies that are above the roll-off of the low-pass filter, if needed. However, prescriptive targets should still be matched with frequency lowering over the broadest frequency range that is possible to ensure good audibility of the lowered signal.

## The Situational Hearing Aid Response Profile (SHARP)

The electroacoustic measurements taken during the hearing aid verification process assume that the listener is in quiet, approximately one meter away from the talker of interest. For children, this assumption is rarely reflective of listening conditions in the real world. Infants and toddlers may be held in a cradle position in their parent's arms or on their parent's hip. School-age children may listen in classrooms at distances that are greater than one meter. Being closer or more distant from a particular talker can influence the level of the sound that arrives at the child's ear and has a direct impact on audibility in different listening situations. Average conversational speech at one meter is a good standard to use for comparison, but the child's audibility in different listening situations may be better or poorer than verification measures based on these assumptions would indicate.

The Situational Hearing Aid Response Profile (SHARP) is a free software program (download a copy of SHARP at http://audres.org/rc/sharp/) that was developed to allow audiologists and other professionals to simulate alternative listening situations beyond conversational speech at one meter. Hearing aid verification data can either be manually entered or imported directly from verification equipment that outputs the data in an .XML file format. The SHARP program also calculates the aided and unaided SII for each of the listening conditions that is available in the program, as long as the audiometric thresholds and at least two different input levels (soft, average, or loud) are included. Examples of three different listening situations in SHARP for a child with moderate hearing loss are shown in Figure 4–11.

As a clinical tool, SHARP can be used as an outcome measure to document audibility across different listening situations that a child could encounter in his/her everyday life. Educational personnel may find the different classroom listening situations that are available in SHARP helpful for providing recommendations about the best seating location in the classroom or the need for hearing assistance technologies. Parents have also reported that SHARP is useful as a counseling tool to help them better understand how their child's hearing loss impacts their ability to listen in different situations. In particular, the effects of distance on children with mild hearing loss can lead to dramatic reductions in audibility, compared with the standard conversation at one meter, as most children with mild hearing loss do not have significant reductions in audibility in the standard conversation at one-meter condition. Modeling of the head shadow effect in SHARP can also provide information about audibility of sounds from the side of the impaired ear in children with unilateral hearing loss. Overall, there are a number of different applications that SHARP can be used to estimate audibility for nonstandard listening situations.

## Timing of Verification Follow-Up

Verification is not a one-time event that occurs at the initial hearing aid fitting. As noted throughout this text, children grow and develop and outgrow their earmolds, which necessitates a follow-up schedule for verification that takes these changes into account. Regular hearing aid verification will ensure that children have consistent audibility if their ear canal acoustics or hearing change. The period that includes the most significant changes in ear canal acoustics, as well as the need to gather additional audiometric data, is under 12 months of age. For this reason, infants who wear hearing aids should be seen for electroacoustic verification at three-month intervals during the first year

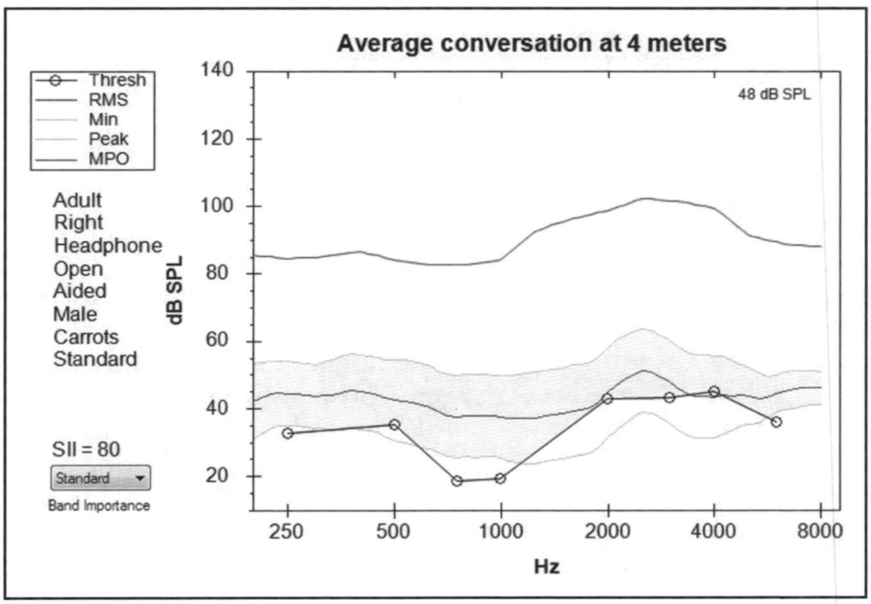


**FIGURE 4–11.** The Situational Hearing Aid Response Profile (SHARP) program can be used to simulate additional listening situations beyond the standard conversational speech at one meter that is used for electroacoustic hearing aid verification.

of life. Earmolds will likely need to be replaced at each appointment to maintain retention and a good acoustic coupling with the ear canal. After 12 months, the frequency of verification can be reduced to every 6 months for children without risk factors for progressive hearing loss. Children with risk factors for progressive hearing loss, such as a history of cytomegalovirus infection or confirmed enlarged vestibular aqueduct syndrome, or who require additional audiometric assessment, may require more frequent follow-up. After three years of age, children with stable hearing can be seen for verification annually or as needed if earmolds need to be replaced.

Electroacoustic verification should be completed any time that earmolds are replaced, as new earmolds can alter the acoustics of the coupling between the child's earmold and the ear canal. If hearing aids are repaired, electroacoustic evaluation should be completed to determine if the problems with the hearing aids have been resolved through the repair, and that the hearing aid settings have not changed or can be restored. Many audiologists will keep the child's most recent RECD measurement so that post-repair electroacoustic verification can be completed in the coupler without the child having to return for an appointment. For most children, an RECD that is less than 6 months old can be used for this process with reasonable accuracy. In cases where no recent measured RECD is available, an age-related average RECD may be used, keeping in mind the previously noted limitations in the accuracy of that approach. Regular electroacoustic verification will promote consistent auditory access throughout the years when critical learning of speech and language are occurring.

### Verifying Audibility: Conclusions

Given the importance of aided audibility to the model of cumulative auditory experience, verifying audibility with accurate electroacoustic measurements is a critically important step in the process of providing amplification for children. Steps can be taken to ensure consistent audibility for children regardless of their degree of hearing loss, including referencing the child's measured SII values to the UWO normative range and minimizing the deviation of the fitting to prescriptive targets. The SHARP can be used to estimate audibility for alternative listening conditions beyond the standard conversational speech at one meter that is traditionally used as a reference for hearing aid verification. Regular hearing aid verification will ensure that the child has auditory access over time.

## ADVANCED FEATURE VERIFICATION

As noted in Chapter 3 on Selection of Amplification, audiologists may select some advanced hearing aid features to be activated in the child's hearing aid. Selection of these advanced features requires additional verification to ensure that the features are functioning as expected and do not compromise audibility for speech. Verification for amplitude compression occurs during the verification of audibility, as long as multiple input levels for speech are assessed during that process. Verification for feedback suppression, digital noise reduction, directional microphones, and frequency lowering require additional verification beyond the assessment of audibility. Those specific procedures will be discussed briefly in the sections that follow.

### Feedback Suppression

Verification of feedback suppression must be completed to ensure that feedback suppression systems do not limit the gain of the hearing aid or audibility for speech, particularly in the high frequencies. Fortunately, verification for feedback suppression does not require additional steps beyond those used to verify audibility in general. As long as the feedback management is activated before electroacoustic verification of audibility, the effects of the feedback suppression should be evident during verification. As noted in the previous section on MPO, some feedback suppression algorithms will attempt to suppress the tonal stimulus used to measure MPO, so the feedback suppression must be deactivated in the programming software to accurately measure the MPO. However, speech signals used for verification of audibility have no such limitation and can be used without interference from feedback suppression. Another consideration with verification of feedback management applies to verification completed in the coupler. The same feedback path is unlikely to occur when the hearing aid is attached to a coupler compared to the child's own ear canal. Some manufacturers design feedback suppression routines in the programming software that require testing be completed with the hearing aids in the ear to estimate the feedback path. Those routines should not be completed in the coupler, even if the child's verification occurs in the coupler. Furthermore, feedback may occur if verification is completed in the coupler. The audiologist should confirm that the hearing aids do not feedback after verification has occurred, but before the child leaves the office, to avoid parents and caregivers being annoyed with whistling or buzzing sounds. Performing electroacoustic verification of audibility after the feedback suppression has been initialized allows any changes related to feedback management to be reflected in those measurements with speech.

## Digital Noise Reduction

Digital noise reduction helps to reduce the negative effects of background noise on listening comfort by reducing the amount of gain provided by the hearing aid. Because of this gain reduction, audibility may also be reduced as a side effect. Verification with digital noise reduction should help audiologists to determine: (1) the amount of noise reduction that occurs, (2) the frequencies where audibility is reduced, (3) whether or not the processing is activated by noise or when speech and noise are both present, and (4) the length of time the hearing aid has to be in noise prior to activation. Basic verification methods can be used to assess all of these aspects of digital noise reduction in a short period of time.

A review of several manufacturers' digital noise reduction algorithms on these metrics was recently published, along with a clinical protocol that is elaborated here (Scollie et al., 2016). One method of verifying digital noise reduction signal processing involves presenting unmodulated noise signals, such as pink noise or speech-spectral-shaped noise, to the hearing aid in the coupler. By comparing these measurements with the digital noise reduction activated and deactivated, audiologists can determine the extent to which noise reduction is occurring, which frequencies are affected, and how much time is required for the processing to activate. Using this type of noise verification, Scollie and colleagues indicated that the average amount of noise reduction was approximately 21 dB. An example of digital noise reduction verification using noise signals is shown in Figure 4–12.

Another option is to simultaneously present speech and noise to the hearing aid to determine whether or not digital noise reduction systems will reduce the gain to the hearing aid when speech and noise are both present. This listening situation represents a potentially larger concern for children, as reducing audibility for speech in noise is unlikely to have positive effects on speech understanding (but recall studies that have indicated no change in speech recognition with digital noise reduction, e.g., Stelmachowicz et al., 2010). Scollie and colleagues found that the average reduction for this type of verification was approximately 15 dB across different manufacturers' noise reduction algorithms, highlighting the need to use this feature judiciously, given the potential negative impacts on audibility.

The verification protocol recommended by Scollie and colleagues addresses all of the key clinical questions needed for digital noise reduction. First, the audibility of the hearing aid must be established with standard verification procedures. Next, a speech signal is presented to the hearing aid, in quiet, at a high input level (75 dB SPL) to determine if the digital noise reduction system attenuates speech in quiet. The high-level speech signal should be identical with noise reduction activated or deactivated. If not, the digital noise reduction may impact the audibility of speech at high input levels and should be avoided. Finally, the use of a noise signal at a high input

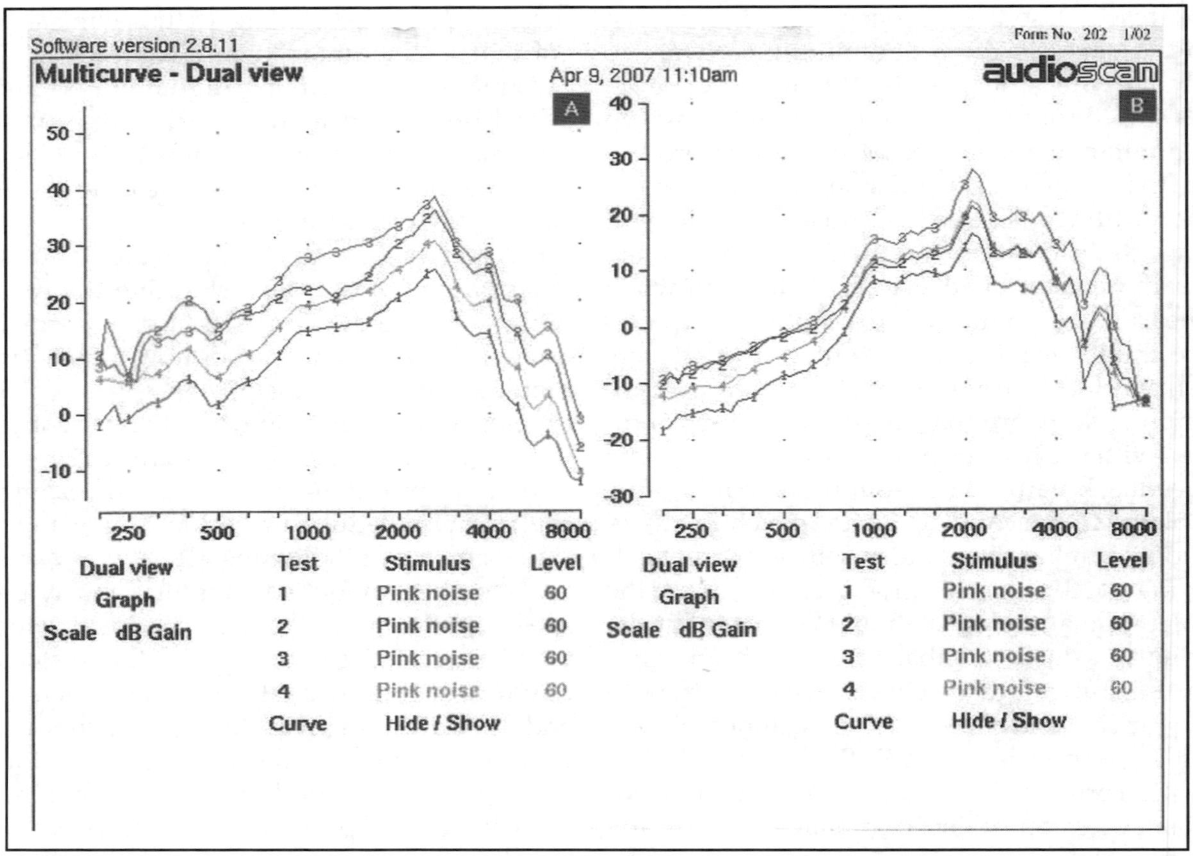


**FIGURE 4–12.** Examples of verification of digital noise reduction using a steady-state pink noise signal for two different hearing aids (*Panels A and B*). Note the changes in the output of the hearing aid with digital noise reduction activated (Line 1), compared to deactivated as a function of frequency (Line 3). Lines 2 and 4 represent the response of each hearing aid with DNR activated at 5 seconds and 15 seconds, respectively.

level (again, 75 dB SPL) should be used to determine the amount of attenuation that occurs with noise only. The strength of noise reduction may be adjusted if needed. Most current hearing aid test systems do not allow simultaneous presentation of speech and noise together to assess the effects of digital noise reduction on audibility for speech in noise, but if this is an option in the future, it may be helpful for clinicians attempting to decide whether or not to activate digital noise reduction for children. Because digital noise reduction is part of the signal processing of the hearing aids, digital noise reduction only needs to be verified at the initial hearing aid fitting or if the digital noise reduction setting is changed.

## Directional Microphones

Directional microphones allow spatial processing of the sound environment by measuring time of arrival differences between microphones on the same hearing aid or microphones on different hearing aids between ears. Because directional microphones are dependent on the function of microphones, which can drift and be affected by debris that accumulates over time, they should be verified on a regular basis if activated in the child's hearing aids. The verification process for directional microphones is not designed to assess adaptive behavior of directional microphones or confirm that the directional microphones will change in their response pattern. Instead, the directional microphone verification process is a fast and easy way to determine that the microphones are directional by comparing an electroacoustic measurement of the hearing aid in the test box from 0 degrees and 180 degrees. This can be accomplished using either a simultaneous recording method in verification test systems with two speakers in the test box or sequentially in verification test systems with a single speaker in the test box.

The simultaneous method requires a single measurement of a speech signal at an average level (65 dB SPL), and a high level (75 dB SPL) with the hearing aid set to a fixed omnidirectional response in the programming software and the same measurements with the hearing aid set to a fixed directional pattern in the software. The results of a simultaneous measure are shown in Figure 4–13.

Note that the response to the front speaker and back speaker are equivalent in the omnidirectional condition, but that the back microphone is reduced relative to the front microphone in the directional condition. In the sequential measurement, the hearing aid is positioned facing the speaker and then a separate measurement is taken with the hearing aid facing away from the speaker. These two measurements are completed

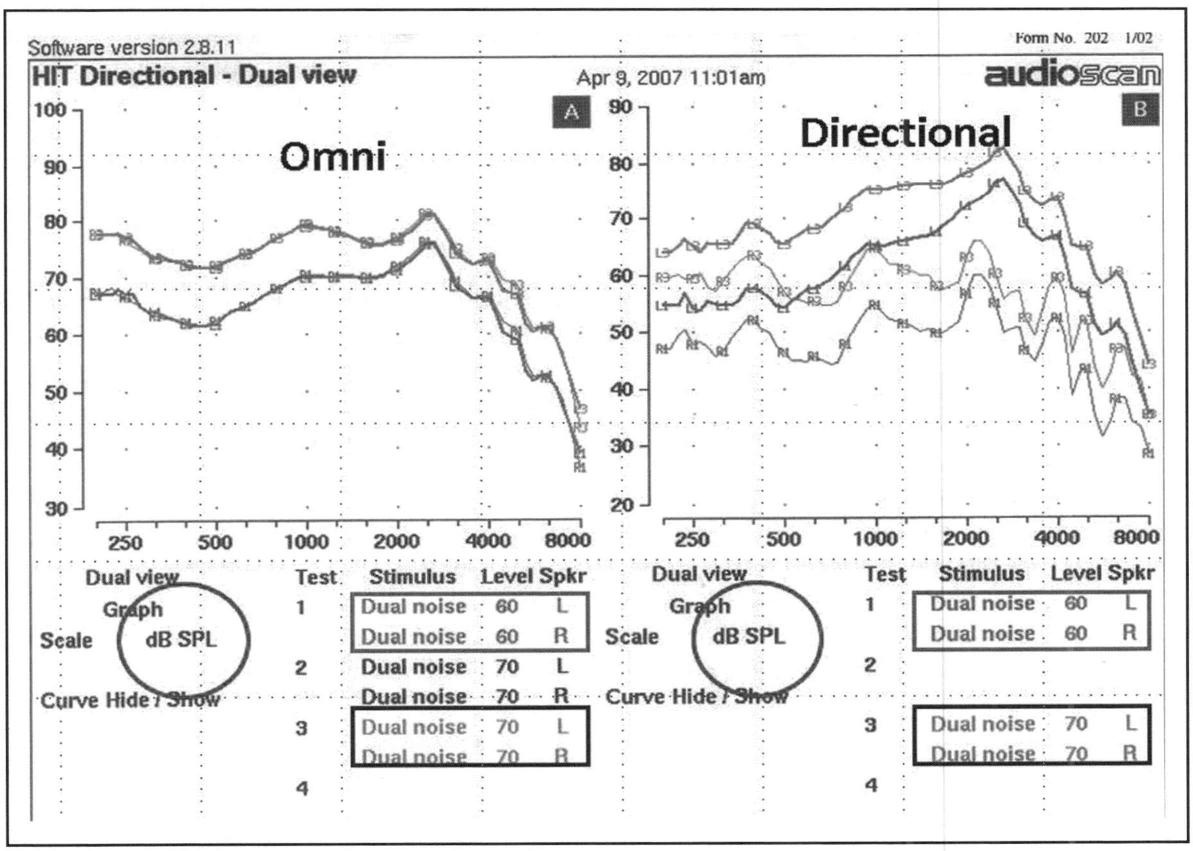


**FIGURE 4–13.** The results from a simultaneous method of directional microphone verification on the Audioscan Verifit. In *Panel A*, the responses of the hearing aid in a fixed omnidirectional mode at 60 dB and 70 dB SPL are plotted as a function of frequency. In *Panel B*, the responses of the hearing aid in a fixed directional pattern at the same intensity levels are plotted. Note the difference between the curves labeled L and R (representing the left and right speakers in the hearing aid test box) in *Panel B*, indicating directional response.

for both omnidirectional and directional settings to achieve the same measurements obtained during the simultaneous method. This approach should demonstrate that the hearing aids are directional when the fixed directional setting is activated. Any changes in the frequency response of the hearing aid with directionality should also be evident from the measurements.

## Frequency Lowering

Frequency lowering can be used to improve the audibility of high-frequency sounds through the hearing aid. Determining whether or not a child needs frequency lowering, and if so, the settings for the frequency lowering that optimize audibility, are both important issues that require specific verification practices. As with the previously discussed issues with manufacturers' default settings for matching prescriptive targets and providing consistent audibility, the manufacturers' default settings for frequency lowering rarely optimize audibility on an individual basis (McCreery, Brennan, Hoover, Kopun, & Stelmachowicz, 2013). Studies that have individually prescribed frequency lowering settings based on the extent to which bandwidth is limited for a specific listener have shown that frequency lowering can result in improvements in speech recognition (McCreery et al., 2014), without sacrificing sound quality for speech or music (Brennan et al., 2014). Other studies have reported that frequency lowering settings that provide too much lowering may offset improvements in audibility, with the distortion of the spectrum leading to null or even negative results for speech recognition (Souza, Arehart, Kates, Croghan, & Gehani, 2013) and sound quality ratings (Parsa, Scollie, Glista, & Seelisch, 2013). Collectively, results suggest that increasing audibility with frequency lowering is an important prerequisite to improving access to high-frequency speech information, but that improvements in audibility must be balanced with increases in spectral distortion that occur when speech is lowered. Traditional electroacoustic verification measures remain an important part of verification for frequency lowering, but current methods do not adequately reflect how much speech information is being lowered or whether that information is interpretable by a person with hearing loss.

To attempt to balance these factors, a protocol was recently published to determine whether an individual patient is a candidate for frequency lowering and the appropriate frequency lowering parameters to maximize audibility without introducing unnecessary distortions (McCreery et al., 2014). As with all advanced signal processing verification procedures, the hearing aid should be well fitted and matched to prescriptive targets prior to frequency lowering verification. Based on the electroacoustic verification of audibility, the audiologist should note the frequencies where the average and peak of the LTASS intersect the patient's audiogram on the SPL-o-gram for an average speech signal. The range of frequencies where the average and peak of the LTASS intersect the audiogram is known as the maximum audible output frequency (MAOF) range (Figure 4–14).

The MAOF range is an estimate of the highest frequencies that are audible to the listening without frequency lowering. Frequencies that are above the MAOF will not be audible without frequency lowering. The frequency lowering setting that is selected should attempt to increase the audibility of sounds above the MAOF with minimal disturbance of frequencies below the MAOF. Depending on the manufacturers' specific implementation of frequency lowering, there may be multiple settings that can provide similar access to frequencies above the MAOF, but the weakest setting that increases audibility above the MAOF range should be selected.

After the frequency lowering setting that maximizes audibility of the MAOF is selected, the hearing aid fitting should be adjusted so that the fitting matches prescriptive targets up to the MAOF (Figure 4–15). If the audiologist fitted the hearing aid to prescriptive targets prior to activation of frequency lowering, most manufacturers' algorithms will require minimal adjustment because the amplitude compression phase of the signal processing occurs after frequency lowering and the gain, and the output should change very little.

The protocol also suggests that narrowband stimuli representing the specific frequency bands

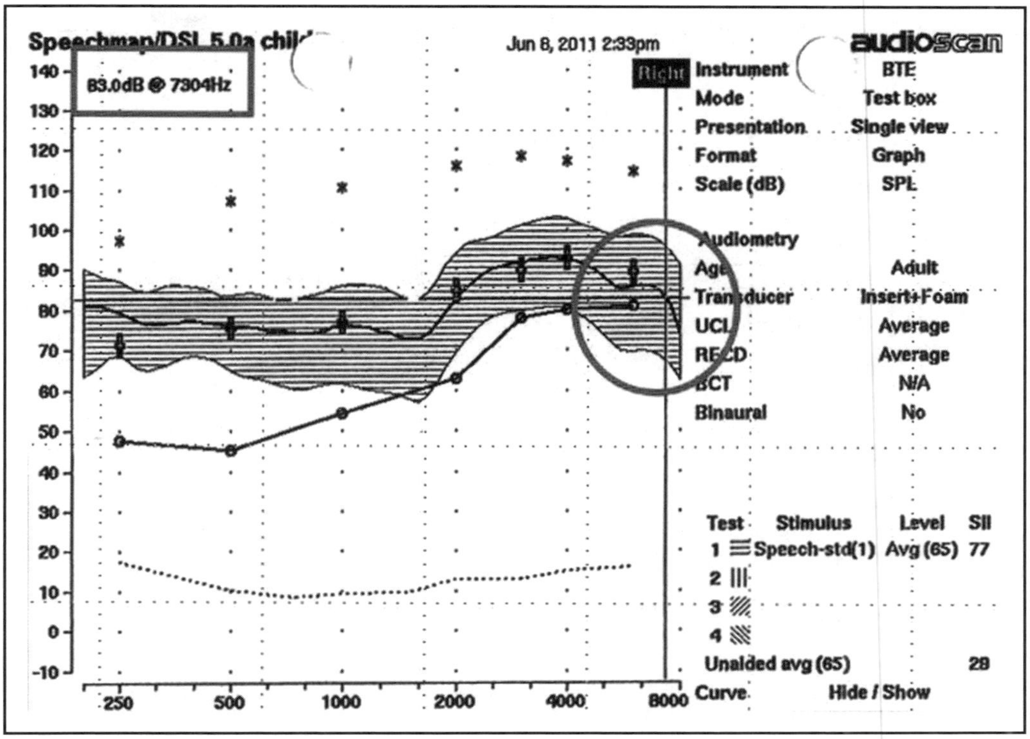


**FIGURE 4–14.** An estimate of the Maximum Audible Output Frequency (MAOF) range from an SPL-o-gram for a child with mild to moderate hearing loss. The MAOF range is defined as the frequencies between where the average and peak of the LTASS intersect the audiogram.

above the MAOF range may be used in some hearing aid verification systems to estimate the location of these frequency bands after lowering and to ensure that the amount of lowering that was implemented is sufficient to bring those sounds into audibility. An example of narrowband speech stimulus from the Audioscan Verifit are shown in Figure 4–16.

Frequency lowering settings may require adjustment as the child grows and the ear canal acoustics and earmolds change. In most cases, the changes that occur with ear canal growth will not be so drastic as to require changes to the amount of frequency lowering, but the MAOF range without lowering should be verified each time the child receives hearing aid verification to ensure that the settings in the hearing aid provide the child with the greatest access to high-frequency speech sounds.

## Advanced Hearing Aid Feature Verification: Conclusions

If advanced hearing aid signal processing features are activated, the impact of those features on the audibility of speech must be verified. In some cases, like feedback suppression, the verification of the advanced feature does not require an additional step, as long as the feature is activated during verification for audibility. In other cases, like directional microphones, the verification does require additional steps, but is essential for ensuring that the advanced feature is functioning and that audibility for speech can be maintained. Though the research on the use of advanced features for children is extremely limited at present, many audiologists will activate these features for children based on the potential benefits that could be achieved in minimizing feedback, improving

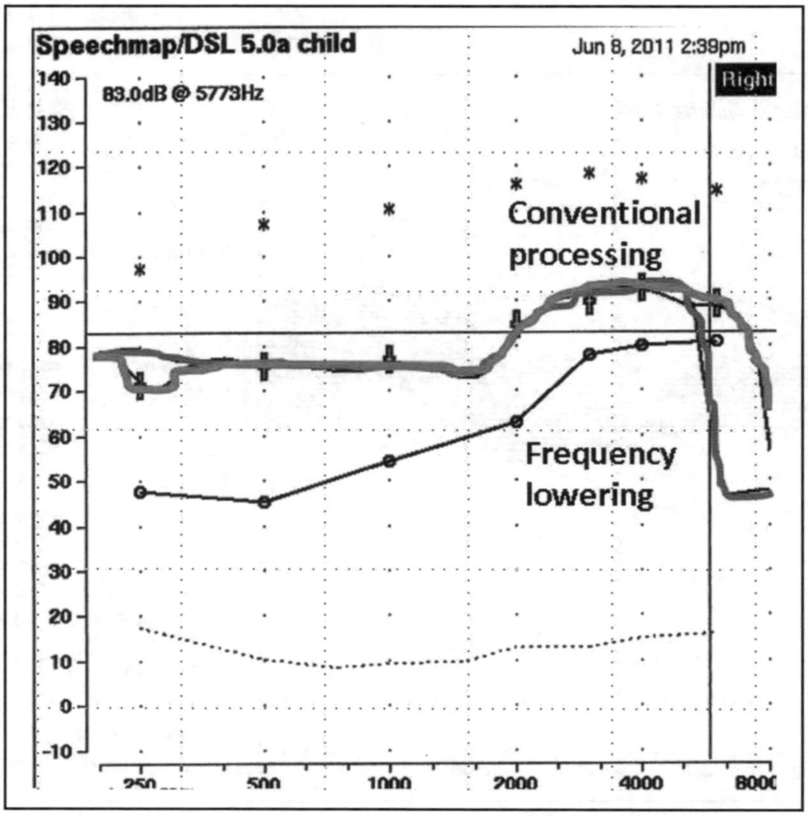


**FIGURE 4–15.** An example of a hearing aid fitting with conventional processing (*Panel A*) and frequency lowering (*Panel B*) for the same audiogram. Prescriptive targets should be matched up to the MAOF.

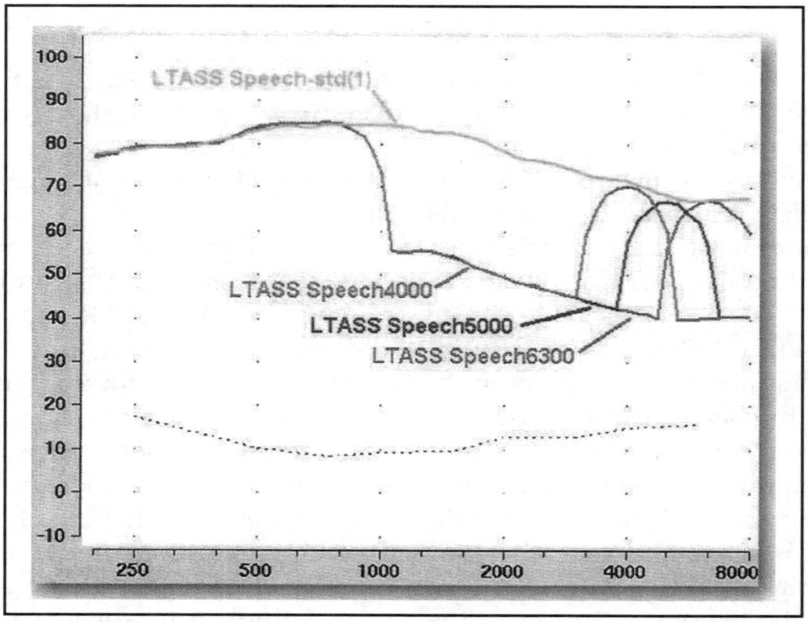


**FIGURE 4–16.** Narrowband speech stimuli from the Audioscan Verifit can be used to estimate the location of speech information above the MAOF.

comfort or speech recognition in noise, or increasing the audibility of high-frequency sounds. These verification procedures can help to avoid unintended negative outcomes with advanced features for children until further clinical evidence to support their efficacy for children.

## CONCLUSIONS

Electroacoustic hearing aid verification is one of the most important steps in the process of providing hearing aids to infants and children because it provides evidence that the hearing aids increase access to speech and language, which will fuel communication development. Audibility is the first outcome measure of the hearing aid fitting process and should be documented at regular intervals during early childhood to ensure the child's access to speech and language remains consistent during this crucial developmental period. Tools like the normative SII range for the UWO PedAMP protocol and the SHARP can help audiologists to determine if the amount of audibility that is provided is sufficient for a child's degree of hearing loss or how distance in different listening situations can affect audibility in everyday listening situations. If advanced hearing aid features are activated, special procedures should be implemented to ensure that these features are appropriately fitted to meet the goals of providing consistent auditory input for children with hearing loss.

## REFERENCES


American National Standards Institute. (1997). Methods for the calculation of the Speech Intelligibility Index. *New York: American National Standards Institute, 19*, 90–119.

Bagatto, M., Moodie, S., Brown, C., Malandrino, A., Richert, F., Clench, D., & Scollie, S. (2016). Prescribing and verifying hearing aids applying the American Academy of Audiology Pediatric Amplification Guideline: Protocols and outcomes from the Ontario Infant Hearing Program. *Journal of the American Academy of Audiology, 27*(3), 188–203.

Bagatto, M. P., Moodie, S. T., Malandrino, A. C., Richert, F. M., Clench, D. A., & Scollie, S. D. (2011). The University of Western Ontario Pediatric Audiological Monitoring Protocol (UWO PedAMP). *Trends in Amplification, 15*(1), 57–76.

Bagatto, M., Moodie, S., Scollie, S., Seewald, R., Moodie, S., Pumford, J., & Liu, K. R. (2005). Clinical protocols for hearing instrument fitting in the Desired Sensation Level method. *Trends in amplification, 9*(4), 199–226.

Bagatto, M. P., Scollie, S. D., Seewald, R. C., Moodie, K. S., & Hoover, B. M. (2002). Real-ear-to-coupler difference predictions as a function of age for two coupling procedures. *Journal of the American Academy of Audiology, 13*(8), 407–415.

Banerjee, S. (2011). Hearing aids in the real world: Typical automatic behavior of expansion, directionality, and noise management. *Journal of the American Academy of Audiology, 22*(1), 34–48.

Brennan, M. A., McCreery, R., Kopun, J., Hoover, B., Alexander, J., Lewis, D., & Stelmachowicz, P. G. (2014). Paired comparisons of nonlinear frequency compression, extended bandwidth, and restricted bandwidth hearing aid processing for children and adults with hearing loss. *Journal of the American Academy of Audiology, 25*(10), 983–998.

Ching, T. Y., Dillon, H., Hou, S., Zhang, V., Day, J., Crowe, K., . . . Flynn, C. (2013b). A randomized controlled comparison of NAL and DSL prescriptions for young children: Hearing-aid characteristics and performance outcomes at three years of age. *International Journal of Audiology, 52*(Suppl. 2), S17–S28.

Ching, T. Y., Johnson, E. E., Seeto, M., & Macrae, J. H. (2013a). Hearing-aid safety: A comparison of estimated threshold shifts for gains recommended by NAL-NL2 and DSL m [i/o] prescriptions for children. *International Journal of Audiology, 52*(Suppl. 2), S39–S45.

Ching, T. Y., Scollie, S. D., Dillon, H., Seewald, R., Britton, L., & Steinberg, J. (2010). Prescribed real-ear and achieved real-life differences in children's hearing aids adjusted according to the NAL-NL1 and the DSL v. 4.1 prescriptions. *International Journal of Audiology, 49*(Suppl. 1), S16–S25.

Crukley, J., & Scollie, S. D. (2012). Children's speech recognition and loudness perception with the Desired Sensation Level v5 quiet and noise prescriptions. *American Journal of Audiology, 21*(2), 149–162.

Gustafson, S., Pittman, A., & Fanning, R. (2013). Effects of tubing length and coupling method on hearing threshold and real-ear to coupler difference measures. *American Journal of Audiology, 22*(1), 190–199.

Holube, I., Fredelake, S., Vlaming, M., & Kollmeier, B. (2010). Development and analysis of an international speech test signal (ISTS). *International Journal of Audiology, 49*(12), 891–903.

Keidser, G., Dillon, H., Flax, M., Ching, T., & Brewer, S. (2011). The NAL-NL2 prescription procedure. *Audiology Research, 1*(1) 88–90.

Kimlinger, C., McCreery, R., & Lewis, D. (2015). High-frequency audibility: The effects of audiometric configuration, stimulus type, and device. *Journal of the American Academy of Audiology, 26*(2), 128–137.

Koehlinger, K., Van Horne, A. O., Oleson, J., McCreery, R., & Moeller, M. P. (2015). The role of sentence position, allomorph, and morpheme type on accurate use of s-related morphemes by children who are hard of hearing. *Journal of Speech, Language, and Hearing Research, 58*(2), 396–409.

Kuk, F., Peeters, H., Lau, C., & Korhonen, P. (2011). Effect of maximum power output and noise reduction on speech recognition in noise. *Journal of the American Academy of Audiology, 22*(5), 265–273.

McCreery, R. W., Alexander, J., Brennan, M. A., Hoover, B., Kopun, J., & Stelmachowicz, P. G. (2014). The influence of audibility on speech recognition with nonlinear frequency compression for children and adults with hearing loss. *Ear and Hearing, 35*(4), 440–447.

McCreery, R. W., Bentler, R. A., & Roush, P. A. (2013). The characteristics of hearing aid fittings in infants and young children. *Ear and Hearing, 34*(6), 701–710.

McCreery, R. W., Brennan, M. A., Hoover, B., Kopun, J., & Stelmachowicz, P. G. (2013). Maximizing audibility and speech recognition with nonlinear frequency compression by estimating audible bandwidth. *Ear and Hearing, 34*(2), e24.

McCreery, R. W., Walker, E. A., Spratford, M., Bentler, R., Holte, L., Roush, P., . . . Moeller, M. P. (2015). Longitudinal predictors of aided speech audibility in infants and children. *Ear and Hearing, 36*(Suppl.) 24S–37S.

McCreery, R., Walker, E., Spratford, M., Kirby, B., Oleson, J., & Brennan, M. (2016). Stability of audiometric thresholds for children with hearing aids applying the American Academy of Audiology Pediatric Amplification Guideline: Implications for safety. *Journal of the American Academy of Audiology, 27*(3), 252–263.

Moodie, S., Pietrobon, J., Rall, E., Lindley, G., Eiten, L., Gordey, D., . . . Folkeard, P. (2016a). Using the real-ear-to-coupler difference within the American Academy of Audiology Pediatric Amplification Guideline: Protocols for applying and predicting earmold RECDs. *Journal of the American Academy of Audiology, 27*(3), 264–275.

Moodie, S., Rall, E., Eiten, L., Lindley, G., Gordey, D., Davidson, L., . . . Scollie, S. (2016b). Pediatric audiology in North America: Current clinical practice and how it relates to the American Academy of Audiology Pediatric Amplification Guideline. *Journal of the American Academy of Audiology, 27*(3), 166–187.

Munro, K. J., & Howlin, E. M. (2010). Comparison of real-ear to coupler difference values in the right and left ear of hearing aid users. *Ear and Hearing, 31*(1), 146–150.

Parsa, V., Scollie, S., Glista, D., & Seelisch, A. (2013). Nonlinear frequency compression effects on sound quality ratings of speech and music. *Trends in Amplification, 17*(1), 54–68.

Scollie, S., Seewald, R., Cornelisse, L., Moodie, S., Bagatto, M., Laurnagaray, D., . . . & Pumford, J. (2005). The Desired Sensation Level multistage input/output algorithm. *Trends in Amplification, 9*(4), 159–197.

Scollie, S., Ching, T. Y., Seewald, R., Dillon, H., Britton, L., Steinberg, J., & Corcoran, J. (2010a). Evaluation of the NAL-NL1 and DSL v4.1 prescriptions for children: Preference in real world use. *International Journal of Audiology, 49*(Suppl. 1), S49–S63.

Scollie, S. D., Ching, T. Y., Seewald, R. C., Dillon, H., Britton, L., Steinberg, J., & King, K. (2010b). Children's speech perception and loudness ratings when fitted with hearing aids using the DSL v. 4.1 and the NAL-NL1 prescriptions. *International Journal of Audiology, 49*(Suppl. 1), S26–S34.

Scollie, S., & Bagatto, M. (2016). Hearing aid verification. In A. M. Tharpe & R. Seewald (Eds.), *Comprehensive handbook of pediatric audiology*. San Diego, CA: Plural.

Scollie, S., Glista, D., Seto, J., Dunn, A., Schuett, B., Hawkins, M., . . . Parsa, V. (2016). Fitting frequency-lowering signal processing applying the American Academy of Audiology Pediatric Amplification Guideline: Updates and protocols. *Journal of the American Academy of Audiology, 27*(3), 219–236.

Scollie, S., Levy, C., Pourmand, N., Abbasalipour, F., Bagatto, M., Richert, F., . . . Parsa, V. (2016). Fitting noise management signal processing applying the American Academy of Audiology Pediatric Amplification Guideline: Verification protocols. *Journal of the American Academy of Audiology, 27*(3), 237–251.

Seewald, R., Mills, J., Bagatto, M., Scollie, S., & Moodie, S. (2008). A comparison of manufacturer-specific prescriptive procedures for infants. *Hearing Journal, 61*(11), 26–28.

Souza, P. E., Arehart, K. H., Kates, J. M., Croghan, N. B., & Gehani, N. (2013). Exploring the limits of frequency lowering. *Journal of Speech, Language, and Hearing Research, 56*(5), 1349–1363.

Stelmachowicz, P., Lewis, D., Hoover, B., Nishi, K., McCreery, R., & Woods, W. (2010). Effects of digital noise reduction on speech perception for children with hearing loss. *Ear and Hearing, 31(3),* 345–355.

Tomblin, J. B., Harrison, M., Ambrose, S. E., Walker, E. A., Oleson, J. J., & Moeller, M. P. (2015). Language outcomes in young children with mild to severe hearing loss. *Ear and Hearing, 36,* 76S–91S.

# 5

# Hearing Aid Use and Orientation

*Elizabeth A. Walker and Ryan W. McCreery*

## INTRODUCTION

Early intervention includes early fitting of hearing aids, with the assumption that appropriately fit hearing aids will provide access to acoustic-phonetic information during the critical years of language acquisition. This assumption is based on the premise that early auditory access will have long-term positive consequences for children with hearing loss. It would be shortsighted to solely focus on early hearing aid fitting, however, and presume that merely being fit with hearing aids at very young ages will directly lead to optimal outcomes. It is also necessary to promote high-quality management. Consistent hearing aid use is one aspect of high-quality management, in combination with high-quality linguistic input from caregivers (Chapter 1) and appropriately fit hearing aids (Chapter 4).

As pediatric audiologists, we advocate for the goal of full-time hearing aid use in children. As any parent or caregiver knows, however, this goal can be difficult to achieve. Nevertheless, it is an important goal, and not one that should be dismissed, even for children with milder degrees of hearing loss. The current chapter will cover the importance of establishing and maintaining consistent hearing aid use for achieving optimal outcomes for children with hearing loss. We will also describe some of the barriers that families may encounter, how to identify which children may be at risk for inconsistent hearing aid use, and how to circumvent those barriers.

## WHAT EVIDENCE DO WE HAVE FOR THE IMPORTANCE OF CONSISTENT HA USE ON OUTCOMES?

Surprisingly, we know very little about the impact of daily hearing aid use on outcomes for children with hearing loss. It is universally acknowledged that auditory access is critical to spoken language development. As a result, the standard clinical recommendation is that children should be encouraged to wear hearing aids during all waking hours. Instead of looking at the relationship between hearing aid use and outcomes, however, the majority of outcome studies have focused on the influence of degree of hearing loss on language, psychosocial, or academic achievement. These studies are critical to our knowledge base because they establish that any degree of hearing loss puts a child at risk for language delays. At the same time, little if any information is available regarding the amount of daily hearing aid use in children or if daily hearing aid use plays a role in outcomes. Because we are advocating that daily hearing aid use is a *malleable* factor in intervention (i.e., a factor that is amenable to change), it is still important to understanding the effects of hearing aid use on language and academic outcomes. This knowledge may have a positive influence on clinicians' and parents' attitudes toward consistent hearing aid use and their willingness to persist when they encounter reluctance on the part of the child to wear the device.

There are many examples of studies that examined the role of degree of hearing loss on outcomes, but few of these studies accounted for the amount of time children wore their hearing aids. For example, Davis, Elfenbein, Schum, and Bentler (1986) examined psychoeducational outcomes of 40 school-age children with mild-to-severe bilateral hearing loss. They found no relationship between pure-tone average and measures of vocabulary, articulation, grammar, mathematics, and reading. They noted that 38 out of the 40 students wore hearing aids monaurally or binaurally, and that parent and child reports indicated consistent use at home and school, but no additional information about hearing aid use was provided. Gilbertson and Kamhi (1995) described 20 children with mild- to moderate-hearing loss. All of the children had been fit with binaural amplification, although the authors did not report age at fitting or if the amplification was used on a regular basis. They reported that 10 of the children showed no delays compared to children with normal hearing who were matched on vocabulary size, while the remaining 10 children performed significantly more poorly on language, phonological processing, and novel word learning. Degree of hearing loss did not affect which children showed delays; therefore, Gilbertson and Kamhi concluded that there is a subset of children with specific language impairment in addition to hearing loss, but mild to moderate hearing loss does not, in itself, result in language delays in children. Although this may be construed as positive evidence that children who are hard of hearing are fairly resilient to the effects of reduced audibility, Gilbertson and Kamhi did not take into account how long individual children had been wearing hearing aids or whether they wore amplification on a consistent basis.

To summarize, both the Davis et al. (1986) and Gilbertson and Kamhi (1995) studies are influential to the pediatric aural habilitation field because they draw attention to the fact that even children with mild hearing loss can experience delays in language acquisition. Although it seems intuitive that children with greater degrees of hearing loss would have poorer outcomes, the mixed results in these studies reinforce the notion that there is more going on than just audibility. The impact of hearing loss on language outcomes cannot be reduced to a single variable—audibility—because each child is a complex, dynamic system. As such, multiple factors may interact with one another to influence outcomes. To understand the relationship between degree of hearing loss and outcomes, we need evidence of how other factors, such as amount of daily hearing aid use, interact with audibility.

Two recent reports from large-scale, longitudinal studies have tried to address the question of how daily hearing aid use influences outcomes for children with hearing loss. Marnane and Ching (2015) examined patterns of hearing aid use and its effect on outcomes in children who were 3 years old or younger. Participants were enrolled in the Longitudinal Outcomes of Children with Hearing Impairment (LOCHI) study, a population-based study in Australia (Ching et al., 2013). One hundred ninety-four children wore hearing aids, and 101 children used cochlear implants. Children in the LOCHI study were evaluated at 6 and 12 months after their initial hearing aid fitting, and again at 3 years of age. At every testing visit, examiners administered the Parent's Evaluation of Aural/Oral Performance of Children (PEACH; Ching & Hill, 2007). One of the questions on the PEACH asked parents to rate how often their child wore their hearing aids using a five-point scale (0%—Never; 1 to 25%—Seldom; 26 to 50%—Sometimes; 51 to 75%—Often; 75 to 100%—Always). In addition, researchers accessed demographic data from an Australian national hearing health care database, which provided parent-report information on the average number of hours per day children wore their devices. This report of device usage was divided into categories: never worn, less than one hour per day, one to four hours per day, four to eight hours per day, and more than eight hours per day. The data from the PEACH and the database were combined. In cases where a child had data from the PEACH and the database at the same visit and there was a difference in hearing aid usage between these two measures, the higher value was reported. The majority of children were categorized as wearing hearing aids either Always (65% of the children) or Often (20% of the children). Only 15% of children were reported to wear hearing aids less than 50% of the time.

Marnane and Ching (2015) investigated the association between consistency of device use and outcomes, using the PEACH total standard score as an outcome measure. The PEACH consists of a parent-report questionnaire that asks about functional, everyday performance in typical listening situations. For reported device use, children with hearing aids and children with cochlear implants were combined into one group. The authors found a significant positive relationship between device use and PEACH standard scores at age 3 years, but after accounting for factors such as maternal education level, additional disabilities, and use of sign language, the relationship was no longer significant. Although this would appear to indicate that increased device use is not associated with better outcomes, these results should be interpreted with caution. The inclusion of children with cochlear implants might explain the lack of significant findings: this group had reduced variance in device use, making it difficult to see an association between hearing aid use and outcomes. Thus, this study provides preliminary data on the impact of hearing aid use on outcomes, but further research is still needed.

A recent prospective, longitudinal study in the United States has also evaluated the influence of hearing aid use on outcomes. The Outcomes of Children with Hearing Loss (OCHL) study consisted of 317 children who were hard of hearing, followed over a period of up to four years (Moeller & Tomblin, 2015). The sample was more homogeneous than the LOCHI study, in that participants in the study were all learning spoken English as their first language and did not have additional disabilities, profound hearing loss, or cochlear implants. This allowed the researchers to focus on the impact of bilateral, mild to severe hearing loss and hearing aids on outcomes, without having to account for additional variables known to affect performance on spoken language measures, such as development delays, learning English as a second language, or using a manual form of communication. A limitation of the OCHL study was that it consisted of a clinical sample, rather than a population-based sample. Although the researchers attempted to recruit all children with hearing loss in the recruitment areas, the OCHL participants were largely recruited based on referrals from service providers or public health officials (audiologists, educators, or early hearing detection and intervention state coordinators). Therefore, children who were not receiving audiological services were unlikely to have been recruited, and the absence of single government-funded, national hearing service providers restricted the ability to recruit a population-based sample.

One of the benefits of longitudinal research designs, as opposed to cross-sectional data, is that researchers are able to track language growth over time, and compare relative progress across children (Tomblin, Harrison et al., 2015). In other words, we can see if children with hearing loss are (1) maintaining the same rate of development over time, compared to typically developing children, (2) catching up to typically developing children over time, or (3) falling further behind in terms of development. For children who are typically developing, we expect to see steady growth in language skills over time, making one year of language growth over a 12-month period. In the case of children with hearing loss, we may see initial delays compared to children with normal hearing, due to the reduced auditory access. By using longitudinal data and examining growth trajectories over time, we can see whether children with hearing loss are closing the gap between themselves and their hearing classmates. Tomblin and his colleagues looked at these growth trajectories based on how often children wore hearing aids on a daily basis. At each research visit, parents reported how many hours per day children wore their hearing aids. These parent reports of hearing aid use were averaged together for each child, and the children were grouped into categories based on average daily hearing aid use. Figure 5–1 shows the growth trajectories in language scores for children with hearing aids, across ages 2 to 6 years. The language scores consisted of a combination of expressive and receptive language measures, determined through principal components analysis to be measuring the same language trait (see Tomblin, Harrison, et al., 2015, for more information on specific language tests). Children who wore hearing aids more than 12.5 hours per day showed an increasing growth rate over time. As shown on the y-axis, a standard score of 100 represents average performance for a typically developing child. Therefore, the consistent HA users were essentially catching up to their same-age peers with normal hearing by 6 years of age. Children who wore hearing aids less than 10 hours per day showed a flat trajectory, decreasing slightly over time. This trend would suggest that children who are inconsistent hearing aid users are at risk for falling further behind children with normal hearing as they get older. This study is the first to report that consistency of hearing aid use contributes to long-term language outcomes. As a related point, 12.5 hours per day is longer than a typical school day of 6 to 8 hours. Parents and children may feel that it is sufficient to only wear hearing aids during the school day, based on an assumption that this is where learning is primarily occurring. The results from the OCHL team suggest that hearing aid use outside of the classroom is also important for language development, perhaps because of the incidental learning that takes place at home and in social settings. This is important evidence for audiologists and related professionals to convey to families, as it supports our efforts to promote full-time hearing aid use in children.

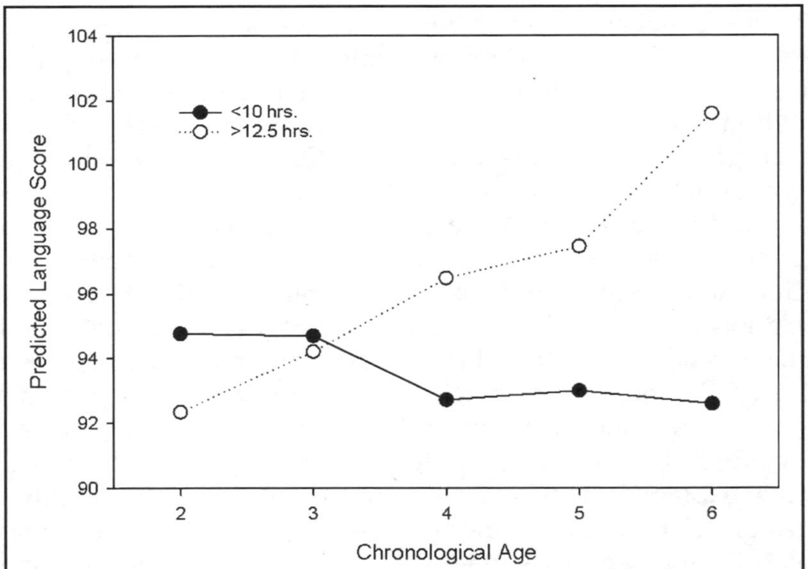


**FIGURE 5–1.** Longitudinal patterns in language growth for children who wore hearing aids less than 10 hours per week (*black circles*), and more than 12.5 hours per week (*white circles*). Modified from a figure in Tomblin et al. (2015).

## HOW DO WE MEASURE HEARING AID USE?

Because we have data to support consistency of hearing aid use in children with mild to severe hearing loss, a question arises as to what is the best way to go about measuring hearing aid use. When it comes to children, especially very young children, we cannot just ask them to tell us how often they are wearing their devices. Fortunately, there are a number of subjective and objective ways to get at this question. One simple approach is to ask parents to estimate how many hours per day their child wears their hearing aids. Although this approach seems like the most straightforward, however, there is a limitation regarding the accuracy with which parents can provide an estimate of daily use time. This limitation has to do with the validity of self-report or parent-report measures of hearing aid use.

Two studies by Walker and colleagues (Walker, Spratford, et al., 2013; Walker, McCreery, et al., 2015) addressed the question of parent accuracy in reporting hearing aid use by comparing subjective, parent-report measures to objective, data logging values. Data logging is a feature built in to most modern hearing aids. Audiologists can connect the hearing aids to the programming software via a cable. As shown in Figure 5–2, within the programming software there is a report that details the total number of hours the battery door is closed and the battery is activated, since the last time the hearing aids were connected and the data were saved. The report also provides an average number of hours of use per day, by taking the total number of hours the battery was activated, divided by the number of days since the last connection to the hearing aid software. Walker and her colleagues compared the parent estimates to the data logging for 133 children. They found a strong, positive correlation (r = .76) between the two measures, but as Figure 5–3 shows, most parents tend to overestimate daily use by several hours. To illustrate this point, the rectangular box in Figure 5–3 shows parents who reported 12 hours per day of use. Data logging varied between 3 and 15 hours for these children. Another way to interpret these data is that the relative distance between parent report and data logging is consistent (as parent-report measures increase, data logging tends to increase as well), but the absolute values differ. In terms of clinical implications, it is important for audiologists to recognize that asking for a ballpark estimate of how often a child wears hearing aids may be a difficult question for parents to answer. There are always going to be situations during a typical day where the hearing aids are not being worn, and parents may provide a best-case scenario when estimating use, rather than an average day's usage.

Fortunately, there are better alternatives to establishing how often children are wearing hearing aids than just relying on parent estimates of all day usage. One option is the aforementioned data logging capacities available in most modern hearing aids. In addition to capturing data logging information at each clinic visit, another strategy for tracking ongoing hearing aid use is to ask parents to rate frequency of use across different situations. Moeller, Hoover, Peterson, and Stelmachowicz (2009) and Walker et al. (2013) both used informal tools to collect situational assessments of hearing aid use. Parents rated the consistency of hearing aid use across multiple contexts: (a) car, (b) preschool/school, (c) daycare, (d) meal time, (e) playing alone, (f) book sharing, (g) playground, and (h) public (e.g., store, zoo, restaurant). Situations were rated on a 5-point Likert scale of never (0), rarely (1), sometimes (2), often (3), and always (4). This rating scale complements information the audiologist obtains from data logging or asking the parent to estimate hours of daily use. Furthermore, rating scales may identify situations that are challenging for families and may help families and audiologists recognize which contexts are easier for achieving consistent hearing aid use. For example, Moeller and colleagues found that parents reported less success when they could not directly supervise their infants, such as in the car or at daycare. On the other hand, parents reported better success in situations when they could monitor their infant closely, such as playing together, shared book reading, and mealtimes. In those contexts, infants achieved frequent hearing aid use by around 1½ years of age. Given that some

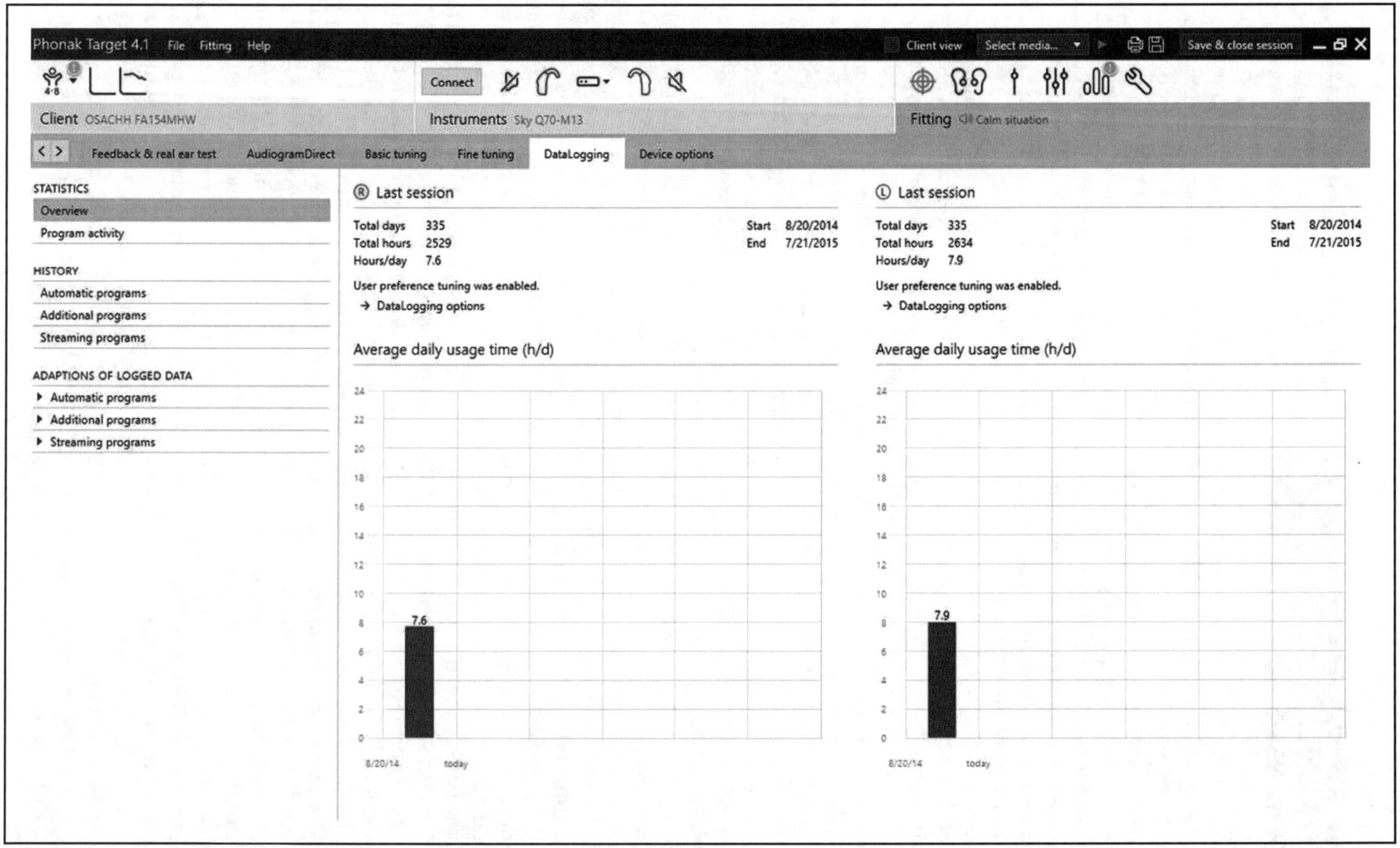


**FIGURE 5–2.** Example of hearing aid data logging. Phonak hearing aids are shown. Image courtesy of Sonova AG, © 2017.

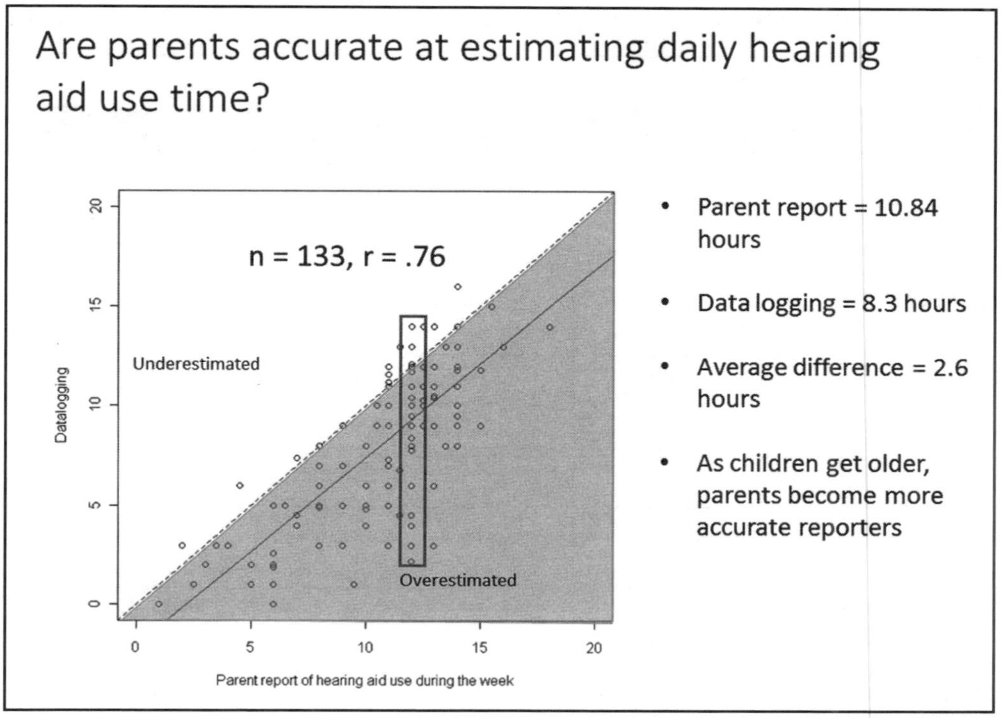


**FIGURE 5–3.** The association between parent report of hearing aid use and data logging. Modified from a figure in Walker et al. (2013).

situations are clearly more difficult than others, we encourage audiologists to utilize situational rating assessments during hearing aid visits. Administration takes very little time and can be an effective, non-confrontational way to address difficulties that parents are having with getting their young child to wear hearing aids. Situational ratings can be used as a counseling tool and may help to build rapport and trust between audiologists and parents. Table 5–1 shows a version of the situational rating assessment, which can be adapted for audiologists' own use, depending on the age range with which they work.

## HOW OFTEN ARE CHILDREN WEARING HEARING AIDS?

Now that we have described various tools that capture the consistency of hearing aid use, we will review the evidence related to how often children are wearing hearing aids. There are only a handful of peer-reviewed articles that have described how often children wear hearing aids. Most of these articles relied on parent-report measures (Fitzpatrick, Durieux-Smith, & Whittingham, 2010; Marnane & Ching, 2015; Moeller et al., 2009; Muñoz & Hill, 2015; Muñoz et al., 2015; Muñoz, Preston, & Hicken, 2014; Weston, Muñoz, & Blaiser, 2014), while a few others have included parent report and data logging (Klein et al., in press; Muñoz et al., 2014; Walker, Holte, et al., 2015; Walker, McCreery, et al., 2015; Walker, Spratford, et al., 2013). To the best of our knowledge, only one study has employed direct observation of children (Gustafson, Davis, Hornsby, & Bess, 2015).

Moeller and her colleagues (2009) reported on a non-validated assessment tool called the "Amplification in Daily Life" questionnaire. They interviewed seven mothers of infants with mild to moderately severe hearing loss, using this tool. The interviews were conducted across a series of three to four visits, spaced four to six months apart, starting when the infants were around 11 months old. The interview procedure involved

**Table 5–1.** Situational Rating scale for Assessing Consistency of Hearing Aid Use Across Different Contexts

Put an X in the boxes below to indicate how consistently your child uses has in the situations listed:

| Situation | Never (0) | Rare (1) | Sometimes (2) | Often (3) | Always (4) | N/A |
|---|---|---|---|---|---|---|
| Car | | | | | | |
| Preschool/School | | | | | | |
| Daycare | | | | | | |
| Meal Time | | | | | | |
| Playing Alone | | | | | | |
| Book Sharing | | | | | | |
| Playground | | | | | | |
| Public (store, zoo, restaurant) | | | | | | |

situational ratings of consistency of use (described above); given concerns about the validity of estimates of daily use time, parents were not asked to report on average hours of use per day. Results from the rating scales indicated that infants had difficulty achieving full-time hearing aid use (i.e., during all waking hours) until about 28.5 months.

Marnane and Ching (2015) used a parent-report questionnaire, the PEACH (Ching & Hill, 2007), to assess amount of daily hearing aid use. One of the questions on the PEACH asks parents to report, "How often has your child worn his/her hearing aids?" Parents responded using a Likert scale: "Never" (0%), "Seldom" (1 to 25% of the time, or less than one hour per day), "Sometimes" (26 to 50% of the time, or one to four hours per day), "Often" (51 to 75% of the time, or four to eight hours per day,) and "Always" (75 to 100% of the time, or more than eight hours per day). As part of the LOCHI study, parents of 252 three-year-old children who wore hearing aids received the PEACH. Results indicated that 65% of parents reported consistency of use as "Always" and 20% reported "Often." In contrast, 15% of parents reported that their child wore hearing aids less than 50% of the time. Thus, these results would suggest that while most children are consistent hearing aid users by age 3 years, approximately one out of six children had difficulty achieving consistent use by preschool. These results should be interpreted with caution, however, because the authors relied entirely on parent report measures. By categorizing the amount of daily hearing aid use into five levels, rather than looking at hearing aid use as a continuous variable, it is also challenging to see the individual differences in daily use across the sample of children.

Other researchers have found lower amounts of daily hearing aid use in children, compared to the findings by Marnane and Ching (2015). Muñoz et al. (2014) collected data logging on 29 children between the ages of 7 months and 6 years of age. Approximately half of the children who were 5 years old or younger wore hearing aids six hours or less per day. In a follow-up study, Muñoz et al. (2015) collected anonymous surveys from 37 parents of children with hearing loss (mean age of children = 22 months). Parents estimated the number of hours per day their child usually wore hearing aids. Approximately one third of parents indicated that their child wore hearing aids during all waking hours (11 or more hours per day), whereas another one third of parents reported inconsistent usage (less than five hours per day). Taken together, these results indicate that hearing aid use may be more of a challenge in younger children than Marnane and Ching's results would suggest.

Walker, McCreery, et al. (2015) collected data on a larger sample of children, including 290 children who were hard of hearing between the ages of 6 months and 9 years of age (*M* = 3.3 years; SD = 1.8 months). A combination of parent-report and data logging measures were used. Parents estimated that children wore their devices for 10.6 hours per day, on average, while data logging indicated that children wore their devices an average of 8.4 hours per day. When data logging was divided by age, infants (6 to 24 month olds) wore hearing aids an average of 4.4 hours per day, preschoolers (2 to 4 year olds) wore hearing aids an average of 7.8 hours per day, and school-age children (5 to 9 year olds) wore hearing aids an average of 10.2 hours per day. Figure 5–4 shows the distribution of hearing aid use in these three age groups. Because this is the largest peer-reviewed study that utilized data logging information as a metric for daily hearing aid use, the data shown in Figure 5–4 may be considered as benchmark values for average hearing aid use by children in the United States under the age of 9 years. At the same time, these values should not be considered best-practice recommendations, particularly for infants and preschoolers. These early years of life are a sensitive period in development, in which auditory access is critical for spoken language acquisition. Thus, the goal for families and service providers should be to help children achieve consistent hearing aid use during all waking hours, in order to maximize auditory access. It should also be noted that parents in the OCHL sample tended to have higher education levels than the U.S. population, when the educational levels of the mothers and fathers who participated in the study were

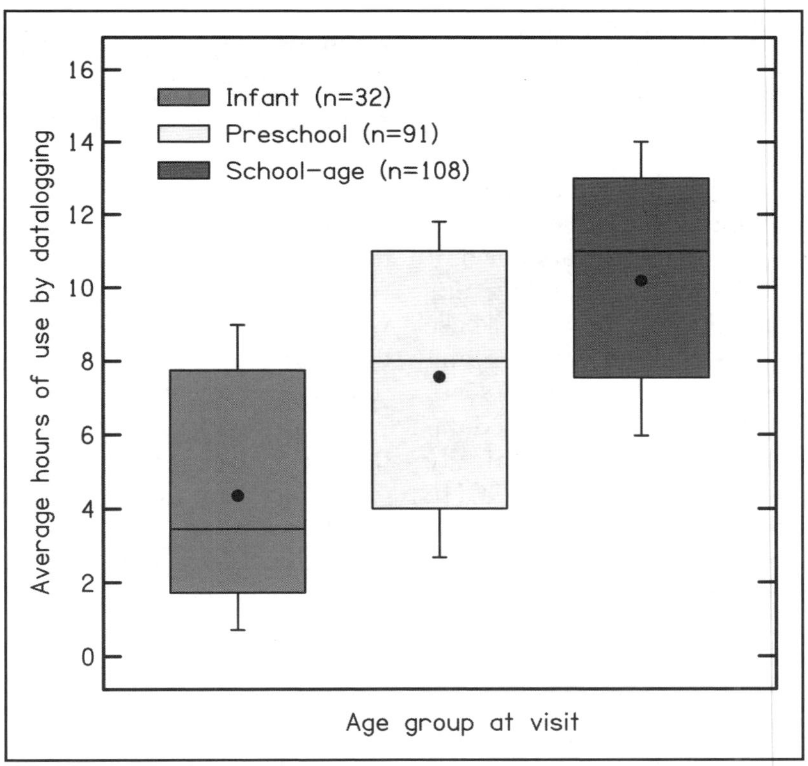


**FIGURE 5–4.** Comparison of hearing aid data logging by age groups (infants: 6 months to 18 months; preschool: 2 to 4 years; school age: 5 to 9 years). The central lines represent the median values, the black dots are the mean values, and the box limits are the 25th and 75th percentiles. The lower fence is from the 10th to the 25th percentile, and the upper fence is from the 75th to the 90th percentile.

compared to the 2012 U.S. Census data (Tomblin, Walker, et al., 2015). Thus, the income and educational status of the participants was not representative of the U.S. population as a whole. This bias toward higher socioeconomic status is common in longitudinal research studies that recruit on a volunteer basis. Furthermore, children who spoke English as a second language were excluded from participation, resulting in reduced cultural and linguistic diversity in the OCHL sample. As a result, the levels of hearing aid use across different ages may not apply to children from culturally diverse backgrounds or less-advantaged families.

Two reports from conferences proceedings have provided further information on data logging across a wide age range of birth to 18 year olds. Jones and Launer (2010) and Jones and Feilner (2013) reported on data obtained from the Cuper project, in which data were collected from hearing aid fitting sessions at more than 60 audiology clinics in the United States. This project recorded data logging information from nearly 5000 participants, whenever audiologists connected their patients' hearing aids to the Phonak programming software. To protect confidentiality, only information on patients' ages and gender were included in the database. On average, patients under 19 years of age wore hearing aids 5.5 hours per day. The 0- to 4-year-old age group wore hearing aids the least often, averaging 5 hours per day. These values are lower than the average data logging values reported for preschoolers in the OCHL sample. However, it is likely that the Cuper database includes a more culturally and economically diverse sample of participants than the OCHL project and other studies.

To date, only one peer-reviewed study has focused specifically on hearing aid use in older children. Gustafson et al. (2015) visited the classrooms of 38 children who were hard of hearing, in grades 1 through 7. The researchers observed whether or not children were wearing their hearing aids on four separate visits, during regular classroom instruction. Parents were also asked to estimate how often their child was wearing hearing aids in school. Nearly a quarter of the children (24%) were not wearing their hearing aids at either of the school visits. Furthermore, parents were likely to overestimate school hearing aid use time, particularly for students in the older grades. While the sample size is small, the results of this study suggest that some children are at risk for limited hearing aid use in the educational setting. Although there is no published evidence that specifically supports the use of hearing aids on a regular basis in school, there is clear evidence that there are negative consequences to having reduced access to academic instruction (Dockrell & Shield, 2006). In addition, Dockrell and Shield (2012) have reported that children in classrooms with poor acoustics benefit from improved access to sound with classroom audio distribution systems, specifically on listening comprehension measures. Clinically, these findings have important implications for audiologists, teachers, and parents, in that increased monitoring of hearing aids is important not just for infants and toddlers, but also for school-age children.

## WHAT FACTORS INFLUENCE HEARING AID USE?

As discussed, there is a great deal of variation in how often children wear hearing aids. Throughout the course of our research, we have seen children who do not wear their hearing aids at all, children who wear amplification for the majority of the day, and even some children who wear amplification when they sleep. The reasons for these individual differences vary, but being able to identify the reasons why some children wear hearing aids more than others can be important for counseling families who are new to the hearing aid process. Recent studies have identified several factors that may play a role in hearing aid use.

### Chronological Age

Not surprisingly, the age of the child can influence how often hearing aids are worn. Walker and colleagues (Walker, Spratford, et al., 2013; Walker, McCreery, et al., 2015) found age to be a significant factor in hearing aid use, in that younger children wore hearing aids less often than older children. Figure 5–5 shows this trend of increasing

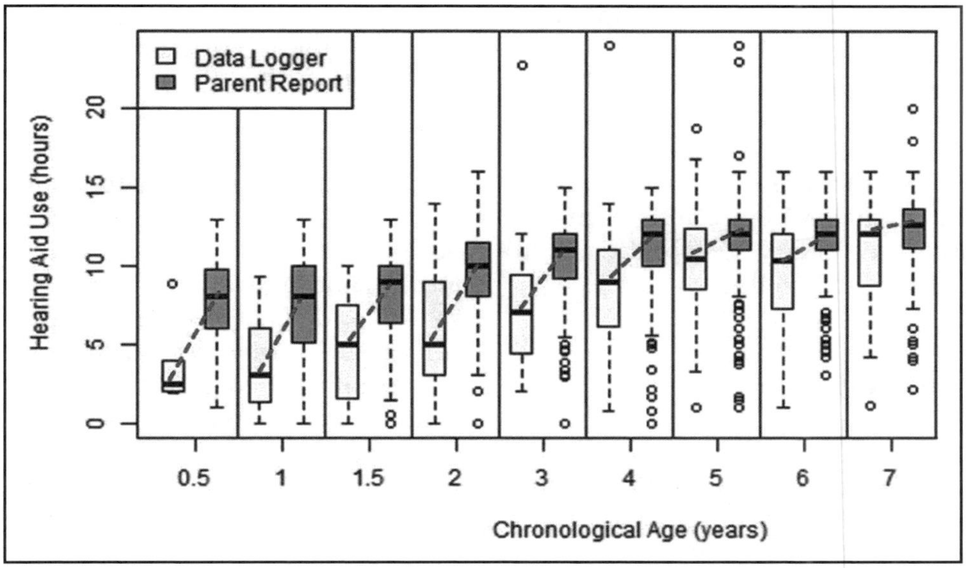


**FIGURE 5–5.** Comparison of data logging and parent report measures of daily hearing aid use over time. The central lines represent the median values and the box limits are the 25th and 75th percentiles. The lower fence is from the 10th to the 25th percentile, and the upper fence is from the 75th to the 90th percentile. The circles represent outliers at the upper and lower 10th percentiles.

hearing aid use with age, based on both parent report measures and data logging. As the figure shows, by age 7, children are wearing hearing aids approximately 10 hours per day, although the confidence intervals and outliers show that there is still wide variability during the early elementary years. The dashed lines connecting the box plots in the figure show how the difference in median values between data logging and parent report measures decreases with age.

Gustafson et al. (2015) also found that chronological age influenced hearing aid use as children get older. Gustafson and her colleagues examined children between first and seventh grade. Children in grades 1 through 4 displayed a pattern of consistent hearing aid use in the classroom, with 89.5% wearing hearing aids during all four visits (only two children, 11% of the younger children, were not observed wearing hearing aids at any visits). In contrast, children in grades 5 through 7 showed variability with hearing aid use, with only 42% of children wearing hearing aids during all four school visits. Thirty-seven percent (7 out of 19) of the older school-age children were observed without hearing aids at all four visits.

Taken together, the results of the OCHL study and Gustafson et al. (2015) may indicate a general trend of lower use during infancy and preschool, consistent use during early elementary school, and lower use again starting around junior high. The study by Gustafson et al. was a pilot study, and the number of children who participated was small ($n = 38$). Further research with a larger sample size is needed to establish whether a significant number of secondary-age students show a pattern of decreased hearing aid use at school, home, or in social settings. Regardless, pediatric audiologists should be cognizant of the fact that as children enter into secondary grades, they may be at risk for lower device use than when they were in primary grades. Possible reasons for this reduction of device use may be the social pressures students face at this age, accompanied by a desire to fit in with normal-hearing peers (Gustafson et al., 2015). Another underlying reason may be less monitoring of hearing assistive technology by teachers, as students transition to multiple classrooms and become more responsible for their hearing aid equipment. It may be helpful for clinicians and parents to include children in management of hearing aids starting in the primary grades, so that they will be prepared to take over the responsibility in middle school. This personal responsibility may generate feelings of self-efficacy, which in turn, may promote consistent device usage. Thus far, there have been no investigations into factors that influence amount of daily hearing aid use in secondary-age children. Additional research is needed on this topic.

## Degree of Hearing Loss

Another variable that has been found to influence hearing aid use is the severity of the loss. Studies have consistently shown that children with milder degrees of hearing loss wear hearing aids fewer hours than children with more severe hearing loss (Muñoz et al., 2014; Vesterager & Parving, 1995; Walker, McCreery, et al., 2015; Walker et al., 2013). Moeller et al. (2009) also noted that children with mild hearing loss experienced difficulty achieving consistent use. Parents may perceive less benefit from hearing aids in children with more residual hearing, which may lead parents to question the necessity of hearing aid use in children with mild hearing loss. Research by Muñoz et al. (2015) supports this assumption. They did not directly examine degree of hearing loss as a factor, but they did find a significant positive correlation between parents' perception of benefit from hearing aids and amount of hearing aid use. Parents who reported greater benefit also reported more hours of use. It is important to acknowledge to parents that they may not see much difference in auditory behavior with or without hearing aids in the infant and toddler years, particularly for children who have significant residual hearing. However, we can also remind parents that auditory stimulation has a positive impact on brain development. Because hearing aids increase a child's access to acoustic-phonetic cues, increased auditory exposure promotes development in the auditory areas of the brain (Sharma & Dorman, 2006; Sharma, Dorman, & Kral, 2005; Sharma, Dorman, & Spahr, 2002). Audiologists can also emphasize the cumulative effect of consistent auditory access provided by hearing aids. Children with more consistent access to speech will develop stronger language and memory skills in the long term, which has a cascading influence on later development (Werker & Hensch, 2015).

## Socioeconomic Status

Socioeconomic status of the family (i.e., parent income and educational level) is also associated with amount of hearing aid use. Marnane and Ching (2015) reported that family income level was positively correlated with hearing aid use, in that families with higher income levels had children who wore hearing aids more hours per day. Walker, McCreery, et al. (2015) also found a relationship between maternal education level and long-term trends in hearing aid use. Mothers with more education were more likely to provide infants with routine hearing aid use (more than 8 hours per day from first to last research visit) than mothers with less education. This same pattern was found in school-age children; however, there was no significant relationship between maternal education level and long-term trends in hearing aid use for preschoolers. The relationship between maternal education level and reported amount of hearing aid use does not appear to be due to overestimation on the part of mothers with more education. A regression analysis of the amount of overestimation (calculated by determining the difference between data logging and parent report of hearing aid use) did not show a significant relationship between maternal education level and overestimation (Walker et al., 2013).

To date, there has been little investigation into specifically why socioeconomic status plays a role in amount of hearing aid use. Researchers have speculated that it may be due to parents' knowledge and beliefs regarding the connection between auditory stimulation, caregiver linguistic input, and child development (Elfenbein, 1994; Marnane & Ching, 2015; Moeller et al., 2009). Reinforcing the importance of this link may be beneficial, particularly for lower-income families. Regular hands-on training with the hearing aids also may help families become more comfortable with the devices. Finally, lower-income families, particularly single-family homes, may also struggle with hearing aid compliance due to lack of support in other aspects of life (e.g., child care, difficulty getting to and from audiology appointments). It is important for clinical audiologists to be in contact with additional avenues of support for these families, such as social workers, teachers of the deaf/hard of hearing, or speech-language pathologists. Extended family members can also be considered an avenue of support, as grandparents or older siblings may have regular contact with the child and parents. Good communication among service providers and family members may help to overcome barriers related to economic status.

## HOW CAN AUDIOLOGISTS IMPROVE HEARING AID USE IN CHILDREN?

Thus far, we have discussed how consistent hearing aid use provides protection against language delay and supports auditory development. We have also described how audiologists can measure daily hearing aid use and which groups of children are at risk for minimal use. So what can audiologists do to support families in improving consistency of hearing aid use?

One direct strategy is to explore hearing aid retention devices. Many parents report that a barrier to increasing daily hearing aid use in infants and toddlers revolves around safety concerns related to the child removing their hearing aids (Moeller et al., 2009). For example, parents have reported reduced consistency of use during outdoor play and family outings, due to concerns about damage or loss of the hearing aids. Given these concerns, audiologists should discuss options for retention devices. These options include Hanna Andersson caps and bonnets, clips, wig/toupee tape, Ear Gear, SafeNSound, and hearing aid sweatbands (Figure 5–6). Anderson and Madell (2014) recently discussed these many options in an audiology trade journal, *The Hearing Review*. The article included a survey in which parents and audiologists rated which retention devices they found most useful. Parents and audiologists gave the highest ratings to Ear Gear, Hanna Andersson Caps, and SafeNSound. Audiologists also gave high ratings to clips (e.g., Critter Clips, Phonak Junior Kidz Clips, and Otoclips). In contrast, parents gave clips the lowest ratings, which suggests there may be differences of opinion between audiologists and parents on the effectiveness of different retention devices.

Anderson and Madell (2014) also asked parents and audiologists whether they had heard of the various retention products. Most of the 101 audiologists who responded to the surveys indicated that they had heard of all of the retention devices. Parents reported less familiarity with retention devices. Notably, 39% of parents (111 out of 286) said they had never heard of Hanna Andersson caps, even though caps were rated highly by parents who reported using them. The take-home message here is that it is important to familiarize parents with all of the options that are available to them and discuss the relative effectiveness of different devices. Audiologists have a central role in conveying this information to parents, and it is a disservice to parents to omit this potentially valuable information or limit the discussion of retention options to the audiologists' preferred solutions. While much of the information on hearing retention devices is available on the Internet, many parents might not know that these devices exist and, therefore, may not search them online. Karen Anderson's webpage (http://successforkidswithhearingloss.com/) provides downloadable brochures for audiologists and families, tailored to specific age ranges, with information on hearing aid retention devices.

Another counseling strategy for improving hearing aid use is to take advantage of the data logging capacities in hearing aids. Sharing the information provided by data logging may increase transparency and communication between audiologists and families (McCreery, 2013). For this transparency to be successful, however, audiologists need to inform parents about what data logging can and cannot do, starting at the initial hearing aid appointment. Data logging is merely averaging the amount of time the hearing aid battery is in the hearing aid and activated. It cannot record conversations going on in the home and does not have GPS capabilities (although many parents might wish that hearing aids had this capability when a child's hearing aid goes missing in the couch, car, or playground).

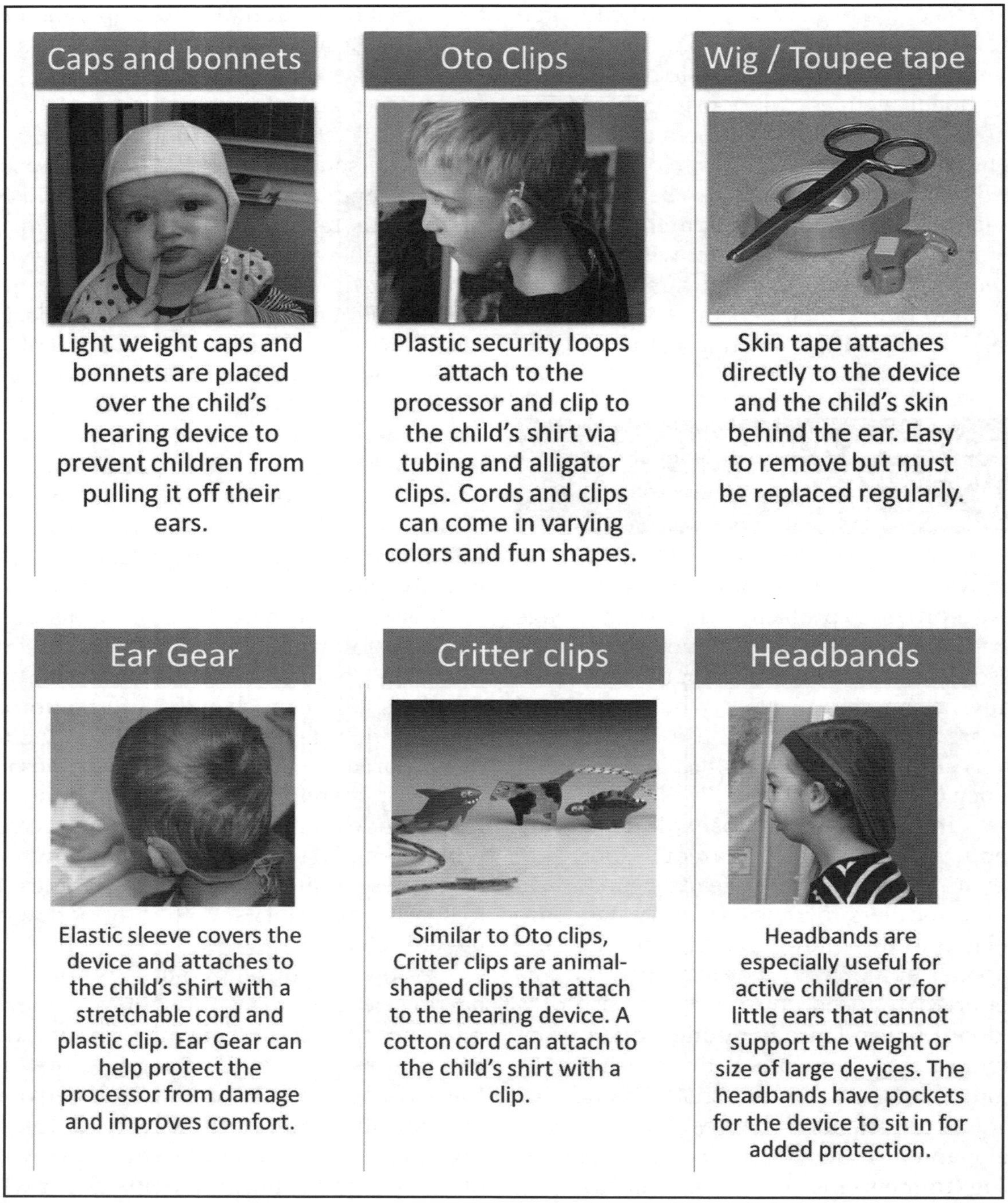


**FIGURE 5–6.** Examples of hearing aid retention devices (*Top L–R:* Caps and Bonnets, Oto Clips, Wig/Toupee Tape; *Bottom L–R:* Ear Gear, Critter Clips, and Headbands).

Why is it important to be transparent about data logging capacities with parents? The primary reason is that parents may feel defensive when their own self-report of their child's hearing aid use is discrepant from what the data logging is reporting. This can create an awkward moment between parents and audiologists and might even damage any trust that has been established in the professional-client relationship. Recent evidence suggests that audiologists encounter this situation of discrepancies regularly. Meibos et al. (2016) conducted a survey with 349 pediatric audiologists regarding clinical management for children with hearing aids. They reported that 90% of the audiologists used data logging to monitor hearing aid use. Over half of the audiologists (57%) indicated that they had encountered defensiveness on the part of the parents after sharing the data logging information. Therefore, it is important for audiologists to manage situations in which the data logging does not match what the parent is saying in a sensitive manner. McCreery (2013) recommends that we approach this situation as an opportunity to have an open and frank conversation with parents about the challenges in achieving consistent hearing aid use. If there is a discrepancy between data logging and parent report of daily hearing aid use, the audiologist can discuss what types of situations are helpful for hearing aid use and what types of situations are difficult. By addressing data logging in a supportive manner, audiologists can increase caregivers' awareness of how often the hearing aids are being utilized. Collaborative problem solving between audiologists and parents may also increase in the course of these conversations. It is also important to acknowledge to the parent that you, as the audiologist, recognize that they are working hard to achieve consistent device use.

Muñoz et al. (2014) describes a clinic protocol for routine sharing of data logging information with parents. Muñoz and her colleagues acknowledge that discussing data logging with parents can be a challenge for clinicians. They suggest talking about data logging at the hearing aid fitting appointment, which will lead to hearing aid use becoming a regular part of the conversation at each visit. In their clinic protocol, data logging is initially discussed as a feature in the hearing aids that shows the amount of hours of hearing aid use. Data logging can be described as a benefit to the parents, given the difficulty in keeping track of situations that get in the way of wearing the hearing aids on any given day. At the follow-up appointments, Muñoz and colleagues suggest that the audiologist first acknowledge something positive that the parents and child have accomplished since the previous visit (e.g., getting comfortable with inserting the hearing aids in the child's ears). After recognizing opportunities for success, they recommend looking at the data logging. If it is discrepant from what the parent is reporting, the audiologist can ask the parent to describe situations that might be getting in the way of hearing aid use, and then problem solve how to deal with those situations. For example, the parent may report that it is difficult to remember to put the hearing aids in first thing in the morning, and the audiologist and parent can come up with a plan to deal with that issue. Finally, it is suggested that the audiologist remind the parents that the goal is for the child to wear the hearing aids whenever he or she is awake. For infants and toddlers who sleep approximately 14 hours a day, this will be about 10 hours per day.

Although it is important to provide information to parents about retention devices and data logging, it is equally important to recognize the challenges in trying to achieve consistent hearing aid use with children. Audiologists will often encounter situations in which retention strategies are not sufficient. It may be tempting for audiologists to assume that if parents are just persistent enough, full-time use will be accomplished. Persistence on the part of the parents is certainly one aspect of increasing usage, but attributing everything to "trying harder" is likely an oversimplification of the situation. As Moeller and colleagues (2009) point out, the process of getting a child to wear hearing aids is complex and bidirectional. In other words, there are parent-specific factors that will influence device use, such as parental adjustment to the diagnosis of hearing loss and hearing aid management. There are also child-specific issues. Some of these include motor development. For example, children begin to develop a pincer grasp around 6 months of age, which allows them to pull out the hearing aids. Cognitive development also undergoes rapid changes in the first year of life. Concepts such as emergence of cause and effect occur around 10 to 12 months of age, which allow the child to become aware that removal of the hearing aids will increase attention from parents. Temper tantrums and other infant-related issues (e.g., teething, ear infections, hunger, etc.) will also emerge as new challenges for parents.

Each of these developmental changes and associated behaviors may require different and flexible approaches in hearing aid management. Although audiologists may be inclined to continue making the standard recommendation of "just keep putting the hearing aid back in," service providers should sensitive to how parent and infant behaviors interact with one another. This is especially true in the case of children with multiple disabilities or additional health concerns. These parents are coping with more than just hearing loss, and audiologists need to be aware of these added difficulties and provide support as needed. Furthermore, behavior management may be an area that audiologists are not trained in or comfortable with. As a result, audiologists may avoid addressing it with parents, or they may assume that other service providers are addressing the issue.

Muñoz and her colleagues have pointed out the importance of supporting families not just in the technical aspects of hearing aid management and care, but in addressing emotional needs (Muñoz et al., 2014). Muñoz et al. (2015) reported reduced hours of hearing aid use with higher incidence of parent-reported challenges, such as feelings of frustration, confusion, and lack of confidence with hearing aid management. It appears that parents who are more confident in their ability to manage their child's hearing aids are successful in getting their children to wear the hearing aids more often. However, it is unclear what it is about self-confidence that influences hearing aid use, or how audiologists and related service providers can go about supporting parents in this domain.

A study by DesJardin (2005) may provide further insight into how audiologists can promote parents' self-confidence. DesJardin (2005) specifically targeted one aspect of confidence and competence—*self-efficacy*—in an investigation of mothers of children with hearing aids or cochlear implants. Self-efficacy is a construct that emerges from social learning theory (Bandura, 1989). It can be described as one's belief that he or she can successfully complete a specific task. Feelings of self-efficacy can support persistence in difficult situations, in that individuals who believe they are knowledgeable and competent will persist in a given task until success is achieved. On the other hand, individuals who lack self-efficacy may give up more easily, due to feelings of self-doubt and limited beliefs that they can carry out intervention goals. DesJardin administered a questionnaire on self-efficacy for mothers of children with hearing aids or cochlear implants called, the Scale of Parental Involvement and Maternal Self-Efficacy (SPISE)(DesJardin, 2003). Mothers of children with cochlear implants rated themselves as more efficacious than mothers of children with hearing aids. They also reported that they were more involved in daily listening checks and more competent in adjusting the device, compared to mothers of children with hearing aids.

> Self-efficacy is the belief in one's ability to successfully achieve goals or accomplish tasks.

Clinically, DesJardin's results have important implications for audiologists and related service providers, as they emphasize the importance in helping parents feel confident in their ability to manage the hearing aids. Unfortunately, not all audiologists routinely provide parents with support in achieving effective hearing aid management, perhaps because of lack of time or lack of reimbursement through insurance. In the Meibos et al. (2016) survey mentioned previously, approximately one-third to one-half of audiologists reported that they did not provide parents with information on how to do hearing aid maintenance (44%), how to do a Ling 6 sound check (52%), or how to teach other caregivers about hearing aid management (38%). A large number of the audiologists who completed the survey also reported a need for additional training in counseling skills. Thus, there is room for improvement in how audiologists work with parents on hearing aid management. During hearing aid orientation and follow-up visits, audiologists should check that parents are comfortable handling the hearing aids on their own. Even more importantly, audiologists should encourage parents to view themselves as advocates for their child and involve the parents in the hearing aid management process. This may involve showing the parents how to troubleshoot equipment and helping parents to feel confident enough in their own skills in order to teach others (e.g., grandparents, daycare providers) how to manage the hearing aids. If parents can make the connection that their knowledge about hearing aids will make a difference in their child's listening and language-learning outcomes, they may be more likely to follow through with recommended goals for hearing aid use. Although teaching parents these skills may require a time investment during the initial fitting process, that time is well spent because parents become more independent in their abilities to take care of their child's hearing aid. As a final note, parent-to-parent support may play an important role in increasing self-efficacy. If audiologists have the ability to connect parents of children with hearing loss to other parents in the same situation, or if your state has programs such as "Guide By Your Side" (http://www.handsandvoices.org/gbys/), a parent-to-parent networking group associated with "Hands and Voices," these options may be extremely helpful to parents.

## CONCLUSIONS

Hearing aid use is a part of cumulative auditory experience that is easy to overlook. Nevertheless, research shows that there is great variability in the amount of time children wear hearing aids, and parents often struggle with getting their child to wear their hearing device on a consistent basis. Common sense tells us that children with hearing loss cannot access sounds if they do not wear their hearing aids. Thus, audiologists should be aware of how to effectively measure daily use, convey that information to parents, explore possible challenges parents will face, support their process of learning how to manage challenges, and monitor the success of their efforts.

## REFERENCES

Anderson, K., & Madell, J. (2014). Improving hearing and hearing aid retention for infants and young children. *Hearing Review, 21*(2), 16–20.

Bandura, A. (1989). Regulation of cognitive processes through perceived self-efficacy. *Developmental Psychology, 25*(5), 729–735.

Ching, T. Y., Dillon, H., Marnane, V., Hou, S., Day, J., Seeto, M., . . . Van Buynder, P. (2013). Outcomes of early- and late-identified children at 3 years of age: Findings from a prospective population-based study. *Ear and Hearing, 34*(5), 535–552.

Ching, T. Y., & Hill, M. (2007). The parents' evaluation of aural/oral performance of children (PEACH) scale: Normative data. *Journal of the American Academy of Audiology, 18*(3), 220–235.

Davis, J. M., Elfenbein, J., Schum, R., & Bentler, R. A. (1986). Effects of mild and moderate hearing impairments on language, educational, and psychosocial behavior of children. *Journal of Speech and Hearing Disorders, 51*(1), 53–62.

DesJardin, J. L. (2003). Assessing parental perceptions of self-efficacy and involvement in families of young children with hearing loss. *Volta Review, 103*(4), 275–298.

DesJardin, J. L. (2005). Maternal perceptions of self-efficacy and involvement in the auditory development of young children with prelingual deafness. *Journal of Early Intervention, 27*(3), 193–209.

Dockrell, J. E., & Shield, B. M. (2006). Acoustical barriers in classrooms: The impact of noise on performance in the classroom. *British Educational Research Journal, 32*(3), 509–525.

Dockrell, J. E., & Shield, B. (2012). The impact of sound-field systems on learning and attention in elementary school classrooms. *Journal of Speech, Language, and Hearing Research, 55*(4), 1163–1176.

Elfenbein, J. L. (1994). Monitoring preschoolers' hearing aids: Issues in program design and implementation. *American Journal of Audiology, 3*(2), 65–70.

Fitzpatrick, E. M., Durieux-Smith, A., & Whittingham, J. (2010). Clinical practice for children with mild bilateral and unilateral hearing loss. *Ear and Hearing, 31*(3), 392–400.

Gilbertson, M., & Kamhi, A. G. (1995). Novel word learning in children with hearing impairment. *Journal of Speech, Language, and Hearing Research, 38*(3), 630–642.

Gustafson, S. J., Davis, H., Hornsby, B. W., & Bess, F. H. (2015). Factors influencing hearing aid use in the classroom: A pilot study. *American Journal of Audiology, 24*(4), 563–568.

Jones, C., & Feilner, M. (2013). What do we know about the fitting and daily life usage of hearing instruments in pediatrics? In R. C. Seewald & J. M. Bamford (Eds.), *A Sound Foundation through early amplification: Proceedings of the 2013 International Conference* (pp. 97–103). Chicago, IL: Phonak AG.

Jones, C., & Launer, S. (2010). Pediatric fittings in 2010: The Sound Foundations Cuper project. In R. C. Seewald & J. M. Bamford (Eds.), *A Sound Founda-*

*tion through early amplification: Proceedings of the 2010 International Conference* (pp. 187–192). Chicago, IL: Phonak AG.

Klein, K.E., Walker, E.A., Kirby, B., & McCreery, R.W. (in press). Vocabulary facilitates speech perception in children with hearing aids. *Journal of Speech, Language, Hearing Research.*

Marnane, V., & Ching, T. Y. (2015). Hearing aid and cochlear implant use in children with hearing loss at three years of age: Predictors of use and predictors of changes in use. *International Journal of Audiology, 54*(8), 544–551.

McCreery, R. (2013). Data logging and hearing aid use: Focus on the forest, not the trees. *Hearing Journal, 66*(12), 18–19.

Meibos, A., Muñoz, K., White, K., Preston, E., Pitt, C., & Twohig, M. (2016). Audiologist practices: Parent hearing aid education and support. *Journal of the American Academy of Audiology, 27*(4), 324–332.

Moeller, M. P., Hoover, B., Peterson, B., & Stelmachowicz, P. (2009). Consistency of hearing aid use in infants with early-identified hearing loss. *American Journal of Audiology, 18*(1), 14–23.

Moeller, M. P., & Tomblin, J. B. (2015). An introduction to the outcomes of children with hearing loss study. *Ear and Hearing, 36*, 4S–13S.

Muñoz, K., & Hill, M. M. (2015). Hearing aid use for children with hearing loss: A literature review. *SIG 9 Perspectives on Hearing and Hearing Disorders in Childhood, 25*(1), 4–14.

Muñoz, K., Olson, W. A., Twohig, M. P., Preston, E., Blaiser, K., & White, K. R. (2015). Pediatric hearing aid use: Parent-reported challenges. *Ear and Hearing, 36*(2), 279–287.

Muñoz, K., Preston, E., & Hicken, S. (2014). Pediatric hearing aid use: How can audiologists support parents to increase consistency? *Journal of the American Academy of Audiology, 25*(4), 380–387.

Sharma, A., & Dorman, M. F. (2006). Central auditory development in children with cochlear implants: Clinical implications. *Advances in Oto-Rhino-Laryngology, 64*, 66–88.

Sharma, A., Dorman, M. F., & Kral, A. (2005). The influence of a sensitive period on central auditory development in children with unilateral and bilateral cochlear implants. *Hearing Research, 203*(1), 134–143.

Sharma, A., Dorman, M. F., & Spahr, A. J. (2002). A sensitive period for the development of the central auditory system in children with cochlear implants: Implications for age of implantation. *Ear and Hearing, 23*(6), 532–539.

Tomblin, J. B., Harrison, M., Ambrose, S. E., Walker, E. A., Oleson, J. J., & Moeller, M. P. (2015). Language outcomes in young children with mild to severe hearing loss. *Ear and Hearing, 36*, 76S–91S.

Tomblin, J. B., Walker, E. A., McCreery, R. W., Arenas, R. M., Harrison, M., & Moeller, M. P. (2015). Outcomes of children with hearing loss: Data collection and methods. *Ear and Hearing, 36*, 14S–23S.

Vesterager, V., & Parving, A. (1995). Rehabilitation of hearing-impaired children: Intervention and outcome. *Audiology, 34*(4), 207–217.

Walker, E. A., Holte, L., McCreery, R. W., Spratford, M., Page, T., & Moeller, M. P. (2015). The influence of hearing aid use on outcomes of children with mild hearing loss. *Journal of Speech, Language, and Hearing Research, 58*(5), 1611–1625.

Walker, E. A., McCreery, R. W., Spratford, M., Oleson, J. J., Van Buren, J., Bentler, R., . . . Moeller, M. P. (2015). Trends and predictors of longitudinal hearing aid use for children who are hard of hearing. *Ear and Hearing, 36*, 38S–47S.

Walker, E. A., Spratford, M., Moeller, M. P., Oleson, J., Ou, H., Roush, P., & Jacobs, S. (2013). Predictors of hearing aid use time in children with mild-to-severe hearing loss. *Language, Speech, and Hearing Services in Schools, 44*(1), 73–88.

Werker, J. F., & Hensch, T. K. (2015). Critical periods in speech perception: New directions. *Psychology, 66*(1), 173–196.

Weston, M., Muñoz, K. F., & Blaiser, K. (2014). Monitoring progress for children with hearing loss. *SIG 9 Perspectives on Hearing and Hearing Disorders in Childhood, 24*(2), 74–81.

# 6

# Monitoring Outcomes

*Elizabeth A. Walker and Ryan W. McCreery*

## INTRODUCTION

Audiologists and related professionals agree that appropriate and timely diagnostic and intervention services will lead to more successful outcomes for children with hearing loss. This overarching goal of early hearing detection and intervention (EHDI) can be broken down into several critical benchmarks, known as the "1-3-6" timeline (Figure 6–1).

Meeting these benchmarks puts children with hearing loss on the right path to achieving listening and spoken language skills. At the same time, it is critical to use best practice techniques to verify that children are obtaining appropriate aided audibility from their hearing aids and to monitor device use time to determine if children are wearing hearing aids consistently. There is one more important step in the process that needs to be taken to ensure that these goals are met. It is also necessary for audiologists to monitor developmental progress of their pediatric clients over time, so that they can identify possible "red flags" early on. Some of the measures used to monitor developmental progress fall under the purview of related hearing healthcare professionals, such

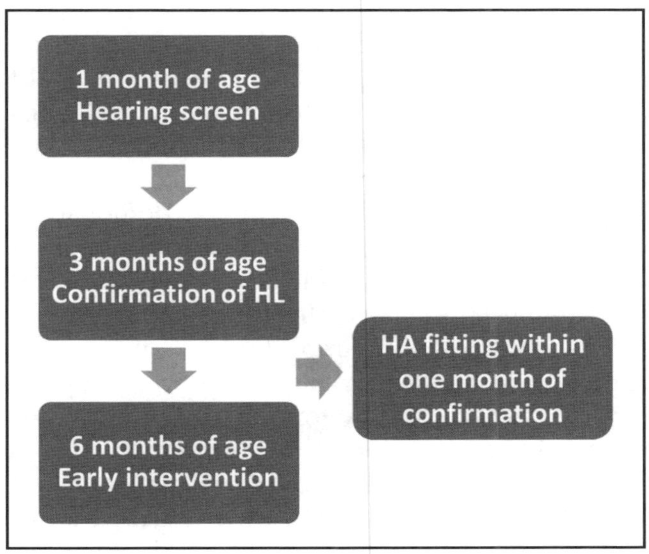


**FIGURE 6–1.** Early Hearing Detection and Intervention "1-3-6" benchmarks for service delivery for children who do not pass the newborn hearing screen, as recommended by the Joint Committee on Infant Hearing (2007).

as speech-language pathologists, teachers of the deaf/hard of hearing, or psychologists. However, audiologists have a responsibility to monitor the developmental progress of their patients, not relying on other professionals to ensure that children who are hard of hearing do not fall behind. There are a number of validated, easy-to-use, outcome measures that are readily available for audiologists who work with children. There are also measures that are more limited in their reliability or validity. Audiologists should be aware of what measures can be of the most use to their clinical practice. This chapter presents an evidence-based evaluation of the available tools for monitoring outcomes in children with hearing loss.

## WHAT ARE "RED FLAGS"?

Before diving into the world of pediatric audiology outcome measures, we will provide an overview of "red flags" and why it is important for audiologists to be aware of them. Red flags are signs of possible developmental delays or additional disabilities. These warning signs may not be readily apparent when children are first identified with hearing loss because the initial focus is on confirming the degree of hearing loss, fitting the child with hearing aids, and getting the child enrolled in early intervention. Many red flags may not emerge until children have missed some developmental milestones. It can also be a challenge to figure out when a child is demonstrating speech or language delays due to the hearing loss and when there is some other developmental issue going on that will affect long-term prognosis. Nevertheless, it is important to note when a child does not appear to making progress in cognitive, language, and motor domains, in order for the child to receive appropriate interventions.

Although estimates vary, reports suggest that 30 to 40% of children with hearing loss have additional cognitive or medical conditions (Holden-Pitt & Diaz, 1998). The Gallaudet Research Institute conducted its annual survey of schools/program for deaf and or hard of hearing students from around the United States in 2009–2010 (2011). The survey included 37,828 students. Thirty-nine percent had one or more additional conditions, including low vision or legal blindness, orthopedic impairment, traumatic brain injury, or autism. Cognitive or behavioral issues had the highest prevalence; 8.3% of students had an intellectual disability, 8% had a learning disability, 5.4% had ADD/ADHD, and 5.3% had developmental delay. Early identification of comorbid developmental conditions is crucial for ensuring that appropriate interventions are undertaken.

It is challenging to identify cognitive and developmental delays during the infant and toddler years. Part of this challenge is due to the fact that it is difficult to distinguish between communication and language delays that are the result of hearing loss and more global delays that are the result of cognitive issues. There are some warning signs that professionals might observe during the first two years of life (Wiley & Moeller, 2007). Figure 6–2 displays these red flags. These early warning signs can be broken into several different areas—gesture development, vocal development, and vocabulary development.

### Gesture Development

By 12 months of age, infants with cognitive skills within the normal range use gestures as an early means of communication, including children with hearing loss (Robinshaw, 1995; Spencer, 1993; Zaidman-Zait & Dromi, 2007). These early gestures include showing (extending the arm to display an object) and pointing (extending the index finger toward an object or event). A key trait with both of these early gestures is that they are coordinated with social interactions with other people (Capone & McGregor, 2004). Delays in pointing or showing may be a sign that a child is having difficulty with social-emotional aspects of language, and may serve as an indicator for conditions such as autism or intellectual disabilities.

### Vocal Development

Canonical babbling is a major milestone in vocal development (Oller & Eilers, 1988). Canonical babbling is the repetition of consonant-vowel syllables. Early in development, these consonant-vowel

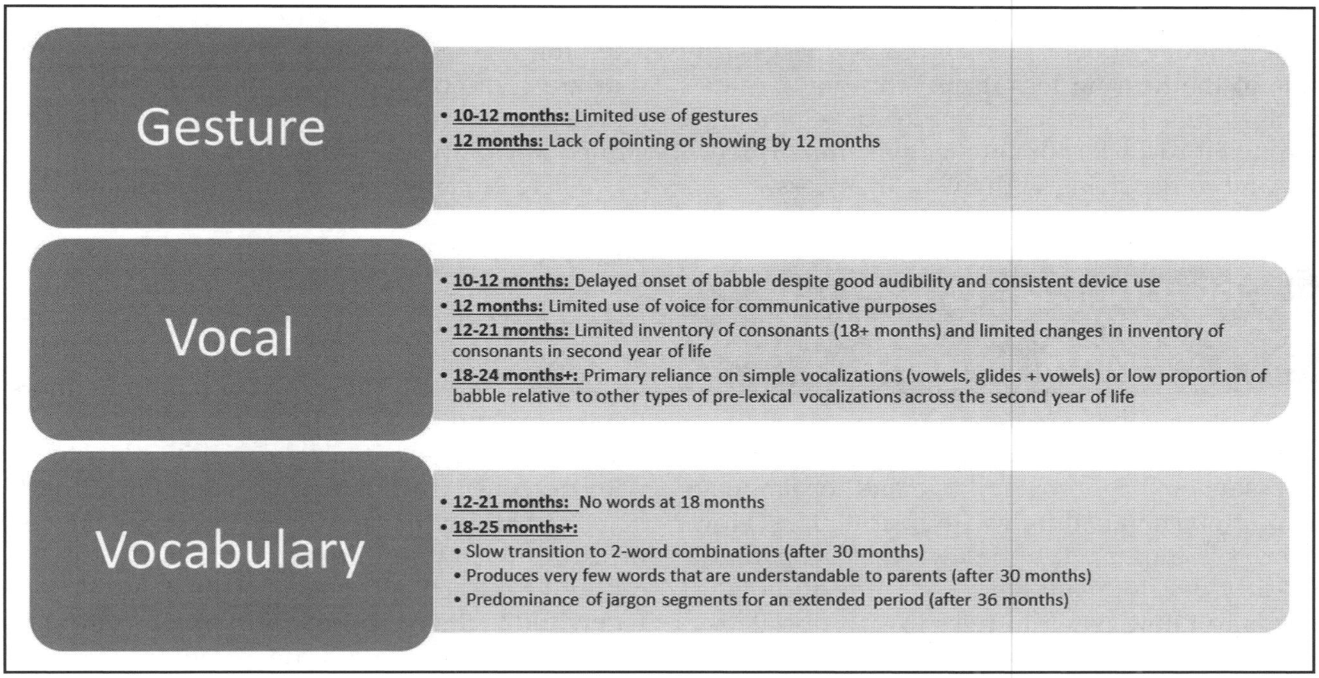


**FIGURE 6–2.** "Red flags" for possible developmental delays in the areas of gesture, vocal, and vocabulary during the first two years of life.

syllables usually consist of /d/, /b/, or /m/ (MacNeilage, Davis, Kinney, & Matyear, 2000). Canonical babbling emerges around 6 to 8 months of age in hearing children. Production may be delayed in children with hearing loss, particularly children with severe-profound hearing loss (Bass-Ringdahl, 2010). Children with mild-moderate degrees of hearing loss who have good access to sound through their hearing aids begin producing canonical babbling between 9 and 12 months of age (Moeller et al., 2007a). Infants (with or without hearing loss) who are delayed in producing consonants in their babble tend to be delayed in later speech and vocabulary outcomes (Stoel-Gammon, 1989; Walker & Bass-Ringdahl, 2008). Vocalizations that consist primarily of vowels or "soft consonants" (e.g., "yayayaya" or "wawawawa") may be indicative of later difficulties with language development.

## Vocabulary Development

After early gestures and canonical babbling emerge, we see production of first words. Hearing children typically produce first words around 12 months of age and will have approximately 50 words in their expressive vocabulary by 18 months, at which point two-word combinations usually emerge. For children who are deaf or hard of hearing, these stages of early language development follow the same developmental pattern, albeit delayed. In a longitudinal study of early vocal and lexical development in 12 children with hearing loss and 21 children with normal hearing, Moeller et al. (2007b) identified six children (two with normal hearing and four with hearing loss) who appeared to be atypical in terms of their rate of language development. One sign that these children were at risk for later problems included absent or limited production of recognizable single words by 2 years of age. Reduced production at the one-word stage has a cascading influence on later vocabulary and grammatical development because it results in delays in two-word combinations. Service providers should be aware of important milestones, such as first word productions and two-word combinations. If a child with hearing aids has no spoken words in their expressive vocabulary by 2 years of age or is not combining two words by 2½ years, this is a red flag for possible language delays, which are not necessarily due to the hearing loss itself. Additional issues, such as autism spectrum disorder, developmental language disorder, or intellectual impairments, may be co-occurring with the hearing loss.

## OUTCOME MEASURES FOR MONITORING AUDITORY DEVELOPMENT

It is outside of the audiologist's scope of practice to assess or diagnose cognitive and/or language impairments in children with hearing loss. However, it is important to be aware of benchmarks in early development because (1) the audiologist needs to know when to refer to appropriate service providers and (2) early auditory development is closely tied to language and cognitive development. As described in this chapter, there are many outcome measures that are available to audiologists. The following section describes some commonly used measures, in an attempt to provide evidence-based guidance on tools for monitoring development in children.

Perhaps in your first audiology course, your professor may have observed that the field of audiology is replete with acronyms. One area where that is patently obvious is with pediatric audiology outcome measures. Pediatric audiology has a plethora of acronyms associated with outcome measures, often with clever names like the LittlEARS, the PEACH, the ELF, or the CHILD, just to name a few. Because there are so many different outcome measures available to pediatric audiologists, it can be a legitimate challenge to determine which measures are valid, reliable, and appropriate for a specific age range or patient population (i.e., children who are deaf or hard of hearing, have cochlear implants or hearing aids, have bilateral or unilateral hearing loss). Our learning objective is for the reader to have a more complete understanding of the relative utility of some of these measures, so that pediatric audiology tests are no longer a laundry list of acronyms for the audiologist to sort through. Given the number of pediatric outcome measures that are available to audiologists, it is beyond the scope of this textbook to review all that are currently available. Therefore, we have chosen to describe measures that are commonly used or measures that may be less familiar to audiologists but have demonstrated reliability and validity.

There are a number of important points that should be taken into consideration when deciding which of these questionnaires or tests to use. Some of these points are practical: *How much does the test cost? Is it readily available and easy for the audiologist to administer and score? Is it available in the family's native language?* Other points are more theoretical, and relate to the psychometric properties of the test. *Is it reliable?* Reliability has to do with the consistency and repeatability of a test. *Is it valid?* Validity has to do with whether the test measures what it says it is going to measure. One can judge the ecological validity (is it valid in the real world?), the concurrent and predictive validity (does it correlate with concurrent measures or predict future performance?), and content validity (do the individual items accurately reflect whatever construct the test is trying to measure?). *Is there a norm-referenced sample?* Some questionnaires and tests allow the examiner to compare the pediatric client's score to the scores obtained by other children. Having a norm-referenced sample for a given test can be very informative because it will allow professionals to determine how their clients are doing compared to peers. If a child is performing at a significantly lower level, this can be important information to convey to parents and other service providers. There is one note of caution with normative data, however. When using a norm-referenced measure, audiologists should be aware of who is in the normative sample. These samples may include children with normal hearing, children with hearing loss, or a combination of the two. There may be a normative sample consisting of children with hearing loss, but the sample was obtained before the advent of universal newborn hearing screening, family-centered early intervention, or cochlear implant technology. Therefore, the normative sample would not be a good comparison group for the current generation of children with hearing loss who have access to early identification and intervention services. Test interpretation will differ based on who the child is being compared to, so knowing who is in the normative group becomes critical.

> Reliability refers to the consistency of a test measure. Test-retest reliability should show a consistency across time. If you administer the same measurement several times in close succession, will you get the same score? Interrater reliability is consistency across examiners. If multiple people administer the same measurement, will they get the same scores? Equivalent forms reliability is applicable to measures that have more than one form that can be administered. If a speech perception test has multiple lists, it is important that all lists are equally challenging and a given patient will have similar scores, regardless of which list is administered. Internal consistency has to do with the individual items on a measure. If the odd items are compared to the even items, are they highly correlated with one another (odd-even correlations)? If half of the items are chosen at random and then compared to the other half of the items on that measure, are they highly correlated with one another (split-half correlations)?

> Validity refers to what the test is actually measuring. Ecological validity asks if a measure is valid in the real world. Concurrent validity asks if a measure correlates with other tests, and predictive validity asks if a measure will predict later performance on a different measure. Content validity has to do with whether the individual items accurately reflect whatever construct the test is trying to measure. For example, if a given test is trying to measure improvement over time, do the individual items start off easier and get more difficult in later sections of the measure?

## Questionnaires

The following sections describe questionnaires that are used by audiologists. Questionnaires are typically completed by the parents, either independently or in an interview format by a professional. Questionnaires may be designed to examine auditory behavior, communication skills, or behavior of the child in different listening conditions. Questionnaires will be grouped together based on age (infant/toddler; preschool/school-age). Both practical and theoretical aspects of the tests are discussed.

### *Infants and Toddlers*

Young children (particularly toddlers) are notoriously difficult to test, and audiologists often rely on parent-report questionnaires to assess early auditory development. With children receiving hearing aids and cochlear implants at very young ages, it is critical to have well-validated tools that monitor auditory-verbal development. Table 6–1 summarizes questionnaires that are appropriate for this age range. Two of the more commonly used parent-report measures are described in detail below.

**LittlEARS.** The LittlEARS (Coninx et al., 2009) is designed to track auditory development in children from birth to 24 months, chronological age, or up to 24 months hearing age (time from first fitting of the device). It can be used with children who have cochlear implants or hearing aids. It is published through the MED-EL Corporation. Parents can complete the questionnaire themselves, or the audiologist can administer it via interview format. The questionnaire consists of 35 "yes/no" questions designed to assess receptive and expressive language skills in response to auditory stimuli. Examples of questions include, "Does your child respond to a familiar voice?" and "When somebody is speaking, does your child turn his/her head toward the speaker?" The number of "yes" responses are added together to obtain the total score, which corresponds to expected values based on the child's age.

**Table 6–1.** Parent-Report Questionnaires for Infants/Toddlers

| *Parent/Teacher-Report Questionnaires* | *Age Range* | *Description* |
|---|---|---|
| LittlEARS Auditory Questionnaire (Coninx et al., 2009) | Birth to 2 yrs. | These are 35 "Yes/No" questions that assess auditory development and expressive language skills. |
| IT-MAIS: Infant Toddler Meaningful Auditory Integration Scale (Zimmerman-Phillips & Osberger, 1997) | Birth to 3 yrs. | This is a parent report scale interview with ten questions used to assess the child's spontaneous responses to sound in his/her everyday environment. |

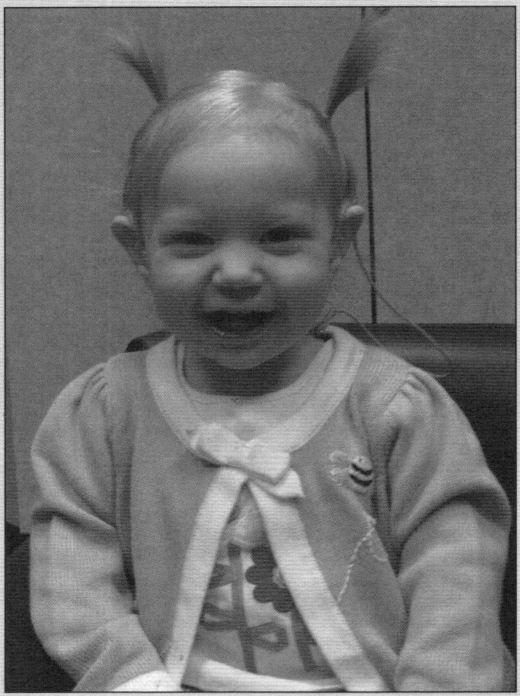

One of the major strengths of the LittlEARS is that it has been validated both internally by the authors, Coninx et al. (2009), in 15 different languages and externally by outside sources (Bagatto, Brown, Moodie, & Scollie, 2011). These peer-reviewed studies have indicated that the LittlEARS questionnaire is highly reliable and valid. Another strength of the LittlEARS is that there are normative scores available in the test manual. As a result, individual children can be compared to the normative curve to determine if they are achieving appropriate skills based on their ages. Figure 6–3 shows the English-speaking norm curve and the minimum 95% confidence interval from the Canadian-derived norms (Bagatto, Brown, et al., 2011). Children falling below the 95% confidence interval are considered to be at risk for delays in auditory development.

Bagatto, Moodie, et al. (2011) published a critical review of auditory development questionnaires, with the goal of formulating evidence-based outcome evaluation guidelines for young children with hearing loss. Of the 12 questionnaires that were evaluated, the LittlEARS received high scores on a number of factors, including appropriate burden for administrators and respondents

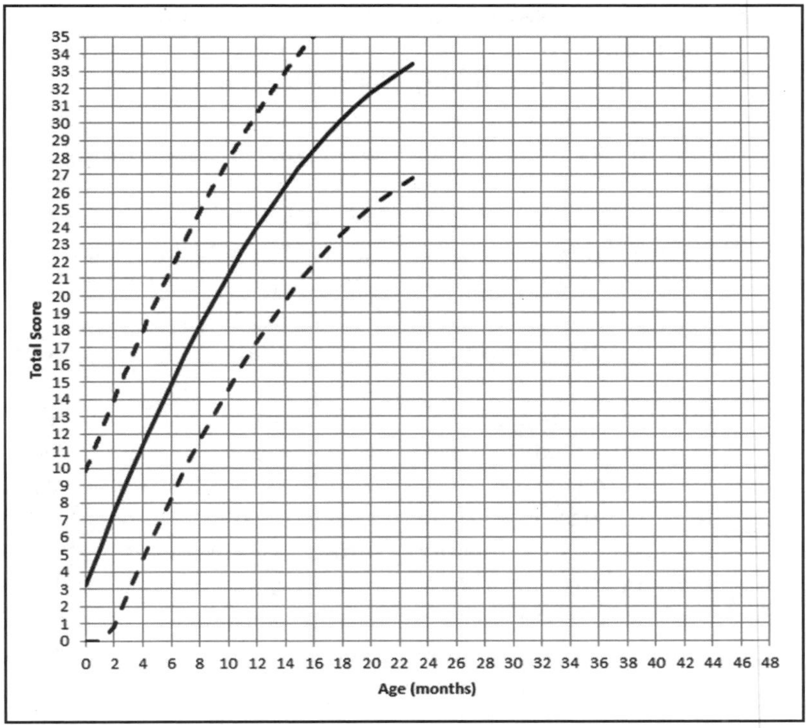


**FIGURE 6–3.** English-speaking normative curve and the minimum 95% confidence intervals from the Canadian-derived norms of the *LittlEARS* parent-report questionnaire (Image courtesy of Marlene Bagatto, AuD, PhD).

(i.e., amount of time to complete the questionnaire, ease of scoring), good reliability and validity, and its availability in a number of different languages. One limitation of the LittlEARS is that many children with hearing loss may reach ceiling levels before 2 years of age (McCreery et al., 2015). Therefore, Bagatto and her colleagues recommend using the LittlEARS as part of a two-stage process by developmental level, in which the LittlEARS is used first. Once an individual child reaches the maximum level of performance on the measure (considered to be a score of 28 or higher), Bagatto and colleagues suggest evaluating the child with the Parents' Evaluation of Aural/Oral Performance of Children (PEACH; Ching & Hill, 2007), which is reviewed in an upcoming section of this chapter.

**Infant-Toddler Meaningful Auditory Integration Scale (IT-MAIS).** The IT-MAIS is intended to measure functional auditory behavior (Zimmerman-Phillips & Osberger, 1997). As its name suggests, it was developed for infants and toddlers with hearing loss. The IT-MAIS is free on the Advanced Bionics website (http://c324175.r75.cf1.rackcdn.com/IT-MAS_20brochure_20_2.pdf). It consists of 10 questions that assess children's spontaneous responses. Unlike the LittlEARS, the IT-MAIS cannot be administered to parents as a written questionnaire. It is designed to be administered only in an interview format, in which the examiner engages the parent in an open conversation about the child's auditory skills. The examiner elicits examples of vocal and listening behaviors from the parent (e.g., "Tell me about the sounds that Jill responds to in her environments) and avoids asking "yes/no" questions. As per the instructions, examples must be from spontaneous situations, not structured contexts (e.g., speech-language intervention sessions). The parent is then asked to rate how often the child demonstrates the specific behaviors, on a 5-point rating scale (never = 0, 1 = rarely, 2 = occasionally, 3 = frequently, 4 = always).

Test administrators are advised that it may be difficult for parents to determine the appropriate ratings. If parents need additional time, the examiner should schedule a phone interview to complete the test, rather than giving the parents the test to fill out at home.

The IT-MAIS is scored by adding up the total points and dividing by 40. Typically, performance is then measured as a percentage and tracked over time. Normative data for children with normal hearing have been published, but these data are for Hebrew and Arabic-speaking families (Kishon-Rabin et al., 2001) and Mandarin-speaking families from China (Zheng et al., 2009). To date, there are no published normative data based on samples of English-speaking children, with or without hearing loss. The IT-MAIS is available in a number of languages (English, German, Polish, Mandarin, Arabic, and Hebrew). The authors of the IT-MAIS suggest that it has good predictive validity, based on results showing that MAIS scores (the older version of the IT-MAIS, intended for children ages 3 years and older) are correlated with open-set speech perception scores in children with hearing loss (Robbins, Svirsky, Osberger, & Pisoni, 1998). Thus, it may be a means for monitoring auditory development in very young children who receive cochlear implants, but are too young to participate in speech perception measures.

There are some limitations with the IT-MAIS that are worth mentioning. The caregiver response format is somewhat cumbersome and may be unreliable across examiners, given that the examiners must elicit responses from parents and then determine scores based on those responses (although the inter-rater reliability has not been verified empirically). Normative data are not available for English-speaking children. Finally, the test is designed to measure benefit in children with cochlear implants, which limits its applicability to children with mild to severe hearing loss who use hearing aids. Similar to the LittlEARS, many children with hearing loss may reach a maximum scores on the IT-MAIS prior to age 2 years. Although the IT-MAIS is widely used, other measures such as the LittlEARS and PEACH rating scale (described in the next section) have demonstrated better evidence-based utility in published literature, including reliability, validity, ease of administration, and appropriate normative data. These factors should be kept in mind when determining appropriate tools to monitor auditory outcomes.

### *Preschool and School-Age Children*

As children enter more formal educational settings, their attention spans and language competency improve. Audiologists and speech-language pathologists are able to administer direct assessments, rather than relying on parent-report measures to monitor progress. Nevertheless, questionnaires may still provide useful information to supplement the information that is gained from standardized testing or speech perception scores. This is particularly true for teacher-report surveys, which give us insight into how children are using their functional auditory skills in the educational setting. Table 6–2 summarizes questionnaires that are appropriate for evaluating children ages 3 and older. It should be noted that we are referring to children who are in this range in terms of cognitive and linguistic development, not chronological age. For children who demonstrate significant developmental delays, audiologists may be able to obtain more information about auditory progress from the questionnaires described in the previous section, such as the LittlEARS. Communication with other service providers becomes critical because knowledge about the cognitive and language levels of pediatric clients will aid audiologists in test selection.

**PEACH Diary and Rating Scale.** The PEACH is an auditory development measure that is appropriate for children ages birth through school age (Ching & Hill, 2007). There are no guidelines specifying the upper age limit of the PEACH, but it should be noted that children with normal hearing appear to plateau on the measure around 30 months of age, and children with hearing loss without additional developmental issues reach maximum levels of performance around 48 months (Bagatto et al., 2011). It is intended to be a measure of effectiveness of amplification in everyday life. The PEACH is free from the National Acoustics Laboratory webpage (http://outcomes.nal.gov.au/peach.html). The measurement tool consists of a parent-report diary and rating scale. In the diary,

**Table 6–2.** Parent and Teacher Report Questionnaires for Preschool and School-Age Children

| *Parent/Teacher Report Questionnaires* | *Age Range* | *Description* |
|---|---|---|
| PEACH: Parents' Evaluation of Aural/oral performance of Children (Ching & Hill, 2007) | 2 to 7 yrs. | This contains 13 questions filled out by a parent designed to evaluate the effectiveness of the child's amplification and assess the child's functional performance in everyday life situations. |
| TEACH: Teachers' Evaluation of Aural/oral performance of Children (Ching & Hill, 2007) | 2 to 7 yrs. | This contains 11 questions taken from the PEACH completed by the child's teacher. The questionnaire accomplishes the same goals as the PEACH. |
| CHILD: Children's Home Inventory for Listening Difficulties (Anderson & Smaldino, 2000) | 3 to 12 yrs. (Best for 7 to 12 yrs.) | This is a 15-item parent report questionnaire that rates their child's understanding of speech in various listening conditions. |
| COW: Children's Outcome Worksheets (Williams, 2004) | 4 to 12 yrs. | The child, parent, and teacher complete a worksheet that identifies five situations where improved listening is desired. Improvement is tracked 4 to 6 weeks later. |
| SIFTER: Screening Instrument For Targeting Educational Risk (Anderson, 1989) | 6+ yrs. | This is a 15-item teacher report questionnaire similar to the Preschool SIFTER with adaptations for older children |

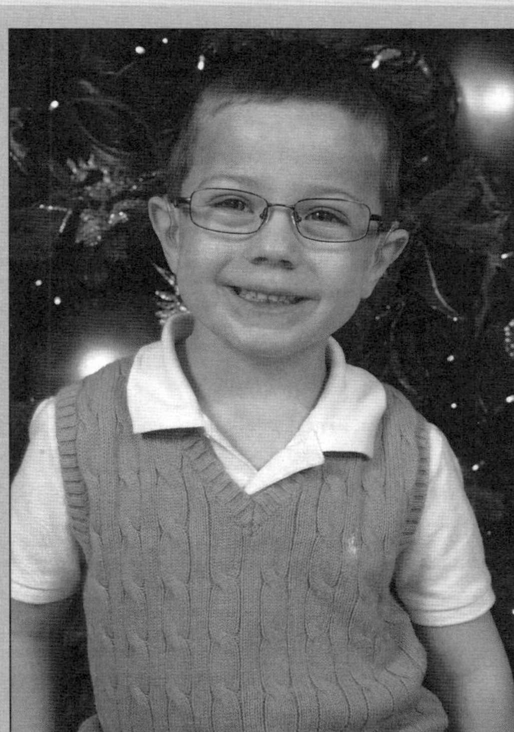

parents are instructed to observe their child for a week, write down examples of how their child is listening in quiet and noisy situations, and then discuss the examples with their service provider. The service provider interviews the parent and then rates how often the child is demonstrating specific behaviors. The diary has been criticized for being difficult to administer due to the challenges in obtaining consistent observations of children across families. Furthermore, the interview process may be inconsistent across examiners (Bagatto, Moodie, Seewald, Bartlett, & Scollie, 2011; Bagatto & Scollie, 2013; Golding et al., 2007).

If the diary portion of the measurement tool is not used, there is a PEACH rating scale (based on questions from the diary) that can be used instead. The scale consists of 13 parent questions that rate how often certain behaviors occur on a 5-point rating scale (never = 0, seldom = 1, sometimes = 2, often = 3, always = 4). Sample questions include, "How often does your child initiate/participate in conversation in a quiet situation?" or "How often does your child understand what you say in the car/bus/train?" A total score is obtained for the last 11 items (the first two items are related to hearing aid use, and are not included in the total score). Subscales for items related to listening in quiet and in noise are also available.

Ching and Hill (2007) demonstrated that the PEACH Diary had good interrater reliability (r = .95) and test-retest reliability (r = .93). The PEACH appears to be valid, as statistical analyses suggest that all the individual items appear to measure the same construct (functional auditory behavior), and early PEACH scores predicted language abilities at 3 years of age (Ching et al., 2010). Ching and Hill also published normative data for the PEACH Diary with a sample of 180 children; 90 children (ages 0.25 to 46 months) had normal hearing, and 90 children (4 months to 19 years) had hearing loss. While the developers of the PEACH have not reported on normative data for the PEACH rating scale, Bagatto and Scollie (2013) administered the English version of the PEACH to 59 children with normal hearing and found high correlations (r = .98) between Ching and Hill's normative data for the PEACH diary and Bagatto and Scollie's smaller sample for the PEACH rating scale. Thus, the norms provided by the PEACH Diary are appropriate for use with the PEACH rating scale. Based on the relative ease in administering the rating scale compared to the diary, researchers have recommended using the PEACH rating scale over the diary format (Bagatto, Moodie, et al., 2011; Moodie et al., 2011). Like the LittlEARS, the PEACH is available in multiple languages. There is a teacher-report version of the scale, called the Teacher's Evaluation of Aural/Oral Performance in Children (TEACH). In summary, evidence shows that the PEACH is a reliable, valid instrument that is easy to administer and score. Used in combination with the LittlEARS, the two measures capture functional auditory skills from birth through preschool.

One potential limitation of using the LittlEARS questionnaire followed by the PEACH was apparent in data from the Outcomes of Children with Hearing Loss longitudinal study (McCreery et al., 2015). In that study, some of the children were administered both the LittlEARS and PEACH questionnaires at the 2-year visit, if the child had reached a criterion score equivalent to maximum performance on the LittlEARS. Many of the children with hearing loss who were well within the normal range on the LittlEARS were found to be in the at-risk or outside of the normative range on the PEACH at the same study visit. In examining the PEACH normative data from Ching and Hill (2007), children under 30 months of age often had lower scores on the PEACH than the older children. The PEACH normative data do not vary as a function of age, unlike the normative data for the LittlEARS (as shown earlier in Figure 6–3). In other words, the scoring guidelines of the PEACH do not account for age of the child. As a result, clinicians may conclude that younger children (less than 24 months of age) are at risk for delays in auditory development based on PEACH scores, when they may actually be making age-appropriate gains. Thus, clinicians should use caution interpreting PEACH scores in children under 24 months who fall into the at-risk range, as the PEACH scores are lower and more variable in this age range.

**Children's Home Inventory for Listening Difficulties (CHILD).** The CHILD was developed by Karen Anderson and Joseph Smaldino (Anderson

& Smaldino, 2000). It can be used with children who are 3 years and older, although it is most appropriate for children between 7 and 12 years of age because children can complete the inventory themselves, starting at around age 7 years. It is available free on Karen Anderson's webpage (http://successforkidswithhearingloss.com/wp-content/uploads/2011/09/CHILD_pgs3-4.pdf). The CHILD is a 15-item parent-report questionnaire, in which parents rate how well their child understands speech in different listening situations (e.g., listening in restaurants, watching television). The child's ability to understand speech is rated on a scale of 1 to 8 (1 = didn't understand any of the message; 8 = heard and understood everything that was said). The measure is scored by adding up the ratings for each question and dividing by 15, to obtain an average of the responses. Subscale scores can be obtained by adding up and calculating the average for items related to five specific listening situations: quiet, noise, distance, social, and media. The 15 items are easy to understand and require little administrative burden on the part of the parent or the service provider. The scope of the CHILD is broad and can be used with children who have mild to profound hearing loss or who use cochlear implants or hearing aids. The CHILD is available in English, Spanish, Arabic, and French. Limitations of the CHILD include a lack of published evidence regarding the reliability or validity of the measure and the fact that there is no normative sample.

**Children's Outcomes Worksheet (COW).** The COW was developed by Gail Whitelaw and Michael Wynne and is intended for use with children between 4 and 12 years of age (Williams, 2004). It is free on the First Years webpage (http://firstyears.org/tests/funclang.htm). The COW was designed as a pediatric version of the Client Oriented Scale of Improvement (COSI; Dillon, James, & Ginis, 1997). The COSI is a validated, reliable adult aural rehabilitation tool, in which clients identify five situations in which they would like to improve in their listening abilities. After the client has undergone aural rehabilitation, he or she revisits the situations with the audiologist and subjectively rates how much ease of listening has improved in those contexts and how well he or she can hear in those situations with amplification. The COW represents a modified version of the COSI. Instead of only the client (in this case, the child) completing the measure, parents and teachers are asked to fill out the survey and set goals for the child.

The administration of the COW is fairly simple. Prior to fitting of new amplification, the child, parent, and teacher each identify five categories related to listening from a list of 15 options, such as during conversations with groups in noise, hearing family members in the home, and hearing the teacher in the classroom. There is an additional or "other" option for situations that were not identified on the list. After identifying the five categories, the child/parent/teacher then notes a specific situation related to each category, such as having a conversation at the child's favorite restaurant. The situations are also ranked in order of importance. Approximately four to six weeks after the fitting of the new device, each member reevaluates their identified target situations and makes two judgments. The first judgment reflects how much change has occurred in the given situation as a result of the new hearing instrument. Degree of change is rated on a scale of 1 to 5 (1 = worse, 2 = no difference, 3 = slightly better, 4 = better, 5 = better). The second judgment is a subjective report of the ability to hear with the new device, in the identified situation. This is also rated on a scale of 1 to 5 (1 = hardly ever, 2 = occasionally, 3 = half the time, 4 = most of the time, and 5 = almost always). The primary intent of the COW is to provide an opportunity for a child, parents, and teachers to identify needs and expectations during the aural habilitation process. In doing so, all parties have "buy in" during transition periods, such as fitting of new hearing aids, use of a school's FM system, or initial stimulation of a second cochlear implant. Although the COW is easy to administer and has good ecological validity, it has not been thoroughly evaluated for its psychometric properties. It is unclear whether the COW correlates with other evidence-based measures of functional auditory skills (concurrent validity) or if it predicts later performance with amplification (predictive validity). The COW appears to have some promise as a counseling tool for families and teachers, but further research is needed to validate this measure.

**Screening Inventory for Targeting Educational Risk (SIFTER).** The SIFTER was developed by Karen Anderson (Anderson, 1989). It is available free on Karen Anderson's webpage (https://successforkidswithhearingloss.com/uploads/SIFTER.pdf). The SIFTER is a popular teacher-report measure with educational audiologists. It consists of 15 questions within five categories (academics, attention, communication, class participation, school behavior). Teachers rate the child's behavior on a scale of 1 to 5, with the meaning of the ratings changing depending on the question. For example, one question asks the teacher to rate the student's class standing relative to other students in the classroom. In this context, 5 represents the upper level of performance and 1 represents the lower level. Another question asks how distractible the student is compared to classmates, with a score of 5 indicating "not very" distractible and 1 indicating "very" distractible. The scores in each content area are added together and the total score within content areas is categorized as a "pass," "marginal," or "fail." The administration booklet emphasizes that the SIFTER is meant to be a screening tool only, and additional testing will be necessary if a child is categorized as failing in any of the content areas. Children in the marginal range should be monitored over time.

Like the CHILD measurement (which has the same author), the SIFTER is easy to understand and takes only a few minutes for the teacher to fill out. Both the CHILD and the SIFTER have been recommended for use with children who have "minimal" hearing loss (i.e., unilateral hearing loss or bilateral hearing loss in the 15 to 40 dB HL). Tharpe (2007) suggests using these tools with this specific population of children with hearing loss as a functional auditory assessment. Children with minimal hearing loss may have subtle behavioral or academic problems that will not show up on standardized assessments. Because the SIFTER is designed to assess real-world listening skills, audiologists and related service providers may be able to identify potential problem areas and formulate management plans. Unfortunately, there is a lack of published psychometric data on the SIFTER, as is the case with the CHILD and the COW. Because we do not know about the reliability or validity of this measure, or have access to current normative data, the SIFTER should only be used in combination with other validated measures and not as the sole assessment tool.

## Speech Perception Measures

As described in this chapter, there are a number of auditory questionnaires that are at the disposal of audiologists. These questionnaires provide insight into the functional listening skills of young children with hearing loss and are valuable tools for tracking progress. Once children are able to provide reliable responses on word recognition measures, however, best-practice guidelines recommend that audiologists should obtain this information during clinic visits. Speech perception testing can inform the audiologist about how children are using their listening skills to discriminate, identify, and comprehend spoken language, with and without amplification. This information is therefore critical in assessing whether children are making appropriate progress with their devices. Many children who have been identified with hearing loss at birth can participate in speech perception tests by age 3 years, unless the child presents with severe developmental delays. Unfortunately, studies suggest that approximately 25% of audiologists working with preschool-age children do not administer aided speech perception tests as part of their routine clinical practice (Muñoz, 2012).

Similar to auditory questionnaires, there are many pediatric speech perception measures that are available to audiologists. These measures vary in terms of how thoroughly they have been validated and how the tests can be administered. Table 6–3 summarizes different test variables of pediatric speech perception measures. Specific measures are appropriate for certain developmental ages or specific populations of children with hearing loss. These tests are reviewed based on the age ranges proposed by the American Academy of Audiology Pediatric Amplification guidelines (2013), but audiologists should always be aware of individual children's performance levels when selecting speech perception tests. If a child is at or close to ceiling performance on a measure that is appropriate for his or her age, the audiologist

**Table 6–3.** Speech Perception Tests for Infants Through School-Age Children

| *Pediatric Speech Perception Measures* | *Age Range* | *Description* |
|---|---|---|
| Open and Closed Set Test (Ertmer, Miller, & Quesenberry, 2004) | 18 mos. to 2 yrs. | These are short word lists that measure speech perception and/or production skills. In the open-set task, the child repeats the spoken word. In the closed-set task, the child identifies the target word from a choice of three pictures. |
| ESP: Early Speech Perception Test (Moog & Geers, 1990) | 3+ yrs. | This is a closed-set test for children with severe to profound hearing loss. It includes a low-verbal and standard version. |
| LNT: Lexical Neighborhood Test & MLNT: Multisyllabic Lexical Neighborhood Test (Kirk et al., 1995) | 3 to 5 yrs. | These open-set tests consist of two 50-word lists, each controlled for the lexical characteristics of the words. LNT includes single-syllable words and the MLNT includes two- and three-syllable words. |
| PBK: Phonetically-Balanced Kindergarten Lists (Haskins, 1949) | 5 to 9 yrs. | These are four 50-word lists composed of kindergarten vocabulary presented in an open-set format. The child is asked to verbally repeat the presented word. |
| CASPA: Computer-Assisted Speech Perception Assessment Test (Mackersie, Boothroyd, & Minniear, 2001) | 5 yrs.–Adult | This test consists of 20 ten-word lists that each contains one of the same 30 phonemes (isophonemic). The lists can be presented in quiet, noise, or with multitalker babble. |
| Pediatric AzBio Sentences (Spahr et al., 2014) | 5 yrs.–Adult | This tests consists of 16 age-appropriate lists of 20 sentences each that can be presented in quiet or with multitalker babble. |
| BKB-SIN: Bamford-Kowal-Bench Speech-in-Noise Test (Bench, Kowal, & Bamford, 1979) | 5 yrs.–Adult | The test consists of 18 list pairs with 10 or 8 sentences each. The SNR is decreased by +3 dB after each sentence. |

should consider administering a more difficult metric. Ceiling performance for speech recognition tests is often defined as a score of 84% correct or higher because that percentage is not considered significantly different than 100% based on the binomial theorem for a 25-item list (Thornton & Raffin, 1978). Conversely, if a child scores close to floor level, the audiologist should consider administering an easier test. Floor performance for a speech recognition test with 25 items is considered anything less than 16% or below chance on a forced-choice or point-to-picture task (50% for two-item choice, 33% for three-item choice, or 25% for a four-item choice).

The degree of difficulty of speech recognition tests can be modified in several ways. One common way of making a speech recognition test more difficult is adding background noise. Not only does adding background noise lower performance on the speech recognition test, but it provides a metric of the child's listening abilities that has been correlated with real-world listening conditions (Hillock-Dunn, Taylor, Buss, & Leibold, 2015). The difficulty of the test can also be modified by adding or taking away linguistic context in the stimulus. Generally, children are able to recognize simple sentences at lower signal-to-noise ratios than monosyllabic words. However, lengthening sentences can also increase the load on a child's working memory and make the task more challenging. Using nonsense words or syllables can force the child to rely on phonemic decoding, which can increase the difficulty of the task relative to real words. Thus, test selection can be individualized to children. This tailored approach ensures that audiologists are obtaining sensitive data that will inform caregivers and professionals about the appropriateness of intervention procedures and the benefits from amplification.

### *Infants and Preschool-Age Children*

In the infant and preschool age range (6 months to 5 years), initial speech perception tests consist of closed-set measures. In order to administer these closed-set tests, children must be able to choose between a limited number of alternatives by pointing. As a child gets close to 100% correct on these closed-set measures, increasingly challenging open-set tests may be introduced. Audiologists may present speech perception tests via monitored live voice (MLV) or recorded speech stimuli. Recorded materials have better reliability than MLV, both within and across clients and test administrators. If a test is delivered via MLV, then the child's score is tied to that specific audiologist's presentation on a given date. The audiologist's presentation will vary from day to day, as well as from other audiologists' presentations. This results in variable scores that weaken the ability to interpret performance scores. The significant variability in scores obtained from MLV administration means that any change in performance cannot be interpreted as an improvement or decrement from previous tests. Although MLV does provide flexibility for the audiologist, recorded speech stimuli are recommended whenever possible.

**Aided Ling 6 Sounds.** The Ling 6 sounds are typically used by speech-language pathologists and auditory-verbal therapists at the start of therapy sessions to determine whether a child's hearing aids or cochlear implants are functioning appropriately. The Ling sounds also have clinical utility for audiologists, however, as they can be used during the validation process as a quick metric for speech sound reception (Scollie et al., 2012). In its most basic format, the Ling sounds consist of three vowels (/i/, /a/, and /u/), representing the corners of the vowel quadrilateral, and three consonants (/m/, /s/, and /ʃ/) that cover the range of speech frequencies in English (Figure 6–4). The therapist will present the sounds one at a time via live voice, often covering his/her face with a *speech hoop* (Figure 6–5). Use of a speech hoop is preferable to covering one's mouth behind one's hand, a piece of paper, or a clipboard, which may reduce the intensity of the speech signal. The sounds are often presented to evaluate listening skills at one of the first three stages in Erber's hierarchy of listening skills (Erber, 1982), depending on the ability level of the client: at the *detection* level, in which the client indicates whether he or she heard the sound; at the *discrimination* level, in which the client determines if two sounds are the same or different; or at the *identification* levels,

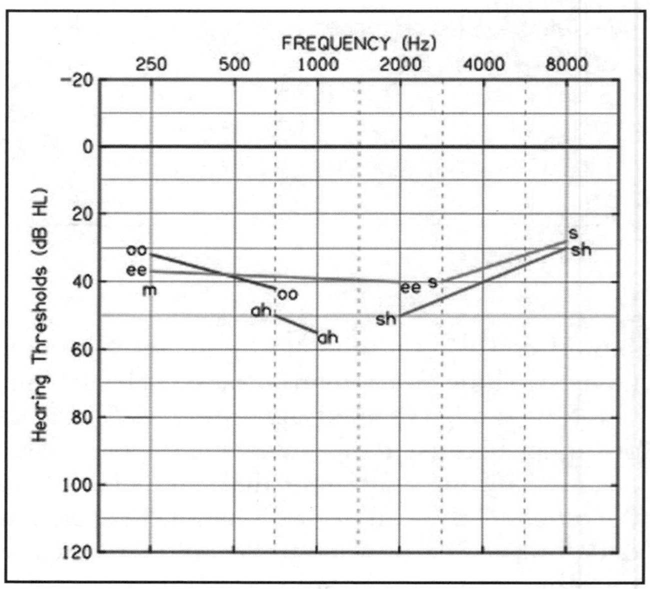


**FIGURE 6–4.** Audiogram showing the frequency and intensity of the Ling sounds that cover the range of speech frequencies in English at a conversational level of speech at 3 feet from the speaker.

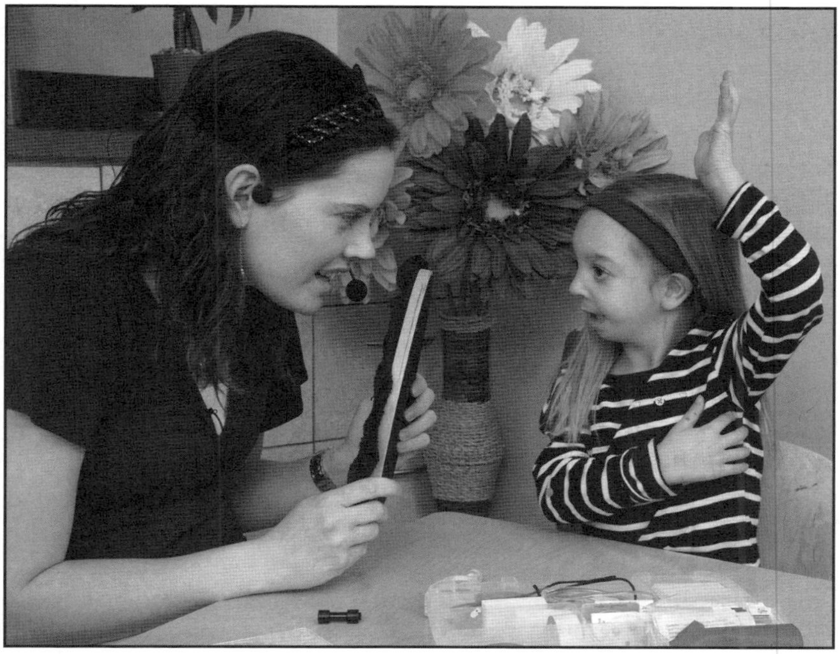

**FIGURE 6–5.** A clinician administering the Ling 6 sound test with a speech hoop.

in which the client repeats the sound. Figure 6–6 depicts a visual representation of Erber's listening hierarchy.

> A speech or listening hoop is a specially designed barrier so the examiner can present sounds to the client without speechreading cues and distortion. Speech hoops are made out of embroidery hoops and two layers of acoustic cloth

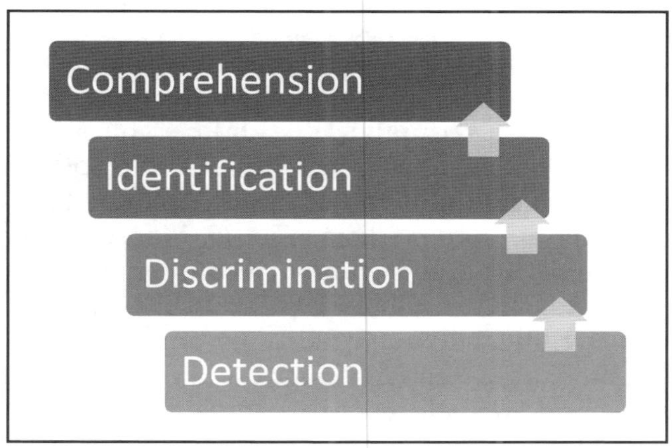


**FIGURE 6–6.** Erber's hierarchy of listening skills (Erber, 1982).

The live voice method of the Ling 6 sounds is often used to assess whether the speech spectrum is audible to a listener. As discussed in earlier chapters, real-ear measures are the best-practice method for determining hearing aid gain and frequency response. For children who wear cochlear implants or bone conduction hearing aids, real-ear measures are not an option for device verification. Instead, audiologists rely on aided sound field thresholds (i.e., functional gain) to verify the hearing devices. There are a number of limitations with using this approach with acoustic hearing aids, however. First, functional gain can be quite time-consuming because multiple thresholds must be obtained across frequencies, both with and without amplification. Most infants do not have the attention span needed to obtain these measures in a single clinic appointment. Second, the stimuli used to measure functional gain (warble tones or narrow band noise) are not encountered in real-world situations and lack ecological validity. Third, hearing aid signal processing strategies may interact with pure-tone stimuli in ways that make results difficult to interpret. For example, feedback suppression algorithms may assume that warble tone sounds used for functional gain assessment are feedback and may adaptively reduce gain for those sounds, negating the validity of the test.

To address these challenges, Scollie et al. (2012) developed a calibrated version of the Ling 6 sounds, called the Ling 6 (HL) test. This version of the Ling sounds was designed to provide audiologists with a reliable means of assessing aided speech perception with infants and young children, but using speech as the stimulus instead of warble tones. The test CD and scoring sheet is available to clinicians on the DSL webpage (http://www.dslio.com). The task is based on the lowest level of Erber's hierarchy, detection. The stimuli consist of a recorded female speaker producing the six Ling sounds. The stimuli are calibrated in dB HL in sound field, to allow for presentation through the audiometer. There are 64 repetitions of the recorded Ling sounds, which can be presented as a standard audiometric threshold detection task (5 dB step sizes, in a two-down, one-up bracketing procedure). Scollie and her colleagues found good test-retest reliability in adults for the recorded version of the Ling 6 (HL) sounds. In a follow-up study, Glista, Scollie, Moodie, and Easwar (2014) found similar results in children ages 3 to 9 years. Glista and her colleagues further investigated test validity by administering questionnaires to nine pediatric audiologists. The questionnaires addressed the quality and clinical utility of the Ling 6 (HL) test. Results indicated that the majority of audiologists surveyed reported that the measure had good clinical utility, was easy to administer, and easy to interpret. The measure takes approximately 2 to 5 minutes to administer. Glista et al. acknowledged that the number of audiologists surveyed was small and further research is needed to validate the measure, particularly with infants. Despite these limitations, the Ling 6 (HL) test has potential value in pediatric audiology as an evidence-based measure of aided speech detection. It can be utilized as a hearing device validation tool for young children who have low attention spans and/or minimal verbal abilities or for clients who cannot be assessed with electroacoustic measures during the verification process (i.e., cochlear implant or bone conduction hearing aid users).

**Open and Closed-Set Test (O & C).** The O & C test measures both speech production and speech perception skills (Ertmer, Miller, & Quesenberry, 2004). It was originally developed as an early articulation measure for younger preschool-age children with hearing loss, but can be used as a word recognition task. It is available on the MED-EL website (http://www.medel-bridge.com). It consists of an open-set task in which the parent or examiner says a target word (e.g., "key") and the child is expected to repeat it back. Next, the parent shows the child a set of three pictures (the target word and two foils) and asks the child to "show me." Figure 6–7 shows an example of the closed-set stimuli. The child is then expected to point to the target picture (the closed-set task). There are 10 monosyllabic target words, selected because they are within the vocabulary of hearing 2-year-olds. The task is scored in three ways: phonemes correctly produced, words correctly approximated from the open-set task, and words correctly identified in the closed-set task.

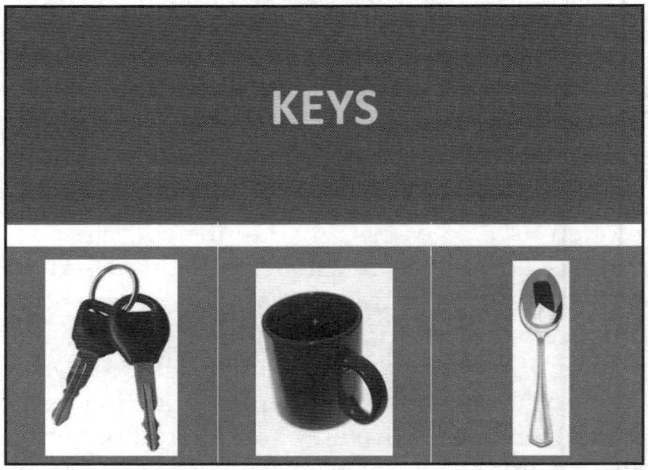


**FIGURE 6–7.** Stimuli from one trial of the *Open and Closed-Set* task (Ertmer, Miller, & Quesenberry, 2004).

A strength of this measure is that it is easy to administer, and parents can be involved in the testing (which may be an advantage with reluctant toddlers). In addition, Ambrose et al. (2014) demonstrated that the O & C at age 2 years had good predictive validity with later articulation skills, and McCreery et al. (2015) found that 2-year-old children with mild-severe hearing loss show a range of word recognition skills on the measure. The child's accuracy on the O & C was associated with their audibility, hearing aid use, and language abilities, suggesting that it is a sensitive measure that reflects variance in those important domains. Additional research is needed to validate this measure and to examine test-retest and interrater reliability.

**Early Speech Perception (ESP) Test.** The ESP is designed for use with children who have severe to profound hearing loss (Moog & Geers, 1990). It is often one of the first speech perception tests administered to young children who utilize cochlear implants. The ESP can be ordered through the Central Institute for the Deaf website. It is a closed-set test that can be administered by MLV or using recorded stimuli. There is a low-verbal version and standard version based on the ability of the child. The low-verbal version is intended for children with minimal vocabulary skills, typically around 2 years of age. The low-verbal version contains 18 toys consisting of monosyllabic words, spondees, trochees, and three-syllable words (e.g., bed, hot dog, baby, ice cream cone, respectively). Figure 6–8 shows some of the toys used in the low-verbal ESP. The objects are presented in closed sets of four items. The standard version is similar, except that the stimuli consist of pictures rather than real objects and are in three sets of 12 pictures. Figure 6–9 displays a live voice administration of the standard version of the ESP. Based on the child's percent correct scores for each of the subtests (pattern perception, spondees, monosyllables), performance is categorized as (1) detection, (2) pattern perception, (3) some word identification, and (4) consistent word identification.

The ESP can be used with children who have varying degrees of hearing loss and children who use hearing aids or cochlear implants, although it may be most informative for children with severe-profound hearing loss who have cochlear implants. A recent study by McCreery et al. (2015) reported on 72 children who were hard of hearing who received the low-verbal ESP at 2 years and 106 children who received the standard ESP at 3 years. Performance was close to ceiling at both ages, suggesting that the ESP may be too easy for

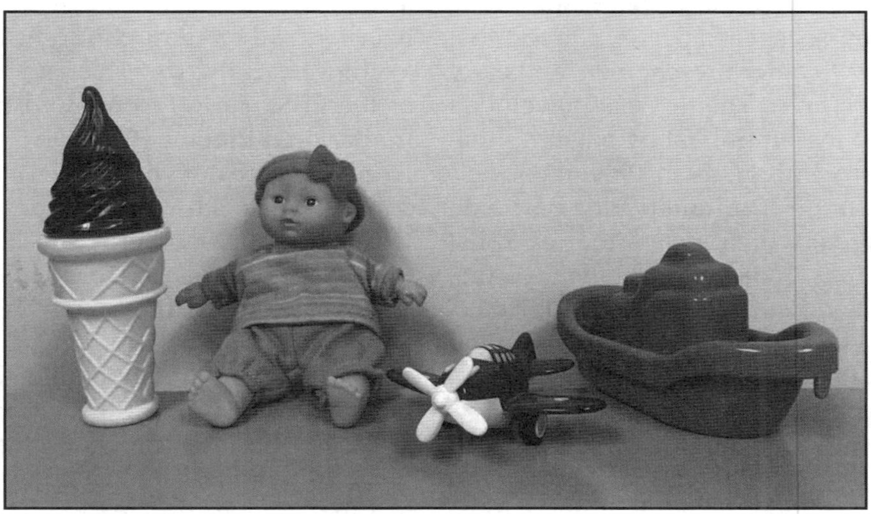

**FIGURE 6–8.** Subset of objects from the low-verbal version of the *Early Speech Perception* test (Moog & Geers, 1990).

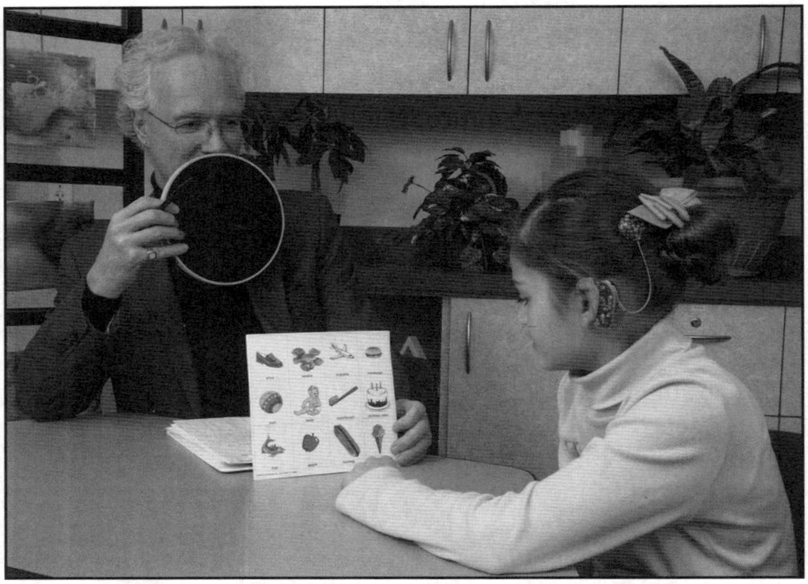

**FIGURE 6–9.** Administration of the *Early Perception Test*—standard version (Moog & Geers, 1990).

typically developing preschool-age children with mild-severe hearing loss (Figure 6–10). In contrast, Eisenberg et al. (2006) tested 2- to 3-year-old children with cochlear implants and found more variability in the scores, which indicates that the ESP may be a sensitive measure for children in the initial period following cochlear implantation.

**Phonetically-Balanced Kindergarten Lists (PBK).** The PBK is an open-set speech perception test that is typically used with older preschoolers and early elementary-age children. The test was developed from Harriet Haskins' unpublished master's thesis at Northwestern University in 1949. It consists of three word lists of 50 phonetically balanced monosyllabic words, which means that each list contained phonemes in approximately the same proportion that they occur in English. A fourth list was included in Haskins' thesis, but was judged to be "more audible" than the other three lists and is not used clinically (Meyer & Pisoni, 1999). It can be administered through MLV or recorded stimuli, usually at 65 or 70 dB SPL. The recorded stimuli consist of a single male talker and can be purchased through Auditec, Inc. During administration, children are instructed to repeat back the words. The measure is scored by calculating whole-word or phoneme recognition.

The PBK is arguably the most commonly used speech perception test for children between the ages of 4 to 6 years old (Muñoz, 2012). Despite its prevalence in clinical settings, researchers have posed valid criticisms of the test. Meyer and Pisoni (1999) pointed out that Haskins tested the equivalence of the PBK lists using adults with normal hearing, rather than children. Kirk and her colleagues have also described additional limitations of the PBK (Kirk, Pisoni, & Osberger, 1995). One limitation is that the PBK lists contain a number of words that are not within the vocabulary of young children, even though it is designed to be used with children. Another limitation is related to the influence of lexical factors on word recognition, specifically word frequency (how often a given word occurs in a language) and neighborhood density (how many phonemically similar words a given word has). The PBK lists were not designed to assess these lexical characteristics. Because of these limitations, Kirk et al. proposed that the PBK lists may underestimate speech perception abilities of children with cochlear implants because they contain unfamiliar words, as well as words that

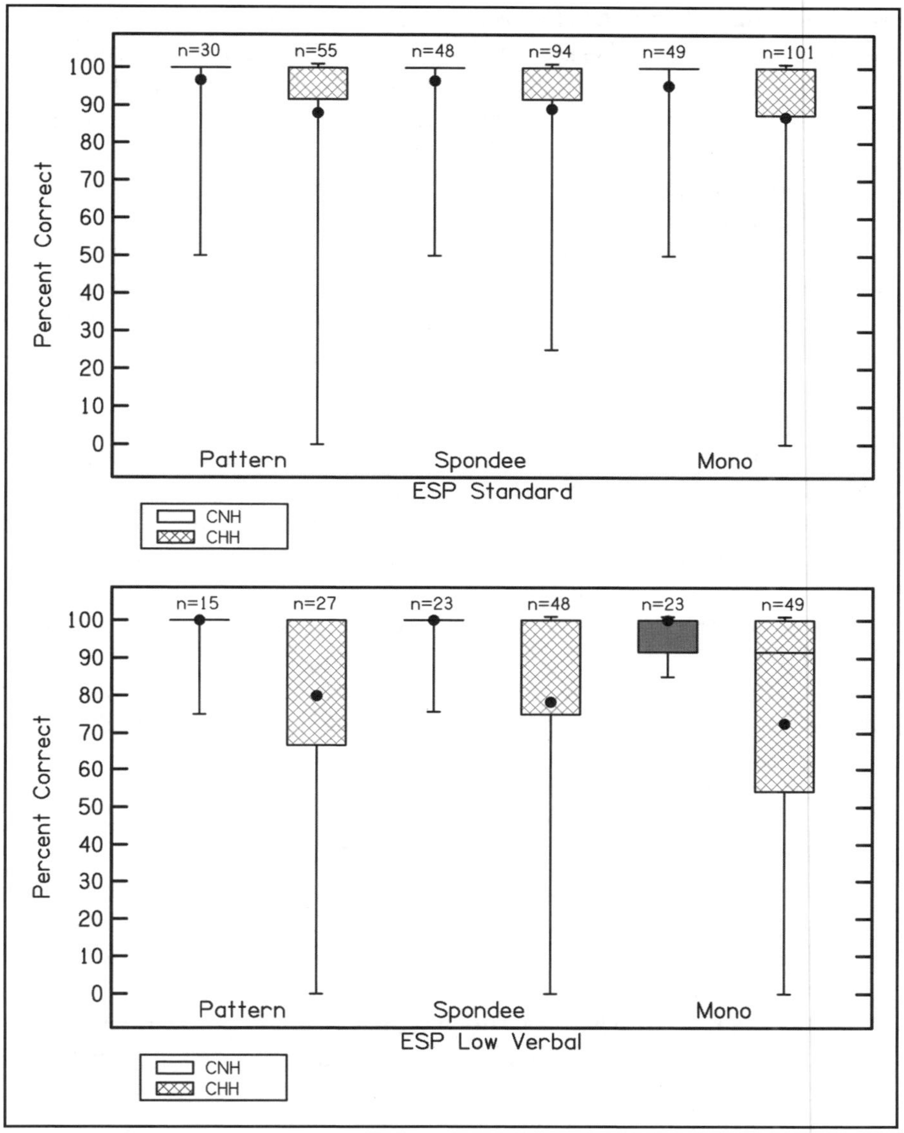


**FIGURE 6–10.** Scores on the standard (*top*) and low-verbal (*bottom*) versions of the *Early Speech Perception* (Moog & Geers, 1990) test for children with normal hearing (*white*) and children who are hard of hearing (*hatched white*). The boxes represent the 25th to 75th percentiles (interquartile range) and the whiskers represent the 5th and 95th percent confidence intervals of the mean. Solid lines display the median and circles are the mean (adapted from McCreery et al., 2015).

are easily confused with similar sounding words. These considerations should be weighed against the positive aspects of the PBK, which are that it is relatively easy to administer and score. Despite these limitations, McCreery and colleagues (2015) found that PBK scores reflected individual differences in aided audibility and vocabulary skills in four and five year-old children with mild-to-severe hearing loss, suggesting that the test is sensitive to differences in these factors.

**Multisyllabic Lexical Neighborhood Test (MLNT) and Lexical Neighborhood Test (LNT).** Karen Kirk and her colleagues at Indiana University developed the MLNT and LNT to address some of the limitations of the PBK (Kirk et al., 1995), specifically the lack of sensitivity in speech perception skills for children with cochlear implants or hearing aids. Like the PBK, the lists can be presented through MLV or a recorded version. The CD can be purchased through Auditec, Inc.

The MLNT and LNT each contain two lists (24 words on each MLNT list, and 50 words on each LNT list). Half of the list is considered "easy" words and half are considered "hard" words, based on the lexical characteristics of the stimuli. These lexical characteristics, word frequency, and neighborhood density, are based on assumptions from a theoretical framework of spoken word recognition, known as the Neighborhood Activation Model (NAM; Luce & Pisoni, 1998). According to NAM, easy words consist of words that are high frequency (frequently occurring in the lexicon) and low density (few similar sounding words, or "neighbors"). Examples of easy words from the MLNT and LNT include *children* and *girl*, respectively. Because they occur often and are not likely to be confused with other words, easy words are recognized faster and more accurately than hard words. Hard words have the reverse characteristics: they are low frequency and have high density. Examples of hard words from the MLNT and LNT include *butter* and *pie*, respectively. Thus, listeners are less likely to identify these words and may confuse the target words with other words. By controlling for the lexical characteristics of the stimuli, Kirk and colleagues were able to create a list of words that was sensitive to the vocabulary levels of children with hearing loss. In addition, the MLNT/LNT lists have good test-retest reliability in children with hearing loss, and the performance across lists is equivalent.

### School-Age Children

Typically, by the time children reach first or second grade, most are capable of completing recorded open-set speech perception tests. Children who are hard of hearing may reach ceiling levels of performance fairly quickly on aided word recognition tests in quiet by this age. McCreery et al. (2015) described results on the PBK and LNT for a group of children (ages 4–8 years) who were hard of hearing, used spoken English as their primary language, and had cognitive skills within normal limits. On average, the participants scored 85% on the PBK and LNT easy and hard lists. The presence of ceiling effects on these open-set tests limits their clinical utility because the measure cannot assess actual variation in performance; thus, the speech perception test loses its sensitivity. Another limitation of speech perception tests in quiet, particularly monosyllabic tests, is that they lack ecological validity. Children will often encounter the deleterious effects of background noise in the real world, particularly in the classroom setting. Testing in quiet does not reflect the challenges of listening in noise, which has an even greater negative impact on children with hearing loss than children with normal hearing (Finitzo-Hieber & Tillman, 1978). The following section reviews some of the available pediatric tests that assess listening in noise.

**Computer-Assisted Speech Perception Assessment Test (CASPA).** The CASPA is a recorded monosyllabic word recognition in noise test (Mackersie, Boothroyd, & Minniear, 2001). The stimuli consist of 20 lists of consonant-vowel-consonant words presented by a female talker, with 10 words in each list. Rather than being phonetically balanced, each list is isophonemic. This means that every list contains one example of the same 30 phonemes. The CASPA software allows for flexible presentation of the stimuli. The examiner can decide whether to use a carrier phrase ("Say the word _____.") or no carrier phrase. Words can be presented in quiet, steady-state white noise, or multitalker babble. When the word lists are presented in noise using the CASPA software, the noise level is fixed at 55 dB SPL and the words can be presented in 5-dB steps, ranging from 45 dB to 75 dB SPL. Thus, the signal-to-noise ratio (SNR) can vary from −10 dB SNR to +20 dB SNR. The software randomizes the order of presentation of words both within and across lists.

Figure 6–11 shows an example of the CASPA computer screen during test administration. The examiner enters the word that the listener says

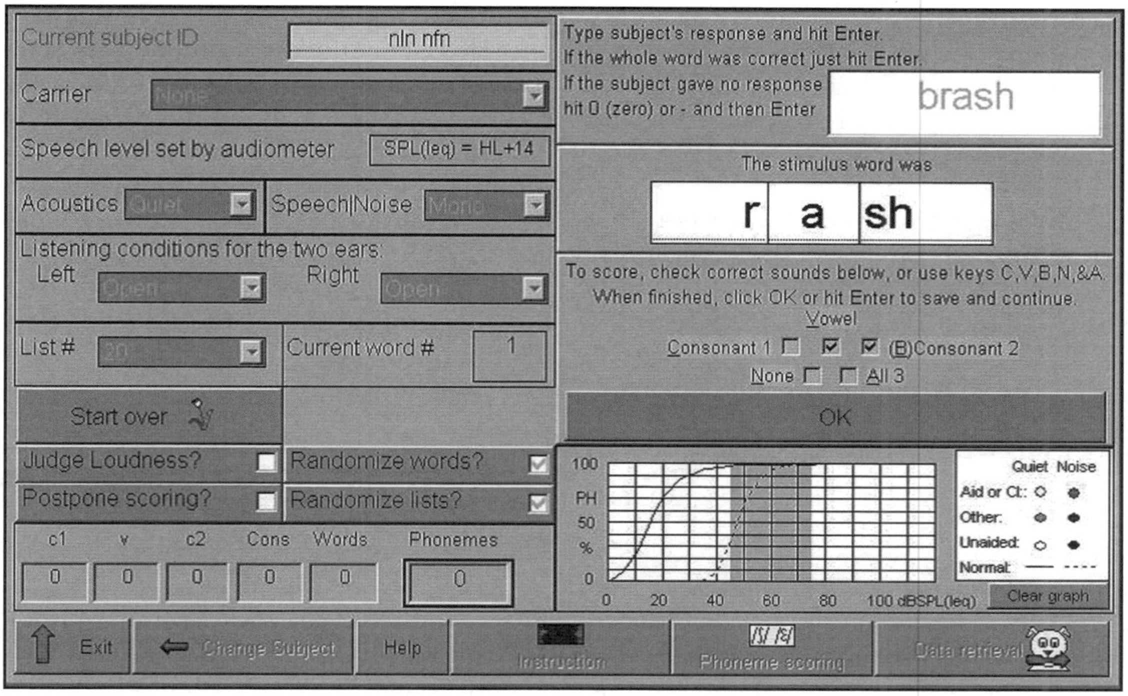


**FIGURE 6–11.** Example of the *Computer Assisted Speech Perception Assessment* (CASPA) computer screen during test administration (Mackersie, Boothroyd, & Minniear, 2001).

and then indicates which phonemes the listener perceives correctly. The software scores performance as percent correct for whole words phonemes, consonants, and vowels, displaying scores in a Microsoft Excel sheet. It will also graph the performance-intensity function, if the examiner presents multiple lists at different presentation levels. It takes approximately one minute to present a single list, so it is not time-consuming to obtain scores across a range of SNRs.

The CASPA can be reliably administered to children as young as 5 years of age (McCreery et al., 2010) and has been studied in 7- to 9-year old children who have hearing loss (McCreery et al., 2015). One limitation of the CASPA is that the scores across lists are not equivalent. Mackersie et al. (2001) tested the equivalency across all of the lists with 20 adults with normal hearing. Four of the lists (lists 3, 6, 7, 16) were found to have significantly higher phoneme correct scores than the remaining 16 lists, leading the authors to suggest excluding these four lists during test administration.

**Pediatric AzBio Sentences.** The Pediatric AzBio Sentences (a.k.a, "Baby Bios") are an adaptation of the adult AzBio sentence lists (Spahr et al., 2012). The sentences are less difficult than the adult version and the content is more age-appropriate. For example, "I'll have a cranberry and vodka, please," a sentence in the adult version, has been excluded from the pediatric version. The Pediatric AzBio lists consist of 16 equivalent lists with 20 unique sentences per list, all presented by a single female talker. The sentences can be presented in quiet or with multitalker babble. Performance variability has been examined in adult and pediatric cochlear implant users to assess the validity of the measure. Results from the validation study suggest that the Pediatric AzBio is appropriate for measuring speech perception performance for children with hearing loss (Spahr et al., 2014). The number of equivalent lists is a strength of the Pediatric AzBio because audiologists can measure progress over time or across multiple conditions (e.g., with or without an assistive listening device) without having to repeat lists. One weakness of the measure is that the performance variability measures were collected in adults and children with cochlear implants. Further validation is needed for children who are hard of hearing and use hearing aids.

**Bamford-Kowal-Bench Speech-in-Noise Test (BKB-SIN).** The BKB-SIN is a speech-in-noise measure (Bench, Kowal, & Bamford, 1979). It is intended for children and adults for whom the QuickSIN is too difficult (Wilson, McArdle, & Smith, 2007). The CDs and test manual are available on the Etymotic webpage. The current version of the test consists of 18 list pairs (e.g., List 1A and List 1B) that are equated for difficulty. The list pairs are presented together. For lists 1 to 8, there are 10 sentences within each list. Lists 9 to 18 have eight sentences per list. The sentences consist of simple vocabulary and grammar. They are derived from language samples of children and are at the language level of a typically developing first grader (Bench et al., 1979). When administering this measure, the SNR automatically decreases in 3-dB SNR steps, starting at +21 dB SNR and ending at −6 dB SNR.

The BKB provides a score that is referred to as the SNR-50 (signal-to-noise ratio for 50% correct). The SNR-50 is calculated by totaling the number of key words correctly identified in a list and subtracting that value from 23.5. The values for the list pairs (List A and List B) are then averaged together to obtain the SNR-50. The goal of the BKB-SIN is to document "SNR loss," which is the dB difference between the SNR that is needed to obtain 50% of key words for a listener compared to normative scores for same-age, hearing peers (Schafer, 2010). For example, a 7-year-old child may obtain an SNR-50 of +5 dB. The average SNR-50 for children between 7 and 10 years of age is +0.8 dB. Therefore, this child's SNR loss is +4.2 dB. The SNR loss can be used to determine whether amplification is providing benefit or if directional microphones or assistive listening devices are warranted.

Schafer (2010) conducted a critical review of several pediatric speech in noise tests, including the BKB-SIN. She reported that this measure showed high validity and reliability, was easy to administer and score, and was highly flexible for audiologists. Another strength was that it was portable and could be administered in classroom settings, where it may be important to measure listening in noise. The noise stimuli consist of multi-talker babble, which simulates real-world listening situations. Schafer noted weaknesses as well, specifically that the vocabulary may be too simple for school-age children. Because of the changing levels of the noise, however, the likelihood of achieving ceiling performance is extremely low.

## FUTURE CONSIDERATION AND DIRECTIONS FOR RESEARCH

Tremendous progress has been made in the past decade to develop new tools that can be used to monitor outcomes in children who have hearing loss and to ensure that they meet appropriate auditory development milestones. Tools developed prior to the advent of newborn hearing screening and early hearing detection and intervention programs may not be appropriate for children who are born with hearing loss today, who have considerable advantages over previous generations of children with hearing loss. We therefore should anticipate that the current tools may eventually not meet the needs as outcomes in children with hearing loss continue to improve. The LittlEARS questionnaire is one current example. More than half of the children who were hard of hearing in a recent study reached a criterion score by 18 months of age (McCreery et al., 2015), suggesting that new tools may be needed to assess the needs of children with hearing loss soon.

A major limitation of current speech recognition tests is that speech recognition is often not testable until 18 months to 2 years of age, which is much later than decisions that are being made about cochlear implantation, which is typically around 12 months. In response to this need, researchers are attempting to develop tools that can be used to assess speech pattern contrast recognition during infancy (Martinez, Eisenberg, Boothroyd, & Visser-Dumont, 2008). Based on experimental paradigms, infants are habituated to a speech sound and then conditioned, using visual reinforcement to turn their head to a novel speech contrast. This approach is still in the early phases of research and not in widespread clinical use, but offers some promise for earlier assessment of speech perception in infants with hearing loss.

Another recent development in the area of pediatric outcome measures is emerging from research related to cortical auditory-evoked potentials. Using electrodes placed on the head, synthetic speech stimuli can be presented to a child, and his or her brain's response to those sounds can be measured objectively while the child watches a quiet video. The ability to objectively assess speech recognition at the cortical level is a major leap forward, not only for infants who may be too young to reliably participate in speech recognition assessment, but also for older children who have significant motor or cognitive delays that prevent them from participating in traditional assessments of speech recognition. More research is needed before this measure can be reliably used in a clinical setting, but feasibility studies have been published with small samples of children with normal hearing and children who wear hearing aids (Golding et al., 2007).

## OUTCOMES VALIDATION: PUTTING IT ALL TOGETHER

The purpose of this chapter thus far has been to provide a list of viable options for monitoring auditory development outcomes in children who wear hearing aids. A wide range of options are available, and we have tried to focus the discussion on measures that are practical in a clinical environment. At each clinical visit, hearing aid verification should be completed, an assessment of hearing aid use using data logging or parent report should be conducted, and age-appropriate speech recognition and auditory development questionnaires should be administered as a validation of the child's current hearing assistive technology. Monitoring these outcomes over time documents the child's progress and helps to identify potential developmental red flags. If speech recognition is assessed at levels used for hearing aid verification, the relationship between the child's aided audibility through their hearing aids and speech recognition abilities can be compared.

## SUMMARY AND CONCLUSIONS

A wide range of outcome measures are available for children who wear hearing aids, including parental questionnaires and measures of speech recognition. As part of the follow-up process after children are fitted with hearing aids, auditory development questionnaires and aided speech recognition assessment should be completed at each visit to document the child's progress with the hearing aids and to help identify potential developmental red flags. If these measures are conducted in a consistent and systematic manner, the information can be useful for parents and other professionals who may serve on the child's plan of care. New tools, such as aided cortical auditory evoked potentials, may be useful in documenting cortical responses to sounds in children who cannot participate in outcomes measurement due to the presence of other motor or cognitive disabilities. Many of these measures have a growing base of research to support their reliability and validity. Measures are now available that cover the range from infancy through the teenage years.

## REFERENCES

American Academy of Audiology. (2013). *Clinical practice guidelines: Pediatric amplification*. Reston, VA: Author

Ambrose, S. E., Berry, L. M. U., Walker, E. A., Harrison, M., Oleson, J., & Moeller, M. P. (2014). Speech sound production in 2-year-olds who are hard of hearing. *American Journal of Speech-Language Pathology, 23*(2), 91–104.

Anderson, K. L. (1989). *Screening instrument for targeting educational risk.* Danville, IL: Interstate.

Anderson, K. L., & Smaldino, J. J. (2000). *Children's Home Inventory for Listening Difficulties (CHILD)*. Retrieved from http://successforkidswithhearingloss.com/tests/

Bagatto, M. P., Brown, C. L., Moodie, S. T., & Scollie, S. D. (2011). External validation of the LittlEARS® Auditory Questionnaire with English-speaking families of Canadian children with normal hearing. *International Journal of Pediatric Otorhinolaryngology, 75*(6), 815–817.

Bagatto, M. P., Moodie, S. T., Malandrino, A. C., Richert, F. M., Clench, D. A., & Scollie, S. D. (2011). The University of Western Ontario Pediatric Audiological Monitoring Protocol (UWO PedAMP). *Trends in Amplification, 15*(1), 57–76.

Bagatto, M. P., Moodie, S. T., Seewald, R. C., Bartlett, D. J., & Scollie, S. D. (2011). A critical review of audiological outcome measures for infants and children. *Trends in Hearing, 15*(1), 23–33.

Bagatto, M. P., & Scollie, S. D. (2013). Validation of the Parents' Evaluation of Aural/Oral Performance of Children (PEACH) Rating Scale. *Journal of the American Academy of Audiology, 24*(2), 121–125.

Bass-Ringdahl, S. M. (2010). The relationship of audibility and the development of canonical babbling in young children with hearing impairment. *Journal of Deaf Studies and Deaf Education, 15*(3), 287–310.

Bench, J., Kowal, A., & Bamford, J. (1979). The BKB (Bamford-Kowal-Bench) sentence lists for partially hearing children. *British Journal of Audiology, 13*, 108–112.

Capone, N. C., & McGregor, K. K. (2004). Gesture development: A review for clinical and research practices. *Journal of Speech, Language, and Hearing Research, 47*(1), 173–186.

Ching, T. Y., Crowe, K., Martin, V., Day, J., Mahler, N., Youn, S., . . . Orsini, J. (2010). Language development and everyday functioning of children with hearing loss assessed at 3 years of age. *International Journal of Speech-Language Pathology, 12*(2), 124–131.

Ching, T. Y., & Hill, M. (2007). The Parents' Evaluation of Aural/Oral Performance of Children (PEACH) scale: Normative data. *Journal of the American Academy of Audiology, 18*(3), 220–235.

Coninx, F., Weichbold, V., Tsiakpini, L., Autrique, E., Bescond, G., Tamas, L., . . . Le Maner-Idrissi, G. (2009). Validation of the LittlEARS® Auditory Questionnaire in children with normal hearing. *International Journal of Pediatric Otorhinolaryngology, 73*(12), 1761–1768.

Dillon, H., James, A., & Ginis, J. (1997). Client Oriented Scale of Improvement (COSI) and its relationship to several other measures of benefit and satisfaction provided by hearing aids. *Journal of the American Academy of Audiology, 8*, 27–43.

Eisenberg, L. S., Johnson, K. C., Martinez, A. S., Cokely, C. G., Tobey, E. A., Quittner, A. L., . . . Niparko, J. K. (2006). Speech recognition at 1-year follow-up in the childhood development after cochlear implantation study: Methods and preliminary findings. *Audiology and Neurotology, 11*(4), 259–268.

Erber, N. (1982). *Auditory training*. Washington, DC: Alexander Graham Bell Association for the Deaf.

Ertmer, D. J., Miller, C. M., & Quesenberry, J. K. (2004). *The Open and Closed-Set Task. Assessment procedure.* West Lafayette, IN: Purdue University.

Finitzo-Hieber, T., & Tillman, T. W. (1978). Room acoustics effects on monosyllabic word discrimination ability for normal and hearing-impaired children. *Journal of Speech, Language, and Hearing Research, 21*(3), 440–458.

Gallaudet Research Institute. (2011). *Regional and national summary report of data from the 2009–10 Annual Survey of Deaf and Hard of Hearing Children and Youth.* Washington, DC: GRI, Gallaudet University.

Glista, D., Scollie, S., Moodie, S., & Easwar, V. (2014). The Ling 6 (HL) test: Typical pediatric performance data and clinical use evaluation. *Journal of the American Academy of Audiology, 25*(10), 1008–1021.

Golding, M., Pearce, W., Seymour, J., Cooper, A., Ching, T., & Dillon, H. (2007). The relationship between obligatory cortical auditory evoked potentials (CAEPs) and functional measures in young infants. *Journal of the American Academy of Audiology, 18*(2), 117–125.

Haskins, H. L. (1949). *A phonetically balanced test of speech discrimination skills for children* (Unpublished master's thesis). Northwestern University, Evanston, IL.

Hillock-Dunn, A., Taylor, C., Buss, E., & Leibold, L. J. (2015). Assessing speech perception in children with hearing loss: What conventional clinical tools may miss. *Ear and Hearing, 36*(2), e57–e60.

Holden-Pitt, L., & Diaz, J. A. (1998). Thirty years of the annual survey of deaf and hard-of-hearing children and youth: A glance over the decades. *American Annals of the Deaf, 143*(2), 71–76.

Joint Committee on Infant Hearing. (2007). Year 2007 position statement: Principles and guidelines for early hearing detection and intervention programs. *Pediatrics, 120*, 898–921.

Kirk, K. I., Pisoni, D. B., & Osberger, M. J. (1995). Lexical effects on spoken word recognition by pediatric cochlear implant users. *Ear and Hearing, 16*(5), 470–481.

Kishon-Rabin, L., Taitelbaum, R., Elichai, O., Maimon, D., Debyiat, D., & Chazan, N. (2001). Developmental aspects of the IT-MAIS in normal-hearing babies. *Israeli Journal of Speech and Hearing, 23*(1), 12–22.

Luce, P. A., & Pisoni, D. B. (1998). Recognizing spoken words: The neighborhood activation model. *Ear and Hearing, 19*(1), 1–36.

Mackersie, C. L., Boothroyd, A., & Minniear, D. (2001). Evaluation of the Computer-Assisted Speech Perception Assessment Test (CASPA). *Journal of the American Academy of Audiology, 12*(8), 390–396.

MacNeilage, P. F., Davis, B. L., Kinney, A., & Matyear, C. L. (2000). The motor core of speech: A comparison of serial organization patterns in infants and languages. *Child Development, 71*, 153–163.

Martinez, A., Eisenberg, L., Boothroyd, A., & Visser-Dumont, L. (2008). Assessing speech pattern contrast perception in infants: Early results on VRASPAC. *Otology and Neurotology, 29*(2), 183–188.

McCreery, R., Ito, R., Spratford, M., Lewis, D., Hoover, B., & Stelmachowicz, P. G. (2010). Performance-intensity functions for normal-hearing adults and children using CASPA. *Ear and Hearing, 31*(1), 95–101.

McCreery, R. W., Walker, E. A., Spratford, M., Oleson, J., Bentler, R., Holte, L., & Roush, P. (2015). Speech recognition and parent ratings from auditory development questionnaires in children who are hard of hearing. *Ear and Hearing, 36*, 60S–75S.

Meyer, T. A., & Pisoni, D. B. (1999). Some computational analyses of the PBK test: Effects of frequency and lexical density on spoken word recognition. *Ear and Hearing, 20*(4), 363–371.

Moeller, M. P., Hoover, B., Putman, C., Arbataitis, K., Bohnenkamp, G., Peterson, B., . . . Stelmachowicz, P. (2007a). Vocalizations of infants with hearing loss compared with infants with normal hearing: Part I–Phonetic development. *Ear and Hearing, 28*(5), 605–627.

Moeller, M. P., Hoover, B., Putman, C., Arbataitis, K., Bohnenkamp, G., Peterson, B., . . . Stelmachowicz, P. (2007b). Vocalizations of infants with hearing loss compared with infants with normal hearing: Part II–Transition to words. *Ear and Hearing, 28*(5), 628–642.

Moodie, S. T., Kothari, A., Bagatto, M. P., Seewald, R., Miller, L. T., & Scollie, S. D. (2011). Knowledge translation in audiology promoting the clinical application of best evidence. *Trends in Amplification, 15*(1), 5–22.

Moog, J. S., & Geers, A. E. (1990). *Early Speech Perception Test.* St Louis, MO: Central Institute for the Deaf.

Muñoz, K. F. (2012). Aided speech perception testing practices for children three to six years of age with permanent hearing loss. *Journal of Educational Audiology, 18*, 53–60.

Oller, D. K., & Eilers, R. E. (1988). The role of audition in infant babbling. *Child Development, 59*, 441–449.

Robbins, A.M., Svirksy, M.A., Osberger, M.J., & Pisoni, D.B. (1998). Beyond the audiogram: The role of functional assessments. In F. Bess (Ed.), *Children with hearing impairments: Contemporary Trends.* Nashville, TN: Vanderbilt Bill Wilkerson Press.

Robinshaw, H. M. (1995). Early intervention for hearing impairment: Differences in the timing of communicative and linguistic development. *British Journal of Audiology, 29*(6), 315–334.

Schafer, E. (2010). Speech perception in noise measures for children: A critical review and case studies. *Journal of Educational Audiology, 16*, 4–15.

Scollie, S., Glista, D., Tenhaaf, J., Dunn, A., Malandrino, A., Keene, K., & Folkeard, P. (2012). Stimuli and normative data for detection of Ling-6 sounds in hearing level. *American Journal of Audiology, 21*(2), 232–241.

Spahr, A. J., Dorman, M. F., Litvak, L. M., Cook, S. J., Loiselle, L. M., DeJong, M. D., . . . Gifford, R. H. (2014). Development and validation of the pediatric AzBio sentence lists. *Ear and Hearing, 35*(4), 418–422.

Spahr, A. J., Dorman, M. F., Litvak, L. M., Van Wie, S., Gifford, R. H., Loizou, P. C., . . . Cook, S. (2012). Development and validation of the AzBio sentence lists. *Ear and Hearing, 33*(1), 112–117.

Spencer, P. E. (1993). Communication behaviors of infants with hearing loss and their hearing mothers. *Journal of Speech, Language, and Hearing Research, 36*(2), 311–321.

Stoel-Gammon, C. (1989). Prespeech and early speech development of two late talkers. *First Language, 9*(6), 207–223.

Tharpe, A. M. (2007). Minimal hearing loss in children: The facts and the fiction. *Sound Foundation Through Early Amplification. Proceedings of the 4th International Conference.* United Kingdom: Cambrian Printers.

Thornton, A. R., & Raffin, M. J. (1978). Speech-discrimination scores modeled as a binomial variable. *Journal of Speech, Language, and Hearing Research, 21*(3), 507–518.

Walker, E. A., & Bass-Ringdahl, S. (2008). Babbling complexity and its relationship to speech and language outcomes in children with cochlear implants. *Otology and Neurotology, 29*(2), 225–229.

Wiley, S., & Moeller, M. P. (2007). Red flags for disabilities in children who are deaf/hard of hearing. *ASHA Leader, 12*, 8–29.

Williams, C. N. (2004). COW—Designed with children in mind. *Hearing Journal, 57*(3), 68.

Wilson, R. H., McArdle, R. A., & Smith, S. L. (2007). An evaluation of the BKB-SIN, HINT, QuickSIN, and WIN materials on listeners with normal hearing and listeners with hearing loss. *Journal of Speech, Language, and Hearing Research, 50*(4), 844–856.

Zaidman-Zait, A., & Dromi, E. (2007). Analogous and distinctive patterns of prelinguistic communication in toddlers with and without hearing loss. *Journal of Speech, Language, and Hearing Research, 50*(5), 1166–1180.

Zheng, Y., Soli, S. D., Wang, K., Meng, J., Meng, Z., Xu, K., & Tao, Y. (2009). A normative study of early prelingual auditory development. *Audiology and Neurotology, 14*(4), 214–222.

Zimmerman-Phillips, S., & Osberger, M. (1997). *Meaningful Auditory Integration Scale (IT-MAIS) for Infants and Toddlers.* Sylmar, CA: Advanced Bionics.

# 7

# Hearing Aid Connectivity

*Meredith Spratford, Ryan W. McCreery, and Elizabeth A. Walker*

## INTRODUCTION

As discussed in previous chapters in this text, we have empirical evidence to support an association between auditory access and language development for children who are hard of hearing (McCreery et al., 2015; Stiles, Bentler, & McGregor, 2012; Tomblin et al., 2014, 2015). Hearing aid fitting is an important first step in early intervention for children who are hard of hearing. However, hearing aids may not be adequate for promoting auditory access in all listening environments encountered by children who wear hearing aids. In situations where environmental noise, distance from the talker, or reverberation from the listening space are barriers to auditory access, audiologists should consider supportive technologies. Hearing assistive technology (HAT), in addition to technologies that promote connectivity between a child's hearing aids and multimedia devices, can increase auditory exposure over time and reduce the risk of speech, language, and auditory delays. The following chapter provides a summary of the factors that may limit a child's auditory access with hearing aids. We also describe different HATs that are appropriate for children with hearing loss and discuss outcomes, challenges, and solutions to using HAT across different age groups.

## HOW REMOTE MICROPHONE HAT AND CONNECTIVE DEVICES CONTRIBUTE TO CUMULATIVE AUDITORY EXPERIENCE

Well-fit, consistently-worn hearing aids support access to linguistic input, leading to improved speech and language development in children who are hard of hearing (Tomblin et al., 2014). However, many children who wear hearing aids remain at risk for delays in language development. One potential source of these persistent delays is related to limitations of hearing aids. It is a challenge for hearing aids to make speech audible in complex listening environments where speech is are presented from a distance, in reverberation, or background noise. Hearing aid features and signal processing strategies, such as directional microphones and noise reduction algorithms, can help to minimize the negative effects of background noise on listener comfort and perception. As discussed in Chapter 3, however, we lack evidence to support the degree to which these advanced hearing aid features benefit children when speakers are at a distance or in noisy and reverberant environments (Ching et al., 2009; Kuk et al., 1999; Pittman, 2011; Stelmachowicz et al., 2010). Remote microphone HAT and connectivity devices may help to increase a child's access in many realistic listening environments above and beyond the benefits of hearing aids alone.

Limited or inconsistent hearing aid use is another potential source of language delays for children who wear hearing aids (Tomblin et al., 2015). If hearing aids provide limited benefit in situations with noise and reverberation, for example, children may be less likely to use their hearing aids in this environment. In the sections that follow, the effects of remote microphone and connective technology on children's cumulative access to linguistic input is detailed.

## Effects of Remote Microphone HAT and Connective Devices on Audibility

The child's degree of hearing loss, background noise, distance from the speaker of interest, and reverberation can limit audibility and subsequently, the child's ability to understand speech or learn with their hearing aids. A brief summary of how each of these factors can limit a child's access with hearing aids. How HAT may resolve these issues is discussed in the following sections.

### *Degree of Hearing Loss*

As noted in Chapters 1 and 3, the child's degree of hearing loss has a significant negative association with aided audibility. Due to constraints of amplification and the child's dynamic range, hearing aid users with greater degrees of hearing loss have poorer audibility with amplification than listeners with mild degrees of hearing loss. Even optimally fitted hearing aids may not provide sufficient audibility for listeners with severe or profound hearing loss. Lack of audibility through hearing aids due to the child's degree of hearing loss may necessitate the use of HAT or other technologies to improve the access a child has to their auditory environment.

Degree of hearing loss can also influence whether a child receives HAT. For example, children with mild hearing loss in the Outcomes of Children with Hearing Loss (OCHL) study were less likely to receive an FM system for home use compared to children who have poorer hearing thresholds (Walker, Curran, Spratford, & Roush, submitted), potentially reflecting professional and parent understanding that children who have poor hearing ability require a cleaner, more audible input signal due to constraints of a reduced dynamic range of hearing and the potential for compression-related distortion from high-gain hearing aids. On the other hand, it may also reflect an underestimation of the need for consistent auditory access for children with mild hearing loss. As discussed throughout the text, children with mild degrees of hearing loss may experience significant disadvantages compared to peers with normal hearing. The use of HAT for children with mild hearing loss may be important in addressing difficulties listening in background noise, or to speech originating from a distance. These areas are not always enhanced with amplification alone.

### *Distance Between Listener and Speaker*

In addition to characteristics of the child's hearing and hearing aid fitting, environmental factors may also impact the audibility of speech through amplification. The distance between the listener and speaker impacts the audibility of speech. The inverse square law dictates that doubling the distance between the talker and listener results in a 6 dB decrease in the intensity of the initial speech signal. Decreased intensity with distance results in reduced speech audibility. Consider how the audibility of a parent or teacher's voice decreases from the front of a quiet room at 1 meter away from the child, to the back of the room at 4 meters away from the child (Figure 7–1). The level of speech decreases from 60 to 54 dB SPL, from 1 meter to 2 meters. From 2 meters to 4 meters, the level of speech further decreases from 54 to 48 dB SPL. The lower speech level results in a corresponding decrease in audibility from .76 to .44, as measured

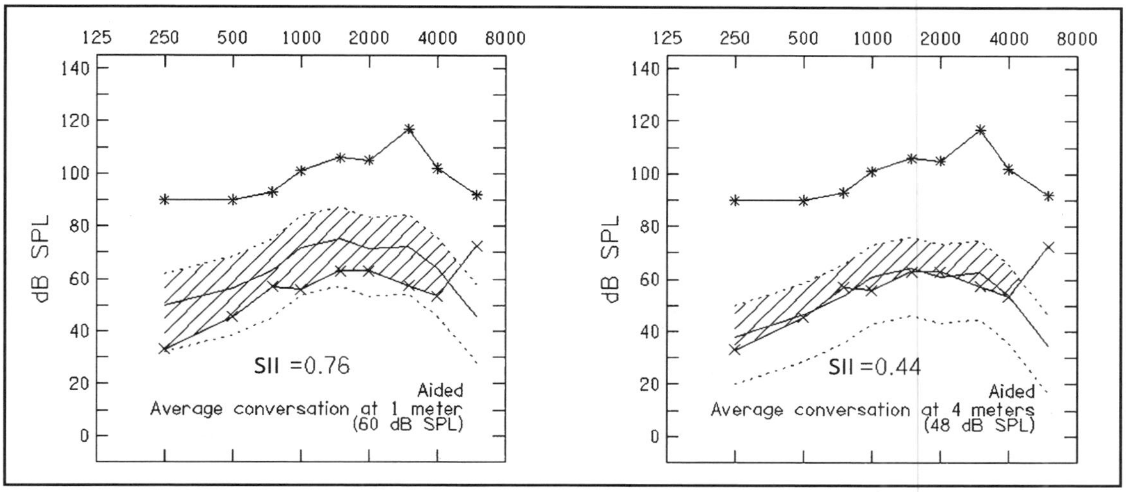


**FIGURE 7–1.** Speechmapping output and Speech Intelligibility Index (SII) for an input level of 60 dB SPL at 1 meter (*left panel*), compared to 4 meters (*right panel*). Hearing thresholds are represented by the connected X symbols. The shaded area represents the region of the aided long-term average speech spectrum that is audible above the hearing thresholds.

by the speech intelligibility index (SII). Speaker-listener distance varies continuously throughout any given day, and implications for resulting changes in audibility should be considered when determining the most efficacious technology to achieve consistent access to speech.

The close placement of the HAT remote microphone to the sound source, approximately 6 inches from the speaker's mouth, minimizes the negative effects of distance on audibility. The level of the speech at the position of the HAT remote microphone remains high, and routing the original signal via HAT to the listener's hearing aids preserves audibility and quality of the original signal. The same can be said of using HAT to connect to electronic media. By routing the audio from the media device to the child's hearing aids via HAT, the original signal level is maintained and processed by the hearing aid for optimal audibility and the best sound quality without the interfering effects of distance or room acoustics.

### *Reverberation*

Reverberation occurs when a sound is reflected off a surface, and the reflected sound wave persists after the original signal has ceased. Reverberation may result in overlapping speech signals in time at the listener's ear due to multiple reflections of sound off a surface or surfaces, distorting the original speech signal in time and intensity. Not only does reverberation introduce energetic masking by overlapping in time and energy with the primary signal of interest, but it can also cause informational masking. The closer a listener is to the speaker in a reverberant environment, the higher likelihood that the listener will receive the direct speech signal. The likelihood that the listener will receive an indirect, or reflected, signal increases the farther the listener is from the source (Figure 7–2). To ensure the best audibility, the listener should be positioned within the room so that he or she has access to the direct speech signal and low interference from the indirect signal. The critical distance, or distance where the direct and indirect signals are equal in level, depends on the physical layout and acoustic characteristics of the room. Critical distance is important to consider when determining types of HAT to use and optimal listening positions in reverberant environments, so that the listener will receive more of the direct signal and less of the indirect, reflected signal that leads to speech distortion and poorer audibility.

The direct transmission of the signal to the listener's hearing aids prevents reflections of the signal in the intermediate distance between the sound source and the listener. In addition, the close placement of HAT remote microphones to the sound

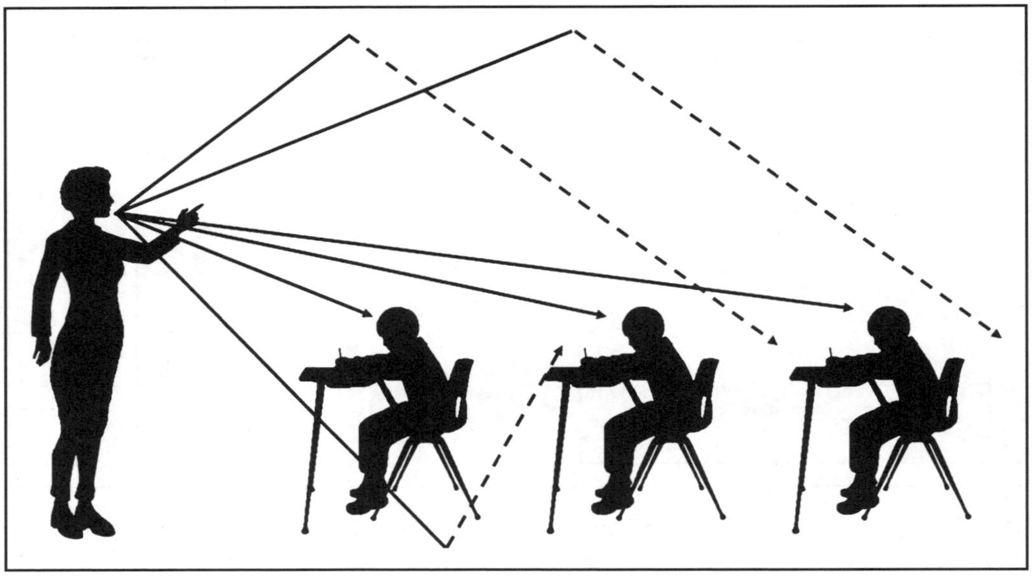

**FIGURE 7–2.** Diagram showing direct propagation (*solid lines*) and indirect reflections (*dashed lines*) of the original sound source within a reverberant classroom environment.

source effectively provides sound quality equal to or better than what would be found within the critical listening distance of the original sound source, regardless of the source and listener's positions in the room. As a result, HAT can help to minimize the negative perceptual consequences of reverberation for children who wear hearing aids.

> Reverberation Time, or RT60, is a measure of the time it takes in seconds for a signal to decay 60 dB. The American National Standards Institute (ANSI; S12.6-2002 Acoustical Performance Criteria in Learning) recommends that primary learning environments have an RT60 of 0.6 s or less.

### Background Noise

The most common acoustic factor that negatively impacts audibility is background noise. There are many types of noise in any given environment that may originate from different sources or locations. Noise may be relatively unchanging in intensity over time, such as the hum of the refrigerator or the heating and ventilation system within a house. Noise can also fluctuate in intensity over time, such as music or electronic media (radio, television), car horns, or other people talking in the background. Following multiple talkers in a conversation may create a complex signal to interpret, requiring additional audibility demands. Regardless of the type or source of the noise, background noise is detrimental to receiving a clear, audible speech signal because it may mask certain speech sounds or even the entire signal of interest. The top panel of Figure 7–3 shows a waveform of a sentence spoken by a male talker in quiet. Some of the acoustic detail is lost when the same sentence is embedded within a background of steady-state noise (middle panel) or multi-talker speech (lower panel). Sources of noise may vary by setting, and the degree of decrement to audibility will depend on the time, intensity, and frequency characteristics of that noise.

> ANSI (S12.6-2002 Acoustical Performance Criteria in Learning) recommends that noise levels in unoccupied classrooms do not exceed 35 dBA and that the teacher's voice is 15 dB above occupied noise levels (+15 dB SNR) in primary learning environments.

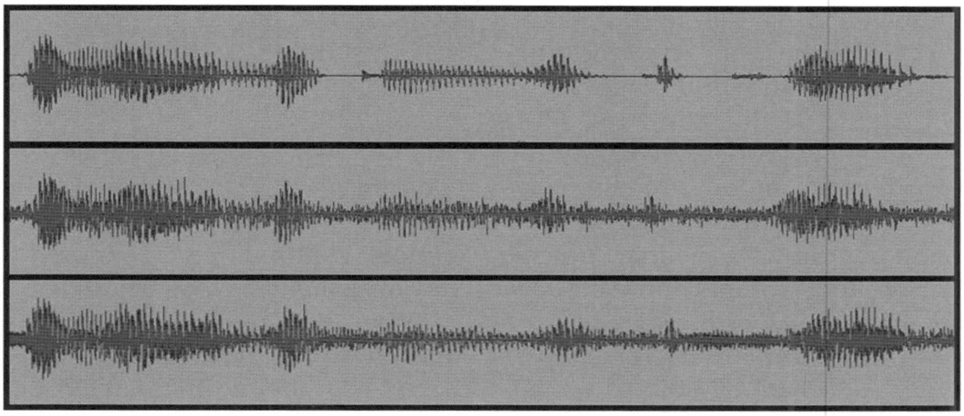

**FIGURE 7–3.** Waveforms of a sentence spoken by a male talker in quiet (*top panel*), with steady-state noise (*middle panel*), and multi-talker babble (*lower panel*).

The type of noise can have differential effects on performance, depending on the processing demands of the task. In a study by Klatte, Lachmann, and Meis (2010), children's performance on a simple speech perception word-picture matching task was more degraded in classroom noise (e.g., chairs and desks moving, tapping pencils and pens, coughing) compared to background speech (one female talker). However, listening comprehension was more degraded in the presence of background speech compared to classroom noise. Classrooms are likely to have both of these sources of noise occurring simultaneously. Bradley and Sato (2008) measured speech intelligibility in classrooms and determined that an SNR of +15 dB, the SNR currently recommended by ANSI for learning environments, may be an underestimation of the actual needs of young children and those with a hearing loss in the classroom. Again, remote microphone HAT and connective devices have the potential to minimize effects of background noise by capturing the input close to the source location and delivering it to the hearing aid(s) without interference of masking from multiple talkers or environmental noise that would otherwise occur in the intermediate distance between the input and listener.

## Developmental Effects of Acoustics

The degree to which distance, noise, and reverberation impact audibility and subsequent understanding may change as children get older and encounter new environments. The transition from home to school is an example of such a transition. These normal transitions that occur with development require audiologists to think about the appropriate use of HAT and connective devices at different developmental stages. Adaptations in the type of equipment or strategies for using HAT should be considered based on the age of the child, listening/processing demands of the task, and acoustics of the child's various listening environments.

When children are very young, infant-directed speech is typically occurring at close distances. For example, while a child is being held in a parent's arms or inside a bassinette, the parent is speaking within close proximity to the child. There is low chance of background noise and reverberation interfering with the audibility of the parent's speech when the parent is close to the child in these situations. As children begin to crawl and walk, distance from the parent typically increases and becomes more variable. This variation in speaker distance leads to varying amounts of speech audibility at the child's ear. Speech sounds that were once audible at a close distance may become inaudible at farther distances, even with optimally fitted amplification. Furthermore, as the child moves away from the parent, the likelihood of also encountering interfering effects of room acoustics, such as background noise and reverberation, increases.

When children enter daycare or preschool, it is important to consider the acoustics of these new environments in regard to the child's ability to listen and learn. Crukley, Scollie, and Parsa (2011) noted that children in daycare were exposed to the highest noise levels compared to children in elementary and high school. In addition, the great majority of time at daycare was spent in speech in noise environments, and extremely little time was spent in quiet or in speech alone listening environments. Instruction may take place in different parts of the classroom, each having unique acoustic characteristics resulting in varying distances from the teacher, levels of noise, and reverberation (e.g., snack time, where children are seated on chairs around a table over a linoleum floor, reading circles where children are seated on a carpeted area at a close distance from the teacher). Compared to adults, children are more prone to the Lombard effect (Whitlock & Dodd, 2008); that is, raising their voices to be heard over background noise. The presence of more competing talkers, especially more children, and reverberation within the room contributes to an overall noisier environment. HAT has the potential to provide more consistent speech input for the child to access fine acoustic details within the speech stream they would otherwise miss in such a noisy environment.

Noise, reverberation, and distance become particularly important factors when considering instructional access in primary and secondary school settings as children are expected to "listen to learn." Crukley, Scollie, and Parsa (2011) measured sound levels of children's instructional and noninstructional activities across their day at daycare, elementary school, and high school. Figure 7–4 shows an example of the varying levels of noise children may be exposed to throughout a day in elementary school based on the activity and location. Varying noise levels across classrooms, activities, and schools may cause inconsistent access to academic material throughout the day.

In reverberant rooms, the presence of background speech and classroom noise (e.g., papers shuffling, desks and chairs being moved) can cause decreases in speech perception performance of approximately 20 to 40% (Klatte et al., 2010). The negative effects of distance on speech perception are exacerbated in the presence of noise and reverberation (Crandell & Bess, 1986). Figure 7–5 demonstrates the detrimental effects of distance on a speech recognition task in a noisy, reverberant classroom compared to a quiet classroom. Moving a student from the first to the second row in a noisy, reverberant classroom could cause a 15 to 23% decrease in the student's word identification. Moving from the first to the third row could cause a decrease of approximately 28 to 30% (Klatte et al., 2010). In addition to decrements in speech recognition, Shield and Dockrell

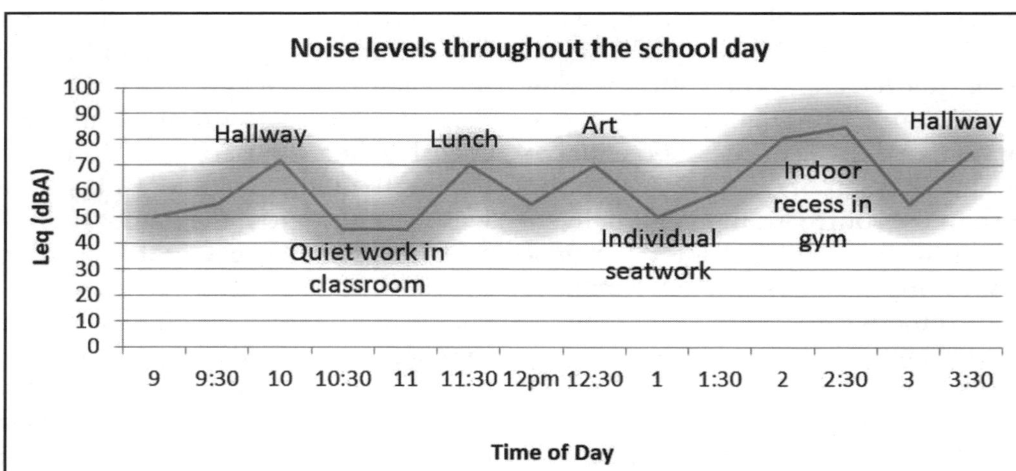


**FIGURE 7–4.** Varying sound levels based on activity throughout a school day of an elementary-aged student. Modification of Cruckley, Scollie, & Parsa (2011) Figure 3c.

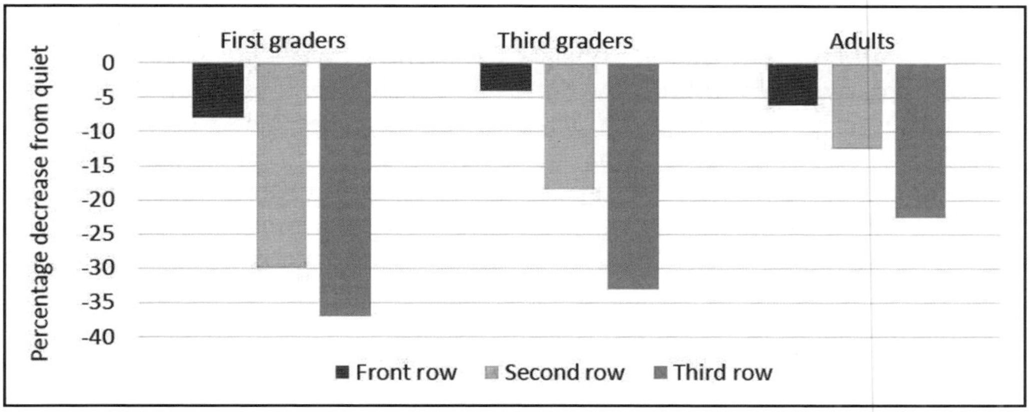


**FIGURE 7–5.** The percentage of reduction in speech recognition ability when in a noisy, reverberant classroom environment, compared to quiet presented by age group (first grade, third grade, adult) and distance from the speaker (front row, second row, third row). Modification of Klatte et al. (2010) Figure 2.

(2008), in a United Kingdom study, documented that environmental noise, whether from inside or outside the classroom, impacted children's academic outcomes on standard achievement tests, with children in noisier classrooms performing more poorly than children in quieter environments. Multi-talker babble within the classroom most affected children's achievement in verbal skills, especially reading and spelling, as well as nonverbal task performance (Dockrell & Shield, 2006). Talker-listener distance, reverberation, and noise levels are high priorities to consider when evaluating students' candidacy for HAT, as these factors compound to detract from the audibility of speech, even when hearing aids are worn.

For children who are hard of hearing (CHH), Picard and Bradley (2001) recommend that background noise in unoccupied classrooms be as low as 21.5 dBA for optimal speech understanding, which is much lower than the ANSI recommendation of 35 dBA. Whitlock and Dodd (2008) propose a reverberation time of 0.4 s, again lower than the ANSI recommendation of 0.6 s, for optimal speech integration for elementary-age children. Crandell and Smaldino (2000) summarized literature on classroom acoustics, and found the majority of classrooms to be much noisier and reverberant than current ANSI guidelines recommend. Larsen and Blair (2008) indicated that the SNR of teacher's voices ranged from +1 to +6 dB in classrooms without the use of HAT, which is significantly poorer than the recommended +15 dB SNR. Improving the layout and acoustics of the classroom is an important first step toward providing a better listening environment for students. Despite a lack of educational preparation regarding teaching children with hearing loss, teachers are amenable to modifying the physical (seating, visual distractions, classroom organization) and acoustic setup of the classrooms, which have been shown to improve academic engagement and reduce disruptive behaviors (Guardino & Antia, 2012). However, any source of background noise, even in an acoustically "favorable" room, may infringe on the audibility of the teacher's voice and impact academic progress. It is especially important to provide a clear signal through remote microphone HATs or connective devices whenever possible and appropriate in the educational environment.

## Summary of HAT and Connective Device Contribution to Audibility

In summary, HATs can improve audibility by minimizing the deleterious effects of distance, background noise, and reverberation. The HAT microphones are placed within close proximity of the speaker's mouth (typically 4–6″), essentially eliminating the negative effects of distance, interfering noise, and reverberation (Madell, 1992). In this way, HATs increase the audibility of the speech signal, resulting in improved speech perception (Davies, Yellon, & Purdy, 2001; Moeller, Donaghy, Beauchaine, Lewis, & Stelmachowicz, 1996) beyond what is achievable with hearing aids alone (Lewis et al., 2004). Crandell and Smaldino (2000, 2001) showed that personal remote microphone systems can improve understanding in noisy environments by 10 to 20 dB compared to the unaided condition. In addition to providing better audibility of live speech, HAT can also be used to connect hearing aids to smart phones, tablets, and personal computers or laptops in noisy environments. This connectivity allows the child to access audio input from electronic devices in acoustic environments where it would otherwise be inaudible or unclear. A child's listening needs and environments are likely to change as they grow and develop, which means the needs for HAT and how it interacts with the child's different listening demands should be regularly discussed with parents and caregivers.

### Effects of Remote Microphone HAT and Connective Devices on Consistency of Hearing Aid Use

Children's hearing aid use may improve if HAT is employed in situations where they would otherwise not wear their hearing aids. Parents of infants and toddlers cite behavior or temperament as the obstacles to their child wearing hearing aids (Moeller, Hoover, Peterson, & Stelmachowicz, 2009; Walker et al., 2013). Using HAT may actually improve hearing aid use, especially in situations of reduced hearing aid use due to low supervision, when the child is bored, or when they are not engaged with the parent. For example, children who would remove their hearing aids during periods of low social interaction (e.g., in the car) would be kept more engaged in their environment due to the better audibility of speech through the use of an FM system and would be less likely to become bored and remove devices. In a longitudinal study of FM use in toddlers, Mulla and McCracken (2014) anecdotally reported better hearing aid use with the adoption of FM for children who would otherwise not wear hearing aids.

As children get older, their use of electronic media increases. Children with hearing loss may remove their hearing aids to use headphones or earbuds in order to access audio from iPods, tablets, video/computer games, apps on smart phones, and so forth. Children also may remove their hearing aids and listen via speakerphone if they have difficulty understanding on the telephone while using their hearing aids. Improper placement of the phone to the hearing aid telecoil or microphone can contribute to difficulty understanding. Holding the phone 1 inch away from the optimal location can decrease the signal by 15 dB (Holmes & Chase, 1985). Furthermore, phone/telecoil programs may not be verified with real-ear, probe microphone verification methods, resulting in poor audibility that contributes to poor understanding and hearing aid nonuse. Because speakerphones and headphones or earbuds do not provide optimal audibility adapted for an individual child's hearing loss, connective technology should be used to route the sound from the electronic device to the child's hearing aids in order to provide the best audio signal possible. Hearing aid use may thus increase because the hearing aids are used in conjunction with the connective device to access a clearer audio signal that supports understanding. Future studies should explore the possibility that HAT and connective device use improves consistency of hearing aid use.

## REMOTE MICROPHONE HAT AND CONNECTIVE DEVICE CANDIDACY CONSIDERATIONS

The Joint Committee on Infant Hearing (JCIH; 2007) recommends fitting amplification within one month of age at confirmation of hearing loss. However, there are no specific guidelines for the timing and provision of remote microphone HAT or connective devices. The American Academy of Audiology (AAA) clinical practice guidelines (2011) recommend consideration of remote microphone HAT once a child spends time at distances away from the talker or in noisy situations. Consideration of HAT should then occur when most babies begin to crawl, between 7 to 10 months of age. Despite these recommendations, little is known about the practice patterns regarding fitting FM systems for use at home and the outcomes of children who use personal FM systems early in life. Having clear access to speech during periods of language acquisition supports the development of phonological, morphological, and preliteracy skills. Taken into consideration with the AAA guidelines, use of remote microphone HAT should begin relatively soon after the child is fit with hearing aids and potentially before one year of age as the child becomes mobile.

Candidacy for the use of connective devices may depend on the age at which children engage with different sources of electronic media and the amount and consistency of exposure. The average age at which children begin interfacing with electronic devices depends on the source of media (Common Sense Media & Rideout, 2011). In 2011, the average age at which children began watching TV was 9 months old, and by 2 years old 96% of children watched TV. Children ages 6 to 23 months spent more time watching TV than reading books per day. By preschool, the majority of children have used a computer, played console video games, and used a cell phone or tablet-type device for games, apps, and videos. The use of electronic media continues into primary and secondary school, where children can use connective technology to have clear access to audio signals for phone and video calls, listening to music, getting directions, social media apps, and when playing games. Children are accessing electronic media at very young ages, and it is important that they have access to audio input from these devices for educational, entertainment, and communication purposes throughout their lifetimes.

The AAA guidelines recommend balancing both acoustic and *psychosocial* factors when determining receipt and use of HAT. For many families of very young children, it can be overwhelming to handle additional equipment at a time when they are just beginning to familiarize themselves with the hearing aids after the initial fitting and orientation. If families are hesitant to pursue HAT while their child is very young, it should be reconsidered and brought up for discussion regularly as their child ages and the family becomes more comfortable with using the hearing aids.

Parent and child buy-in are additional components to consider for candidacy of remote microphone HAT and connective devices. Many factors may relate to motivation to use the equipment: attention and fatigue, self-image, self-advocacy, social acceptance, classroom culture, and family support (AAA, 2011). Providing as much information and experiential training on the benefits of using HAT within the scope of cumulative auditory experience from multiple different professionals and peer supports may encourage use of HAT. Ultimately it is up to the family and child to implement it into their daily lives. If a family is not motivated to use the device or the child refuses, it may not be worthwhile to purchase the expensive equipment.

Within an academic setting, the child's behavior and self-advocacy, educator's teaching strategies and attitude, and classroom acoustics and characteristics should be taken into consideration to anticipate the type of remote microphone technology that would be most beneficial and most likely to be appropriately utilized. Questionnaires focusing on listening and student participation in the classroom (Chapter 6), as well as a functional listening assessment of the child's speech recognition abilities (including recognition in noise and at a distance, aided and unaided) in their typical classroom environment should be performed to help support candidacy decisions in the school setting. Outcome measures, such as questionnaires about the child's performance in classroom environments and speech recognition, can be helpful for assessing candidacy for amplification.

## BASIC DESCRIPTION/ FEATURES OF HATS

After deciding that a child is a candidate for remote microphone or connective technology, the audiologist and the family need to choose the type of devices most appropriate for the needs of the child. Varying configurations of HAT exist, the most popular of which are remote microphone and connective devices. Remote microphone HAT systems are principally used to broadcast speech from a primary speaker to a listener or listeners. The remote microphone HAT system consists of a small microphone placed close to the target speaker's mouth, a transmitter that wirelessly broadcasts the signal, and a receiver that routes the signal to the hearing aids. The remote microphones may be physically connected to a transmitter via a cord, or it may be wireless. Talkers can utilize different types of microphone technology, depending on characteristics of the listening environment.

Connective devices are used to transmit audio from an electronic media source (e.g., iPod, TV) to a listener's hearing aids. At times, the electronic media source may act as the connective device if it has the capability to transmit the audio signal directly to the hearing aid. If not, a separate piece of equipment would be used as an intermediary in routing the audio signal to the hearing aids. The connective device may require a direct, wired connection to the audio source (typically from a headphone port) or may be able to acquire the audio signal wirelessly.

This chapter focuses on HAT devices used for the purposes of transmitting speech or other audio signals, such as music, from electronic media. Other types of HAT exist for environmental awareness (bed shakers, telephone and doorbell alarms, wearable alarms, etc.) that, while important, are beyond the scope of this chapter. The following sections will review remote microphone HAT and connective device technology, methods of signal transmission and reception, as well as signal processing strategies in more detail.

## Remote Microphone HAT Systems

Remote microphone systems are the most common type of HAT. They are popular due to their versatile wireless design, relatively low cost, ease of installation and use, their small size, and the fact that they can be transportable. Remote microphone systems can be used whenever the primary speaker is at a distance from the listener, whether that be inside or outside of a classroom.

### *Types of HAT Remote Microphone Equipment*

Lapel, boom, and mini-mics are best used when there is a primary speaker of interest. These microphones typically can switch the focus of input from the speaker's voice (directional input) to sound coming from in front of the speaker (environmental/omnidirectional input). If the speaker is going to be discussing a private matter or doing a task not directly related to the child, the remote microphone should be muted. Examples of microphones are shown in Figure 7–6. Lapel

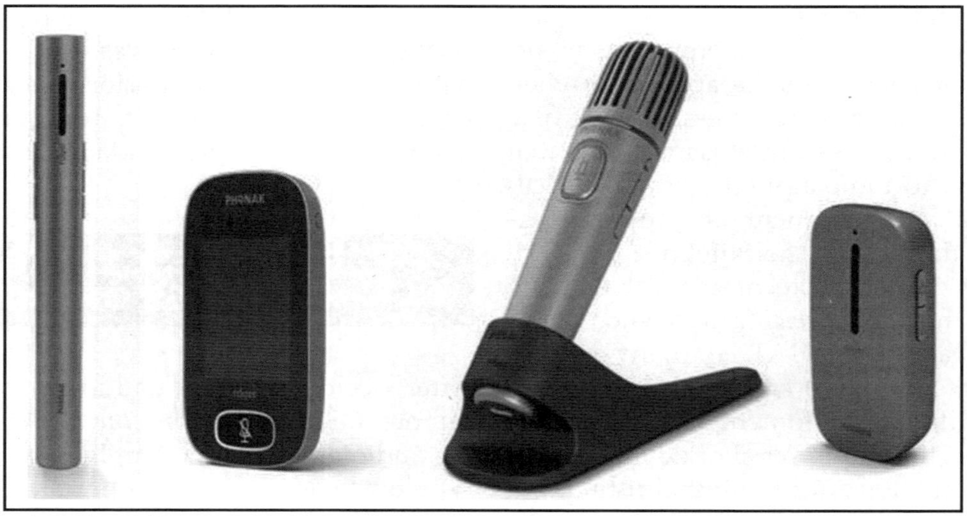

**FIGURE 7–6.** Examples of remote microphones (*left to right:* lapel, touchscreen, pass, manufacturer-specific clip-on microphone/transmitter). Image courtesy of Sonova AG, © 2017.

microphones are clipped to the speaker's shirt or worn on a lanyard around the neck 6 inches from the speaker's mouth. Boom microphones are worn on a headset 3 inches from the speaker's mouth (not pictured in Figure 7–6). Pass or table microphones are typically held 6 inches from the speaker's mouth or set in the center of a table during group discussion. A pass microphone is useful for small group work or in circumstances when more than one or two people will be taking turns speaking. A side benefit is improving thoughtful turn-taking and fewer interruptions during the conversation. "Mini" microphones can be clipped to a shirt or worn with a lanyard around the neck 6 inches from the speaker's mouth. These small devices act as both microphone and transmitter and are housed within a single case.

## Methods of Transmission for Remote Microphone HAT

Remote microphone HAT signals can be transmitted and received by various methods, including Frequency Modulation (FM), Digital Modulation (DM), and infrared transmission. Connective devices may use an induction loop with the hearing aid telecoil, Bluetooth, or other proprietary nearfield communication strategy with a connective streaming device. The method of transmission largely depends on the intended use by the wearer, the size of the area in which it is to be used, the number of potential users, availability of equipment, and the cost of use and installation.

With induction loop transmission, the remote microphone signal is transmitted through a copper wire typically installed within the floor along the perimeter of a venue. The induction loop transmits via magnetic signal that is received by a telecoil, either in a separate receiver or in the hearing aid itself. Induction loops may be smaller in scale and worn around the neck of a listener to transmit signals from a connective device. Infrared transmission uses infrared radiators to transmit signals via infrared light (like a floodlight) to an infrared receiver. The infrared receiver may be integrated into a speaker or be connected to headphones. The range of transmission is restricted by walls or other physical "line-of-sight" obstacles in room, limiting crossover of the transmitted signal between rooms. The integrity of the infrared signal may deteriorate in the presence of bright light. Frequency modulation (FM) uses a small radio transmitter with an antenna to transmit the remote microphone signal via radio frequency to an ear-level receiver or connective device. With digital modulation (DM), the outgoing signal is digitally processed then sent via digital transmitter to a digital ear-level receiver or connective device. The DM has lower noise than FM and better occupancy bandwidth, due to less interference between devices. Thibodeau (2014) showed that adults who were hard of hearing had a subjective preference for DM over FM. The adults also demonstrated better sentence recognition, particularly in the presence of higher levels of background noise, when using DM over traditional FM transmission. Table 7–1 provides additional details and specifications on the different types of transmission used for remote microphone systems.

## Delivery Methods for Transmitted Remote Microphone HAT Signals

After transmission, the signal from the remote microphone must be received and transduced to deliver the signal to the listener. There are various methods of sound delivery, although the most common are through a Classroom Audio Distribution (CAD) system or routing through the listener's hearing aid via a personal device. The CAD system is capable of delivering sound to an entire room of people via a loudspeaker or loudspeakers. Personal devices deliver the sound only to the listener(s) of interest. Further details on the function and benefits of each are described below.

> Classroom Audio Distribution systems were previously called Sound field Amplification systems. The name changed as the capability of remote microphone equipment expanded to provide audio from multiple different sound sources and included adaptive processing of the signal (not just amplification) based on characteristics of the input within the environment, typically a classroom.

**Table 7–1.** Types of Transmission for Remote Microphone Signals

| | *Induction Loop* | *Infrared* | *Frequency Modulation* | *Digital Modulation* |
|---|---|---|---|---|
| Upper range of transmission | Within or near induction loop | 1200 sq. feet | ~ 20 to 50 feet | ~ 30 to 60 feet |
| Carrier/transmitting frequencies | Finite | Unlimited | Finite | Unlimited |
| Line of sight required | No | Yes | No | No |
| Interference from bright light | No | Yes | No | No |
| Crossover between adjacent rooms | Only if adjacent loops are not | No | Yes | No |

*Source:* Adapted from Wolfe et al. (2013) Table 1.

### *Classroom Audio Distribution Systems*

For CADs, the target signal from the remote microphone is transmitted via FM, DM, or infrared to at least one loudspeaker in the room. The goal is to evenly distribute the speech signal across the room so that all listeners have access to the direct signal, within the critical distance from the sound source. The loudspeaker(s) may be mounted on a stand, placed on a structure within the room (e.g., a table or cabinet), or installed in the ceiling. It is important to consider the room's physical and acoustic characteristics when placing or installing loudspeakers. If there is only one in-ceiling speaker for the CAD system, recommended placement of the speaker is in the center of the room. If the single speaker is going to be mounted on a stand or counter, the recommended placement is behind the listeners in order to provide a secondary sound source that allows more people to be within an appropriate critical distance for listening. Room acoustics need to be carefully considered when determining if a CAD system would be an appropriate type of HAT (Nelson & Soli, 2000). The CAD systems can actually cause poorer understanding in rooms with poor acoustics, such as when reverberation and noise levels are high. For example, in a room with a 1.1-s reverberation time, Anderson and Goldstein (2004) reported no improvement in children's sentence recognition when using an infrared CAD system compared to using hearing aids alone. The most benefit from CAD systems occur in acoustically favorable rooms, where background noise and reverberation are low (Crandell & Smaldino, 2000). It is important to measure acoustic characteristics of classrooms and make any necessary physical modifications to the room to ensure effectiveness of a CAD system. When room acoustics are unfavorable and unmodifiable, ear-level HAT should be considered with or over the use of CAD systems. If ear-level HAT is unavailable or when listeners refuse to wear ear-level HAT, CAD systems are certainly a suitable alternative.

### *Personal Remote Microphone HAT*

For personal remote microphone HAT, the target signal from the remote microphone is transmitted via FM or DM to a receiver and then routed to the hearing aids worn by the listener. The transmission for all of these configurations is considered "personal" in that the signal is transmitted only to listeners using receivers synched to the same transmission channel, although multiple listeners can receive the same signal simultaneously. Personal systems are generally considered to have higher signal fidelity than CAD systems alone because they are not susceptible to interference from background noise or reverberation in rooms that have poor acoustics. The personal system may have an integrated receiver or have a receiver that couples directly to the hearing aid; either it has been specifically made for that make and model of hearing aid (dedicated) or will fit multiple devices (universal). Sometimes additional equipment is needed to couple the receiver to the hearing aid. Manufacturer-specific or universal receivers require a shoe, or 3-pin polarized interface device. Some receivers may be integrated into or connected to a streaming device that wirelessly transmits from a personally-worn induction loop to the hearing aid via telecoil. Ear-level receivers provide better bandwidth and signal consistency than induction/telecoil connections (Schafer, Thibodeau, Whalen, & Overson, 2007). Examples of personal HAT receiver configurations are shown below in Figure 7–7.

### *Remote Microphone Technology and Sound Processing Strategies*

Typically, input from the remote microphone is used in conjunction with the input from the listener's hearing aid microphones to differing degrees, depending on the preferred amount of environmental awareness. In many situations, children need to be aware of their surroundings due to safety concerns or for incidental learning purposes. The ratio of input from the HAT and the hearing aid microphones can be balanced or adjusted within the hearing aid software or on the HAT device itself, so that the listener remains aware of sound in their immediate environment, as well as what the primary speaker is saying. Older children may prefer to hear input solely from the HAT, such as when they are watching a movie or listening to music. In this situation, the ratio of input from the HAT is adjusted to be much higher than that from the hearing aids or a dedicated hearing aid program, so input solely from the HAT can be utilized.

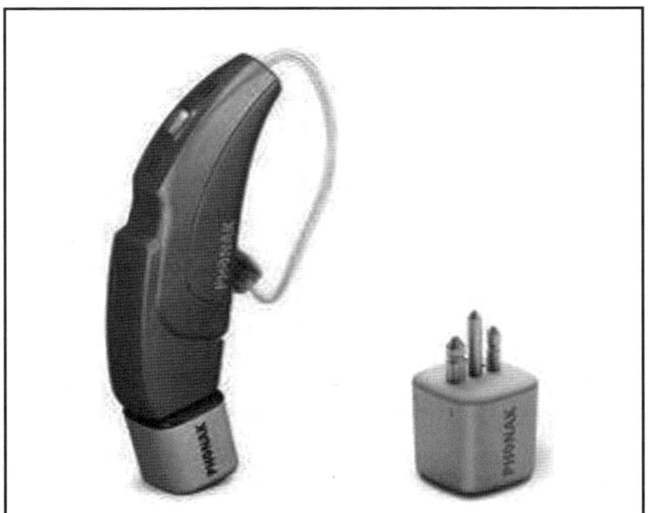

**FIGURE 7–7.** Examples of remote microphone HAT receivers (*left to right:* dedicated, universal). Image courtesy of Sonova AG © 2017.

Relatively recently, algorithms have been created where the HAT microphone(s) monitor ambient noise levels and a processor within the HAT transmitter actively adapts the level of speech input to maintain a positive SNR for the speaker's voice when noise is present. The dynamic SNR strategies can be transmitted via FM or DM in remote microphone HAT systems. Wolfe et al. (2013) showed benefit of speech recognition in noise when using such an adaptive strategy with a single speaker CAD system, compared to a multi-speaker array using a strategy that had fixed-gain input of the speaker's voice. The dynamic SNR technology has been shown to improve sentence recognition, especially when the listener is in environments with high levels of ambient noise (Thibodeau, 2010, 2014; Schafer, Sanders, Bryant, Keeney, & Baldus, 2013; Wolfe et al., 2013).

## Summary of Remote Microphone HAT Features

In summary, no matter the strategy or equipment used, HAT has the potential to benefit children's understanding in complex listening environments over unaided conditions or with hearing aids alone. However, recent advances in technology with dynamic SNR input processing and DM transmission have improved the integrity of the original speech signal, as well as providing accessibility to more listeners with little drawbacks, compared to traditional fixed-gain processing and FM transmission. Ear-level technology relates to better speech understanding compared to CADs in acoustically unfavorable environments and should be used when available.

## CONNECTIVE DEVICE TECHNOLOGY

Children are able to receive input through their hearing aids from multimedia devices for personal, social, and academic purposes with the use of connective technology. Pew Research Center (2015) states approximately three-quarters of teenage children have smartphones that they use to communicate with friends via texting, social media, or through online social games. HAT is advantageous to use with multimedia devices, such as smartphones and tablets because they can provide binaural, appropriately fit audibility with connective devices (Wolfe et al., 2015), privacy for the child using the device (not to mention that their phone call or video game will not interrupt others), and a built-in volume control through hearing aids compared to headphones that are not volume-limiting that may damage hearing. While use of connective technology may increase during the school-age years, connecting to multimedia equipment should be a standard component of the family and provider training, starting when a child begins to engage with electronic media devices, as young as 9 months of age.

Within the academic environment, teachers rely on multimedia equipment to support instruction in the classroom. The Pew Research Center (2013) surveyed 2,462 middle and high school teachers on their use of technology in the classroom and found that almost all educators (96%) were utilizing a laptop or personal computer, smart boards (52%), iPads, and other tablets (43%) of some type to deliver academic material. These new devices come with their own complications for sound delivery for a child who uses amplification. To prevent disrupting classmates, many schools require earbuds or headphones usage with computers and tablets so that students are able to individually listen to instructional modules, videos, and so forth. Removing hearing aids in order to wear earbuds or headphones does not ensure that the child is getting ideal access to instructional material as they would through their hearing aids, which applies frequency-shaped gain to all input. For this reason, it is best for the signal from the multimedia device to be routed through the student's hearing aids, which can be accomplished in a variety of ways. The multimedia device can be: (1) connected to a remote microphone transmitter and then wirelessly routed to the hearing aids, (2) connected to a telecoil headset, which is then positioned next to the hearing aids, (3) connected to a manufacturer-specific connective device (e.g., Oticon Streamer Pro or Phonak Roger Multimedia Hub) that wirelessly send the signal to the hearing aids via induction/telecoil, FM/DM, low power Bluetooth, or proprietary streaming method, or (4) the compatible connective device wirelessly sends to hearing aids directly (Bluetooth 2.0).

Some connective devices may use similar methods of transmission as the remote microphone HAT systems, such as an induction loop routed to the hearing aid telecoil. Manufacturers have created proprietary, nearfield magnetic induction transmission strategies that work similarly to induction loops. Bluetooth and other wireless transmission strategies have become more popular for streaming music and other audio input, at times directly to the hearing aids, without the aid of an intermediary connective device. In collaboration with hearing aid manufacturers, some cell phone companies have developed phones that emit a low power Bluetooth signal (or other proprietary signal) that is received by a separate streaming device or the hearing aid itself. Table 7–2 lists the methods of transmission for connective devices and the technical details for each, including proprietary streaming and low power Bluetooth options that provide optimal sound quality with relatively good battery life.

## RESEARCH ON EFFECTS OF HAT USE

The primary focus of previous research on remote microphone HAT has been on the effects of different equipment and technology on speech rec-

**Table 7–2.** Types of Transmission for Connective Devices

| | *Induction Loop* | *Nearfield Magnetic Induction* | *Bluetooth* | *Proprietary Streaming/Low Power Bluetooth* |
|---|---|---|---|---|
| Number of users | Unlimited | 1 | 2 to 3 | 1 |
| Audio delay | No | No | Yes | No |
| Type of receiver | Telecoil in connective device or hearing aids | Connective device | Connective device | Connective device or hearing aids |

ognition outcomes for school-age children. Many of the studies for school-age children include children either with normal hearing or cochlear implants, and there is limited information on the outcomes of children who are hard of hearing that use HAT. Previous studies on young children's outcomes using HAT are limited in their ability to generalize results due to low numbers of children involved or a lack of a control group. Research on outcomes of children in preschool who use HAT includes subjective, rather than objective, reports of benefit. Few studies explore receipt and use of remote microphone HAT for young children who are hard of hearing who use hearing aids, especially in the home environment.

## Effects of Remote Microphone HAT Use in the Home Setting

Walker et al. (submitted) examined use patterns and factors that predicted receipt of personal FM systems for home use for a young cohort (6 months to 4 years of age) of children who were hard of hearing in the OCHL study. Thirty-six percent ($n$ = 79 out of 217) of children within the OCHL study received a personal FM for home use. On average, children were fitted with a personal FM at 23.4 months (SD = 10.29, range = 6 to 48). When families used the FM system during their daily activities, it was often for short periods of time (1 to 3 hours), and for specific situations or circumstances where audibility was limited by noise or speaker-listener distance, similar to use patterns in other studies (Moeller et al., 1996; Mulla & McCracken, 2014). Children with greater degrees of hearing loss were more likely to receive an FM system for home use compared to children with milder hearing loss. The geographic area also influenced the likelihood of FM receipt at an early age; children in North Carolina were significantly more likely to receive FM systems compared to children from the Midwest. The majority of home FM systems used by families within the OCHL study were purchased using public funding, such as Medicaid or EHDI programs. These programs offer personal remote microphone HAT systems at low or no cost, but vary by state and are not always available.

Only a few studies have been conducted on the impact of FM use on language outcomes for young children who are hard of hearing. Moeller et al. (1996) monitored language progress over a 2-year period for two groups of young children who are hard of hearing. One group used FM plus hearing aids, and a comparison group used only hearing aids. The parents of children within the FM plus hearing aid group reported a range of daily FM device use from approximately 20% to nearly 60% of waking hours. No significant differences emerged in language outcomes between the FM plus hearing aid and hearing aid only groups, although two FM plus hearing aid users had exceptional language growth beyond what was seen for the hearing aid only users. Mulla and McCracken (2014) followed seven families using personal FM systems across a period of 5 to 6 months and analyzed parent-reported language development for their children who were hard of hearing. Overall, parents used the FM for over half of the days in the study, for an average of a couple hours each day. The children in the longitudinal case studies showed no significant growth in language on average over the course of using the FM system, however, some children who were reported to be at-risk for language delays had language scores improving to within the average range after using the FM. It is unknown whether the children in the Mulla and McCracken study made above-expected progress in language, compared to children who did not use FM, because they did not include a control group who did not use FM. These studies are limited by low numbers of participants and/or lack of a control group, however, they both point to improvements in language development for certain listeners (potentially those most at-risk for delays) with the use of FM. More research is needed in this area to generalize results to a broader population of children who are hard of hearing.

Walker et al. (submitted) compared the preschool language outcomes of children who were fit with home FM to children who were not fit with home FM during the birth-to-three period. The authors examined receptive vocabulary, expressive grammar, and discourse language skills for pairs of children with and without FM, matched on predictors that would impact whether they were likely to receive an FM for home use. No significant differences were found between the FM and no-FM groups on vocabulary and grammar measures, although results point toward better understanding of complex language and reasoning ability for the group of preschool children who received FM for home use compared to children who did not have FM for home use. Both the children with and without FM systems generally had a higher socioeconomic status than that of the general population, making it difficult to generalize outcomes to a larger population of children with hearing loss. Even so, it appears that early acoustic access that supports the development of foundational language skills may contribute to better reasoning skills in preschool.

In several studies, nearly all families with an FM system for home use reported that it benefited their child (Moeller et al., 1996; Mulla & McCracken, 2014; Walker et al., submitted). In the Moeller et al. (1996) study, parents anecdotally reported that their children had decreased need for clarification requests, especially in suboptimal listening conditions, as well as increased participation and comprehension of conversations, and development of "pragmatic overhearing." Parents in the Mulla and McCracken (2014) study reported the most benefit from using the FM when listening in noise and at a distance. Parents reported the least amount of benefit of using FM when their child was listening in quiet. Parent responses of situational benefit reflect the expected benefit in outcomes with relation to access to auditory input. Parents reported more benefit in conditions where audibility would be expected to be poor (e.g., noisy; at a distance) compared to conditions where audibility would be expected to be good (quiet environments). These benefits are supported by consistency trends across studies, as well. Similar to Moeller et al. (1996), parents in Walker et al. (submitted) reported relatively high consistency of use in public and at the playground, where audibility would be negatively impacted by distance and interfering noise. The benefit that parents reported likely contributed to continued use of the device in those situations.

## Challenges and Solutions for HAT Use in the Home Setting

Simulations of listening to speech from a distance, in noisy, multitalker environments and in places with high amounts of reverberation, regardless of degree of hearing loss, can be useful in conveying the magnitude of benefit achievable by improving audibility with HAT (Haggard & Primus, 1999). By having clearer access to subtle acoustic details in parent speech and the ability to hear conversations at home, in the car, or at mealtimes, children with any degree of hearing loss may be better prepared to show improvements in language development over the preschool years.

Moeller et al. (1996) reported that the most common parent-reported problem using the FM was that the cords involved with the FM system were inconvenient. Fortunately, much of the current remote microphone technology is moving toward wireless designs that no longer require a cord to connect the microphone and transmitter or a cord to connect the receiver to the hearing aids. Walker et al. (submitted) documented other challenges from families participating in the OCHL study, such as 41% ($n$ = 19 out of 32) of parents reported problems while using the FM system. Other parent-reported problems included difficulty with the connection between the HA and FM receivers, the FM was broken or had to be sent in for repairs, and the battery was quick to drain. Even with current technology, parents seem to be encountering problems when trying to use remote microphone HAT that could impact device function. It is vital that the equipment be evaluated to ensure that it is providing a clear signal and good audibility before use. Parents should continue to do listening checks with the Ling 6 sounds, either with a personal testing stethoset or behaviorally with the child to ensure optimal audibility and transmission from the HAT before each use. Hands-on practice with the technology can support parents' self-efficacy with listening checks and troubleshooting (DesJardin, 2005), and should be integrated into both clinical audiology and routine-based early intervention visits in the home.

As seen in Moeller et al. (1996) and Mulla and McCracken (2014), family preference dictated when and where the FM systems were used. Consistency ratings (see Chapter 5, Table 5–1) may be used to investigate when parents employ HAT. Counseling may be needed on appropriate, strategic use of remote microphone systems if parents utilize it in mostly quiet situations. Some parents may believe more use is always better; however, using HAT consistently throughout the day limits a child's ability to access indirect communication, such as overhearing conversations involving multiple people. As overhearing is important to both the child's vocabulary development and the acquisition of cognitive skills, it is critical not to limit exposure to discourse to only a single talker. Remote microphone systems provide the most benefit when there is a primary speaker of interest and when listening in acoustically unfavorable listening environments.

## Effects of HAT Use in Preschool/Daycare Setting

Two recent studies show variation in the type of HAT used in preschool settings. Nelson, Poole, and Munoz (2013) surveyed teachers of children who are deaf and hard of hearing (TODHH) in private and public preschool programs. Fifty-seven (58%) respondents indicated that they currently use or previously used sound-field systems, now called CAD systems, in their preschool classroom with children who are deaf or hard of hearing. They reported approximately 20 to 25% of students were using personal remote microphone systems in the preschool classroom. Walker et al. (submitted) showed that half ($n$ = 84 out of 168) of preschool-age children in the OCHL study had access to remote microphone technology in their daycare or preschool setting, and the majority of children (80%) had personal, ear-level receivers at preschool and/or daycare. Fewer institutions used a telecoil/neck loop receiver (8%) or CAD system (12%). There are no studies showing the effects of using these different types of HATs on the outcomes of preschool children.

Schafer and Thibodeau (2006) demonstrated up to a 20-dB improvement in children's sentence recognition in classroom noise with the use of FM, although all of the children in the study had cochlear implants, and the sample included school-age students as well as preschoolers. There are no studies showing direct evidence of improved speech, language, or behavioral outcomes with FM use in the preschool setting for children who wear hearing aids. Even so, TODHH report benefits relating to improved academic and language skills and better behavior and attention with the use of classroom HATs (Nelson et al., 2013). The great majority of teachers in the Nelson et al. study recommended the use of a CAD or personal remote microphone system to other teachers.

## Challenges and Solutions to Using HAT in the Preschool/Daycare Setting

Schools and educators have a legal obligation to both use and document hearing aid and FM use in the classroom if it is included in the child's Individualized Education Plan (IEP). However, HAT is not always used in children's classrooms for various reasons. The study by Nelson et al. (2013) provides insight into preschool teachers' obstacles to using FM in their classrooms. When asked why FM was not used in their classrooms, 30% of teachers reported funding or cost as preventive. While CAD equipment and installation and personal HAT equipment can be expensive, there are alternative HATs, such as manufacturer-specific transmitter/receiver units, (e.g., Oticon Voice link/ConnectLine streamer, Signia VoiceTek/EasyTek) that can be purchased at a fraction of the cost and perform similarly, albeit with potentially less functionality. It is possible that more school systems would adopt HAT if given more affordable options.

Approximately 40% of teachers reported not using FM because they believed preschoolers may be too young to report technical difficulties (Nelson et al., 2013). If teachers and interventionists are prepared to perform HAT function checks regularly, this should not be an issue that prevents the use of HAT in the preschool classroom. However, teachers, even those educated specifically to work with children who are hard of hearing, reported wanting more training regarding how FM systems work and on how to troubleshoot the equipment. Indeed, the most frequently reported disadvantages of using the FM included it being uncomfortable to wear and troubleshooting issues. These are areas for audiologists and interventionists to specifically address with educational providers through guided, hands-on practice. Training should also be provided for secondary, itinerant, and substitute teachers so that the child continues to have good auditory access when the primary teacher is unavailable.

In the same study by Nelson et al. (2013), 27% of teachers reported that they did not use the FM because they did not believe the children would benefit enough from the FM technology. Teachers mentioned that using the FM would cause students to be put at a "disadvantage when developing listening skills at a distance." While there may be a rationale for strategically not using remote microphone systems (for example, to help develop spatial listening skills or during small group instruction not involving the child), students are already at a disadvantage when listening at a distance and removing their support for clear access to instruction is inappropriate. Relating the importance of having clear speech audibility during periods of learning, especially preacademic and preliteracy skills, seems to be especially important when teachers do not believe children would benefit from having access to instruction. In addition to hands-on mentoring with the technology, these teachers could benefit from listening to simulations of benefit from use of FM systems in the classroom, especially when speech is at a distance or when room acoustics are suboptimal.

When teachers have trouble remembering to use HAT, it may help if they preplan the use of HAT within their daily routine (e.g., use HAT for group book reading at 10:00 AM, but not independent play time from 11:30 AM to 12:00 PM) and have a daily documentation checklist (Table 7–3) to track the use and function of devices on a daily basis.

> Simply having a functioning remote microphone HAT system within the classroom may not sufficiently meet requirements of the Individuals with Disability Education Act. If it is written in the child's individualized education program (IEP), school districts must also *document* that the student was provided with the functioning equipment on a daily basis. For more information, see: http://successforkidswithhearingloss.com/wp-content/uploads/2014/06/Setting-up-FM-system-does-not-meet-IDEA-documentation-rules.pdf

## Effects of HAT Use in Primary and Secondary School Settings

Rosenberg et al. (1999) completed a 3-year study examining kindergarten through second grade classroom acoustics and the effects of CAD use on student's listening and learning behavior. They also reported child, teacher, parent, and administrator impressions of the utility of classroom FM. Teachers reported a myriad of benefits in using a CAD system: less vocal strain, better student attentiveness, improved comprehension, improved classroom control, assistance managing behavior, and a decrease in the need to repeat instruction. Students also reported benefits of using the classroom FM as easier to hear the teacher, the teacher's voice being loud and clear, and help listening when visual cues were limited. Several studies

**Table 7–3.** Daily Checklist of Hearing Equipment Use and Function

| Date | Hearing Aid Functioning (Y/N/NA) | Explanation | Remote-Mic HAT Functioning (Y/N/NA) | Explanation | Provider Initials |
|---|---|---|---|---|---|
| **Mon** | N | Battery dead in left aid—replaced battery. | N | Corrosion on receiver contacts on hearing aids—cleaned receiver contacts. | TW |
| **Tue** | Y | | N | Microphone intermittent —alerted audiologist, who will send for repair and replace. | TW |
| **Wed** | N | Hearing aid weak due to wax in earmold bore—cleaned earmolds. | N | Microphone out for repair. | TW |
| **Thur** | Y | | Y | | TW |
| **Fri** | NA | Student left hearing aids at home. | NA | Could not use personal remote-mic system without hearing aids. | TW |

have shown objective improvement in performance on speech recognition (Wolfe et al., 2013; Thibodeau, 2010) and listening comprehension (Arnold & Canning, 1999) tasks with the use of FM for school-age children.

## Challenges and Solutions for Using HAT in Primary and Secondary School Settings

Despite the positive outcomes and reported benefits of FM use for school-age children, HAT is not always consistently used in classrooms. Davis, Gustafson, Hornsby, and Bess (2015) documented FM use in the classroom for school-age children at separate intervals on two school days. Thirty-six percent ($n$ = 6 out of 22) of the students were not using their FM systems during the classroom observations. Classroom observations of first through fourth-grade students in the OCHL study revealed that 29% of children who had access to remote microphone systems did not use them (Aunan et al., 2016). The reasons educators or students are not utilizing HAT in the classroom are important to understand, as they provide insight into alternative counseling, training, or approaches that need to be taken to encourage the use of HAT, especially if in the student's IEP.

Reasons for reported nonuse vary depending on personal and professional perspective. Franks (2008) interviewed teachers, interventionists, parents, and school-age children (ages 8 to 18) for their opinion on why HAT was not being used. Most professionals believed children primarily did not use FM due to social concerns, with a secondary reason for mechanical issues (device function). Audiologists also believed users lacked support and thought the FM to be inconvenient. Students agreed that social and mechanical concerns impeded the use of FM. Somewhat surprisingly, they also mentioned the lack of benefit, convenience, and comfort as issues related to why they did not use FM.

Furthermore, some students report that teachers are unwilling to use assistive technology and adaptive teaching strategies or that there were attempts to use outdated technology or damaged devices (Eriks-Brophy & Whittingham, 2013) that did not support clear access to instruction. Just as a parent receives training during initial hearing aid/HAT orientation, teachers should receive training on the remote microphone systems in order to become comfortable with troubleshooting the equipment, understanding its benefits, and using it effectively. This training should include information on the technological components of the devices, including location of microphone, how to turn the devices on and off, the procedure for changing or charging the batteries, and potential sources of dysfunction. Having the appropriate tools for troubleshooting (battery tester, listening tube, cleaning brush/tool, extra batteries, air blower) will also prevent unnecessary downtime of hearing aids and HAT. A troubleshooting guide will help the teacher resolve any issues and decide whether it is necessary to contact the educational audiologist or hearing aid technology support personnel. Furthermore, training on appropriate expectations of benefit from the HAT and how to appropriately use HAT (lecture, small groups, with multimedia devices, etc.) should be included.

Intensive training and support from interventionists that specialize in working with children who are hard of hearing can bolster teacher confidence (Eriks-Brophy & Whittingham, 2013). However, even with training, teachers may feel uncomfortable using HAT independently. Teachers may rely on other professionals in the school, the child's parent, or the child themselves to support their efforts with troubleshooting. This requires students to be able to manage their own technology, as well as support others (e.g., substitute teachers) in its use. It may entail being responsible for transporting equipment from class to class or alerting the teacher when there is an issue with the technology. Some children may not feel comfortable interrupting class to do so out of shyness, a lack of assertiveness, or an unwillingness to stand out among their classmates by drawing attention to their hearing loss. For children with hearing loss who are reluctant users of personal FM due to additional equipment needs or the visibility of FM, the use of a CAD system should be considered. The CAD system ensures access to instruction for every student without singling out the student who is hard of hearing.

## VERIFICATION AND VALIDATION PROCEDURES FOR HAT

The American Academy of Audiology provides guidelines on appropriate verification for HAT, which can be found online (https://audiology-web.s3.amazonaws.com/migrated/HAT_Guidelines_Supplement_A.pdf_53996ef7758497.54419000.pdf). The two main goals of verification of the HAT plus hearing aid are to verify at least 10 dB improvement in speech level and ensure that the same input at both the HAT plus hearing aid and hearing aid microphones results in the same output. This is called "transparency," and ensures that adding the HAT equipment does not detract from or significantly alter the output of the hearing aid. We still want the speech signal to be meeting targets through the hearing aid and do not want to under- or overamplify due to the addition of the HAT.

### Verification of Remote Microphone HAT

A combination of electroacoustic and behavioral measures can be utilized for verification. Because the HAT signal is routed through and processed by the hearing aid, the hearing aid itself will need to be appropriately verified before beginning verification of the HAT plus hearing aid. Verification of the HAT should then be done in the condition the child typically listens in. For example, if the child uses both the HAT plus hearing aid microphones, verification should be assessed using HAT plus hearing aid microphones. For all electroacoustic measurements, the output of the HAT plus hearing aid should be measured through the hearing aid. Similar to verification with hearing aids, it is recommended to verify the output of the HAT using a calibrated, weighted speech signal (i.e., the carrot passage) instead of a speech-shaped/weighted noise. Functional gain measurements (aided audiogram) are not recommended for verification with either hearing aid or HAT systems and should not be considered a verification tool for hearing aid or HAT function. Adjustments in settings based on verification results should be made according to AAA's HAT guidelines. When possible, aided audibility with connective devices should be verified through the hearing aids, using real-ear, probe-microphone speech-mapping measures.

## Validation of Remote Microphone HAT

In addition to electroacoustic verification, it is also recommended to perform behavioral validation of the child's listening performance with HAT. Behavioral validation can be performed to evaluate performance across devices, listening conditions, and over time. The AAA guidelines advise the use of speech perception in noise testing while listening in the child's typical HAT plus hearing aid condition. It is not recommended to test in only the HAT condition because that is not a realistic evaluation of the child's listening ability with potential interference of input from the environmental hearing aid microphone. It is also not advised to use adaptive speech-in-noise tests, such as the HINT, HINT-C, or BKB-SIN test.

The Individuals with Disabilities Education Act requires a functional evaluation in the student's typical environment as part of the validation procedure. This involves an assessment of listening ability in the child's classroom. Self-assessments and observation questionnaires (parent and teacher reports) can be useful tools in validating the efficacy of the FM system in the listening environment, pre and posttreatment. However, caution should be taken when interpreting these questionnaires, especially if they have not been validated against objective outcomes themselves. Results from Spratford, McCreery, and Walker (2016) indicate that parents and school-age teachers may rate listening ability based on students' language skills and potentially other factors (e.g., attention, focus), instead of objective listening capability. A child's own report may not be more accurate, as children may not realize the impact of multitalker speech in the background and the benefit of HAT (Franks, 2008). Objective outcomes from tests such as the Functional Listening Evaluation (Johnson & VonAlmen, 1993) should be relied upon more heavily than results from questionnaires when determining benefit of or eligibility for HAT in the classroom.

> The Functional Listening Evaluation protocol and associated resources can be found online at http://www.adevantage.com/Resources.html

## SUMMARY

In conclusion, the use of remote microphone HAT and connective technology can improve auditory access for children of all ages. Candidacy considerations should include perspectives from the family and audiologist, while also considering potential for objective benefit in the child's development of speech understanding and language learning. Parents, intervention providers, educators, and children should be trained on the appropriate use and maintenance of HAT and connective equipment. It is recommended to use remote microphone HAT and connective technology strategically when audibility of speech is poor, such as when a speaker is at a distance from the listener or noise or reverberation impacts the clarity of the original speech signal. By utilizing remote microphone HAT and connective technology, children's auditory access may be improved not only by increasing the audibility of speech, but also by increasing opportunities to engage with and learn from the surrounding auditory environment.

## REFERENCES

American Academy of Audiology. (2011). *Clinical practice guidelines: Remote microphone hearing assistance technologies for children and youth birth–21 years and Supplement A.* Retrieved from http://www.audiology.org/publications-resources/document-library/hearing-assistance-technologies

American National Standards Institute/Acoustical Society of America. (2010). *Performance criteria, design requirements, and guidelines for schools, Part 1: Permanent schools* (ANSI/ASA S12.60-2010). Melville, NY: Acoustical Society of America.

Arnold, P., & Canning, D. (1999). Does classroom amplification aid comprehension? *British Journal of Audiology, 33*(3), 171–178.

Aunan, J., Walker, E., Spratford, M., & McCreery, R. (2016, November). *Classroom acoustic measures & hearing aid use for school-age children who are hard of hearing*. Poster presented at the American Speech-Language-Hearing Association Conference, Philadelphia, PA.

Bradley, J. S., & Sato, H. (2008). The intelligibility of speech in elementary school classrooms. *Journal of the Acoustical Society of America, 123*(4), 2078–2086.

Ching, T. Y., O'Brien, A., Dillon, H., Chalupper, J., Hartley, L., Hartley, D., . . . Hain, J. (2009). Directional effects on infants and young children in real life: Implications for amplification. *Journal of Speech, Language, and Hearing Research, 52*(5), 1241–1254.

Common Sense Media, & Rideout, V. (2011). *Zero to eight: Children's media use in America*. Common Sense Media. Retrieved from https://www.commonsensemedia.org/research/zero-to-eight-childrens-media-use-in-america-2013.

Crandell, C., & Bess, F. (1986). Speech recognition of children in a "typical" classroom setting. *ASHA, 29*, 87.

Crandell, C. C., & Smaldino, J. J. (2000). Classroom acoustics for children with normal hearing and with hearing impairment. *Language, Speech, and Hearing Services in Schools, 31*(4), 362–370.

Crandell, C. C., & Smaldino, J. J. (2001). Classroom acoustics: Understanding barriers to learning. *Volta Review, 101*(5), n5.

Crukley, J., Scollie, S., & Parsa, V. (2011). An exploration of non-quiet listening at school. *Journal of Educational Audiology, 17*, 23–35.

Davies, M. G., Yellon, L., & Purdy, S. C. (2001). Speech-in-noise perception of children using cochlear implants and FM systems. *Australian and New Zealand Journal of Audiology, 23*(1), 52-62.

Davis, H., Gustafson, S., Hornsby, B. W. Y., & Bess, F. H. (2015, April). *Beyond the fitting appointment: Patterns of hearing aid and FM system use in the classroom*. Poster presentation at Audiology Now! American Academy of Audiology Convention, San Antonio, TX.

Desjardin, J. L. (2005). Maternal perceptions of self-efficacy and involvement in the auditory development of young children with prelingual deafness. *Journal of Early Intervention, 27*(3), 193-209.

Dockrell, J. E., & Shield, B. M. (2006). Acoustical barriers in classrooms: The impact of noise on performance in the classroom. *British Educational Research Journal, 32*(3), 509–525.

Eriks-Brophy, A., & Whittingham, J. (2013). Teachers' perceptions of the inclusion of children with hearing loss in general education settings. *American Annals of the deaf, 158*(1), 63–97.

Franks, J. L. (2008). *Why do students with hearing impairment resist wearing FM amplification?* (Masters theses and doctoral dissertation). East Michigan University, Ypsilanti, MI.

Guardino, C., & Antia, S. D. (2012). Modifying the classroom environment to increase engagement and decrease disruption with students who are deaf or hard of hearing. *Journal of Deaf Studies and Deaf Education, 17*(4), 518–533.

Haggard, R. S., & Primus, M. A. (1999). Parental perceptions of hearing loss classification in children. *American Journal of Audiology, 8*(2), 83–92.

Holmes, A., & Chase, N. (1985). Listening ability with a telephone adapter. *Hearing Instruments, 36*(9), 16–57.

Johnson, C.D. & VonAlmen, P. (1993). The functional listening evaluation. In C. D. Johnson, P. V. Benson, & J. B. Seaton (Eds.), *Educational audiology handbook* (pp. 336–339). San Diego, CA: Singular.

Joint Committee on Infant Hearing. (2007). Year 2007 position statement: Principles and guidelines for early hearing detection and intervention programs. *Pediatrics, 120*, 898–921.

Klatte, M., Lachmann, T., & Meis, M. (2010). Effects of noise and reverberation on speech perception and listening comprehension of children and adults in a classroom-like setting. *Noise and Health, 12*(49), 270–282.

Kuk, F. K., Kollofski, C., Brown, S., Melum, A., & Rosenthal, A. (1999). Use of a digital hearing aid with directional microphones in school-aged children. *Journal of the American Academy of Audiology, 10*, 535–548.

Larsen, J. B., & Blair, J. C. (2008). The effect of classroom amplification on the signal-to-noise ratio in classrooms while class is in session. *Language, Speech, and Hearing Services in Schools, 39*(4), 451–460.

Lenhart, A. (2015). *Teens, social media & Technology overview 2015*. Pew Research Center. Retrieved April 28, 2015, from http://www.pewinternet.org/2015/04/09/teens-social-media-technology-2015/

Lewis, M. S., Crandell, C. C., Valente, M., & Horn, J. E. (2004). Speech perception in noise: Directional microphones versus frequency modulation (FM) systems. *Journal of the American Academy of Audiology, 15*(6), 426–439.

Madden, M., Lenhart, A., Duggan, M. Cortesi, S., & Gasser, U. (2013). *Teens in technology*. Pew Research Center. Retrieved March 9, 2015, from http://www

.pewinternet.org/2013/03/13/teens-and-technology-2013/

Madell, J. R. (1992). FM systems as primary amplification for children with profound hearing loss. *Ear and Hearing, 13*(2), 102–107.

McCreery, R. W., Walker, E. A., Spratford, M., Oleson, J., Bentler, R., Holte, L., & Roush, P. (2015). Speech recognition and parent ratings from auditory development questionnaires in children who are hard of hearing. *Ear and Hearing, 36*, 60S–75S.

Moeller, M. P., Donaghy, K. F., Beauchaine, K. L., Lewis, D. E., & Stelmachowicz, P. G. (1996). Longitudinal study of FM system use in nonacademic settings: Effects on language development. *Ear and Hearing, 17*(1), 28–41.

Moeller, M. P., Hoover, B., Peterson, B., & Stelmachowicz, P. (2009). Consistency of hearing aid use in infants with early-identified hearing loss. *American Journal of Audiology, 18*(1), 14–23.

Mulla, I., & McCracken, W. (2014). Frequency modulation for preschoolers with hearing loss. *Seminars in Hearing, 35*(3), 206–216.

Nelson, L. H., Poole, B., & Muñoz, K. (2013). Preschool teachers' perception and use of hearing assistive technology in educational settings. *Language, Speech, and Hearing Services in Schools, 44*(3), 239–251.

Nelson, P. B., & Soli, S. (2000). Acoustical barriers to learning: Children at risk in every classroom. *Language, Speech, and Hearing Services in Schools, 31*(4), 356–361.

Picard, M., & Bradley, J. S. (2001). Revisiting speech interference in classrooms. *Audiology, 40*(5), 221–244.

Pittman, A. (2011). Children's performance in complex listening conditions: Effects of hearing loss and digital noise reduction. *Journal of Speech, Language, and Hearing Research, 54*(4), 1224–1239.

Rosenberg, G. G., Blake-Rahter, P., Heavner, J., Allen, L., Redmond, B. M., Phillips, J., & Stigers, K. (1999). Improving classroom acoustics (ICA): A three-year FM sound-field classroom amplification study. *Journal of Educational Audiology, 7*, 8–28.

Schafer, E. C., Sanders, K., Bryant, D., Keeney, K., & Baldus, N. (2013). Effects of voice priority in FM systems for children with hearing aids. *Journal of Educational Audiology, 19*, 12–24.

Schafer, E. C., & Thibodeau, L. M. (2006). Speech recognition in noise in children with cochlear implants while listening in bilateral, bimodal, and FM-system arrangements. *American Journal of Audiology, 15*(2), 114–126.

Schafer, E. C., Thibodeau, L. M., Whalen, H. S., & Overson, G. J. (2007). Electroacoustic evaluation of frequency-modulated receivers interfaced with personal hearing aids. *Language, Speech, and Hearing Services in Schools, 38*(4), 315–326.

Shield, B. M., & Dockrell, J. E. (2008). The effects of environmental and classroom noise on the academic attainments of primary school children. *The Journal of the Acoustical Society of America, 123*(1), 133–144.

Spangler, C., & Johnson, C. D. (2013). Audiology Self-Advocacy checklist-Elementary School; Audiology Self-Advocacy checklist-Middle School; Audiology Self-Advocacy checklist-High School; (2013). *Self-advocacy competency guide in guide to access planning.*

Spratford, M., McCreery, R. W., & Walker, E. A. (2016, March). *Predictors of teacher and student perception of classroom listening ability.* Poster presented at the American Auditory Society, Scottsdale, AZ.

Stelmachowicz, P., Lewis, D., Hoover, B., Nishi, K., McCreery, R., & Woods, W. (2010). Effects of digital noise reduction on speech perception for children with hearing loss. *Ear and Hearing, 31*(3), 345.

Stiles, D. J., Bentler, R. A., & McGregor, K. K. (2012). The speech intelligibility index and the pure-tone average as predictors of lexical ability in children fit with hearing aids. *Journal of Speech, Language, and Hearing Research, 55*(3), 764–778.

Thibodeau, L. (2010). Benefits of adaptive FM systems on speech recognition in noise for listeners who use hearing aids. *American Journal of Audiology, 19*(1), 36–45.

Thibodeau, L. (2014). Comparison of speech recognition with adaptive digital and FM remote microphone hearing assistance technology by listeners who use hearing aids. *American Journal of Audiology, 23*(2), 201–210.

Tomblin, J. B., Harrison, M., Ambrose, S. E., Walker, E. A., Oleson, J. J., & Moeller, M. P. (2015). Language outcomes in young children with mild to severe hearing loss. *Ear and Hearing, 36*, 76S–91S.

Tomblin, J. B., Oleson, J. J., Ambrose, S. E., Walker, E., & Moeller, M. P. (2014). The influence of hearing aids on the speech and language development of children with hearing loss. *JAMA Otolaryngology-Head & Neck Surgery, 140*(5), 403–409.

Walker, E.A., Curran, M., Spratford, M., Roush, P. (submitted). RM systems for preschool-age children who are hard of hearing: Access, utilization and impact on language acquisition.

Walker, E. A., Spratford, M., Moeller, M. P., Oleson, J., Ou, H., Roush, P., & Jacobs, S. (2013). Predictors of hearing aid use time in children with mild-to-severe hearing loss. *Language, Speech, and Hearing Services in Schools, 44*(1), 73–88.

Whitlock, J. A., & Dodd, G. (2008). Speech intelligibility in classrooms: Specific acoustical needs for primary school children. *Building Acoustics, 15*(1), 35–47.

Wolfe, J., Morais, M., Neumann, S., Schafer, E., Mülder, H., Wells, N., & Hudson, M. (2013). Evaluation of speech recognition with personal FM and classroom audio distribution systems. *Journal of Educational Audiology, 19*, 65–79.

Wolfe, J., Schafer, E., Mills, E., John, A., Hudson, M., & Anderson, S. (2015). Evaluation of the benefits of binaural hearing on the telephone for children with hearing loss. *Journal of the American Academy of Audiology, 26*, 93–100.

# 8

# Transition to Cochlear Implants

*Elizabeth A. Walker and Ryan W. McCreery*

## INTRODUCTION

Cochlear implants have revolutionized aural (re) habilitation for children and adults with sensorineural hearing loss. Originally, they were intended for individuals with profound hearing loss who had no access to the speech spectrum and demonstrated limited benefit from hearing aids. Cochlear implants have since become the standard of care for children with pure-tone averages greater than 90 dB HL. As more children show substantial benefits from cochlear implants with respect to speech perception, speech production, language, and psychosocial outcomes, there has been increased discussion regarding expanding the audiometric candidacy to include individual with less severe hearing loss. Unfortunately, we do not know the point at which cochlear implants provide better access to sound than hearing aids. Children also show enormous individual differences in outcomes with cochlear implants, making it a challenge to predict how any given child will do with the device (Hyde, Punch, & Komesaroff, 2010). As a result, professionals and parents face the difficult decision of whether to continue with hearing aids or pursue implantation for children who have usable hearing. The following chapter describes candidacy issues related to cochlear implants and provides information for audiologists and families on when it is appropriate to consider cochlear implants as an intervention option.

## HOW DOES A COCHLEAR IMPLANT WORK?

A cochlear implant is a prosthetic device that provides direct electrical stimulation to the auditory nerve, effectively bypassing the damaged hair cells of the cochlea in the inner ear. It is intended to be used with individuals with severe-to-profound hearing loss who do not receive benefit from hearing aids, with the goals of increasing sound awareness and speech perception. In the case of children, additional goals are to improve spoken language, articulation, reading, and academic performance. There are several different cochlear implant manufacturers that are approved by the Food and Drug Administration (FDA) in the United States. These include Advanced Bionics Corporation, Cochlear Corporation, and Med-El Corporation. Each system has its own specific features. They also have components that operate in the same basic fashion. Regardless of the manufacturer, the device itself consists of external and internal components. Figure 8–1 shows the internal components, while Figure 8–2 shows a schematic of the external and internal components. The external components include a microphone that picks up acoustic sounds in the environment, a processor that converts the acoustic signal to an electrical signal, and a transmitter coil that sends the converted electrical signal via radio waves to the internal components. The internal components include a receiver that is surgically implanted under the skin and behind the ear. It receives input from the transmitter coil, which is then sent to an electrode array implanted in the scala tympani and near the spiral ganglion. This electrode array stimulates the auditory nerve.

## HISTORY OF COCHLEAR IMPLANTS

The history of cochlear implants actually dates all the way back to the late eighteenth century. In 1790, Alessandro Volta earned the distinction of being among the first to electrically stimulate the auditory system. He accomplished this feat by connecting a battery to two metal rods. He then inserted the metal rods into his own ears. When he closed the circuit, he reported, "I received a shock in the head, and some moments after I began to hear a sound . . . which I cannot well define: it was a kind of crackling with shock, as if some paste or tenacious matter had been boiling" (Volta & Banks, 1800). Volta mused that the "disagreeable sensation" may have been dangerous. Not surprisingly, scientists were deterred from pursuing follow-up experiments for a number of years. The experiment did provide the first critical evidence that electric stimulation could induce auditory sensations, however.

In the twentieth century, progress toward a functional cochlear implant device proceeded more rapidly. In 1957, Djourno and Eyries implanted an induction coil into the eighth nerve stump in a patient with bilateral temporal bone resections. The patient reportedly could detect environmental sounds but could not discriminate speech sounds or comprehend speech. The device failed after several months and the patient was re-implanted, but this device also failed (Djourno & Eyries, 1957; Djourno, Eyries, & Vallancien, 1957). William House, a surgeon in California, heard about Djourno and Eyries' work, somewhat serendipitously when one of his own patients gave him an article describing the French scientists' experiments. House began intensive work trying to find practical ways to electrically stimulate the cochlea. In 1961, he implanted gold wire single-electrode arrays into the cochleae of two deaf individuals. The patients could hear environmental

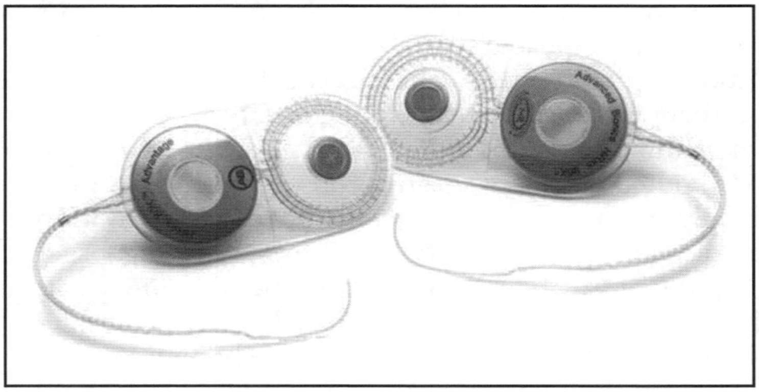

FIGURE 8–1. Advanced Bionics HiRes 90K internal components. Image courtesy of Advanced Bionics, LLC.

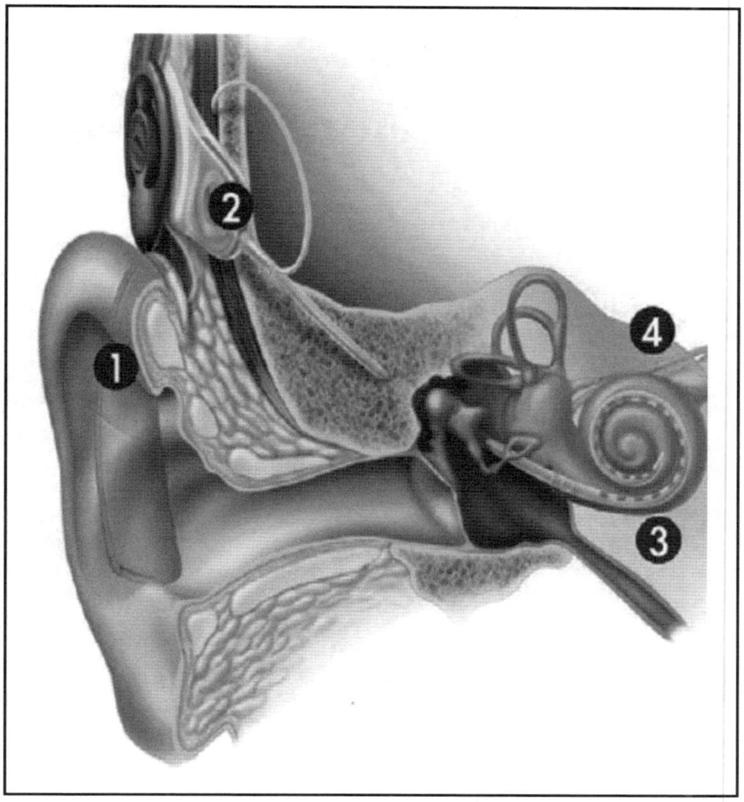


**FIGURE 8–2.** Schematic of the external and internal components of a cochlear implant: (1) the external sound processor picks up sounds in the environment and turns the sounds into a digital code, (2) the transmitter coil sends the converted digital signal via radio waves to the internal components, (3) the internal implant converts the digital code to an electrical signal that is sent to the electrode array implanted in the scala tympani and along the basilar membrane of the cochlea, and (4) this electrode array stimulates the auditory nerve, which sends a signal to the brain that is interpreted as sound.

sounds, but had no speech understanding (Wilson & Dorman, 2008). These early attempts at cochlear implantation were rudimentary, but they laid the foundation for later technological innovations. House's approach of inserting electrode arrays into the cochlea is the same approach used today.

In 1984, the first single-electrode cochlear implant was approved for adults by the FDA. That same year, multichannel cochlear implants were introduced into clinical trials in the U.S., and they were approved the following year. Children have been approved to use multichannel cochlear implants since 1990. The FDA lowered the age at which children can receive cochlear implants several times over the last decade of the twentieth century: from two years of age in 1990, to 18 months in 1998, and finally to 12 months in 2000, where the age cutoff currently stands. Surgeons can and do go "off-label" (i.e., implanting patients outside of the FDA guidelines). As a result, infants have been implanted under 12 months of age, based on the cochlear implant team's discretion. In addition, countries outside of the United States have lower age limits; for example, children as young as 3 months of age are receiving cochlear implants in Australia and Germany. Figure 8–3 shows a timeline of events in the development of cochlear implants.

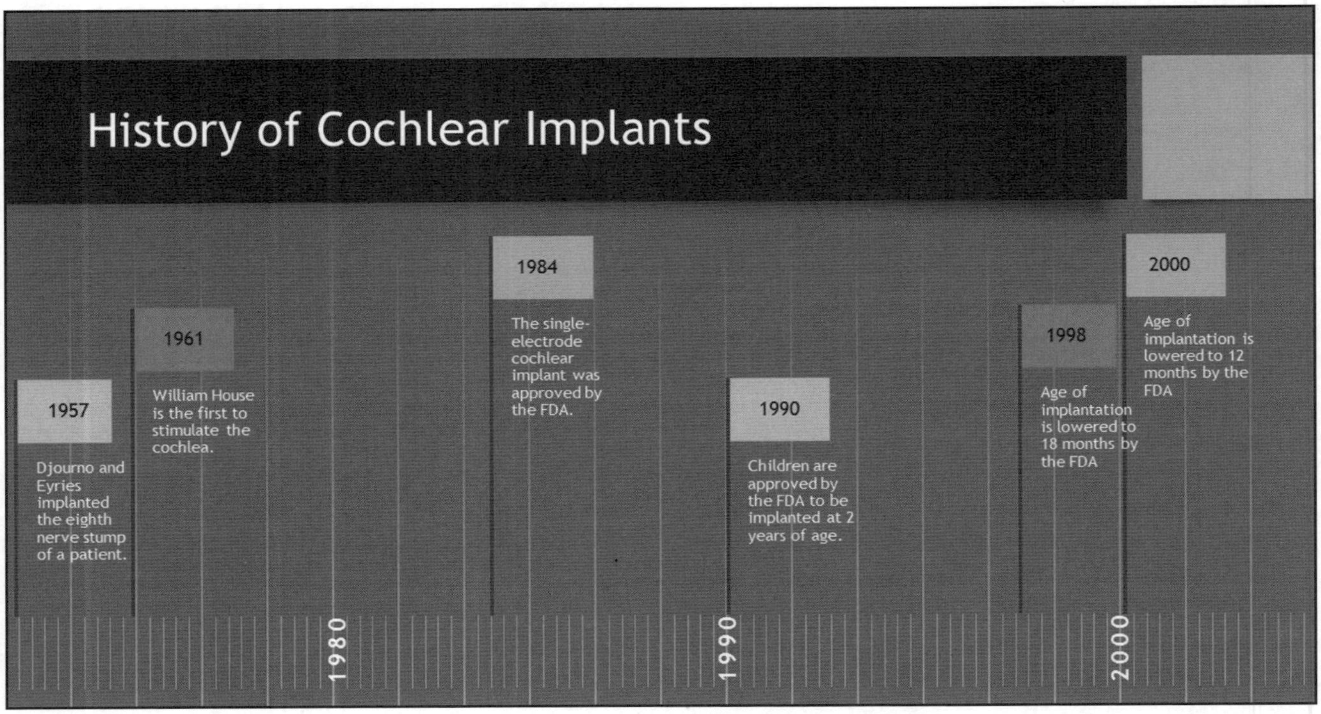


**FIGURE 8–3.** Timeline of major milestones in the history of cochlear implants.

## THE COCHLEAR IMPLANT EVALUATION PROCESS

Candidates must undergo a formal evaluation process to determine if they are medically and audiometrically suitable for cochlear implantation (Heman-Ackah, Roland, Haynes, & Waltzman, 2012). This evaluation process is multidisciplinary and includes otolaryngologists, audiologists, speech-language pathologists, and sometimes psychologists. The otolaryngologist conducts a medical examination of the external, middle, and inner ear to look for indications of infection or abnormality. The physician also attempts to identify the cause of the hearing loss, if the cause has not been already identified. Imaging takes place, involving either computerized tomography (CT)

> Computerized tomography is a cross-sectional image of a section of the human body that is produced by combining many x-rays from different angles (Herman, 2009). Because CT scans use x-rays, they are used to visualize structures within the temporal bone where the cochleae and auditory nerve are located. CT scans cannot be used to visualize soft tissue within the temporal bones, but can be used to infer whether or not the spaces in the bone for those structures are normal.
>
> Magnetic resonance imaging is a three-dimensional image of the human body that uses radio-frequency waves and magnetic fields to excite atoms. The patterns of these atoms display detailed views of internal body organs, muscles, and joints (Edelman & Warach, 1993). Because MRI can be used to visualize soft tissue, MRI may be preferred over CT scans to identify soft tissue anomalies with the cochleae or auditory nerves that cannot be determined from CT scans.

scans or magnetic resonance imaging (MRI), to evaluate the shape and patency of the cochlea and auditory nerve. Figure 8–4A shows an example of a CT scan of an individual's temporal bone and internal auditory canal, and Figure 8–4B displays an MRI scan of an internal auditory canal. The speech-language pathologist assesses speech and language acquisition, while the psychologist evaluates nonverbal cognitive skills, and determines if the patient has developmental delays.

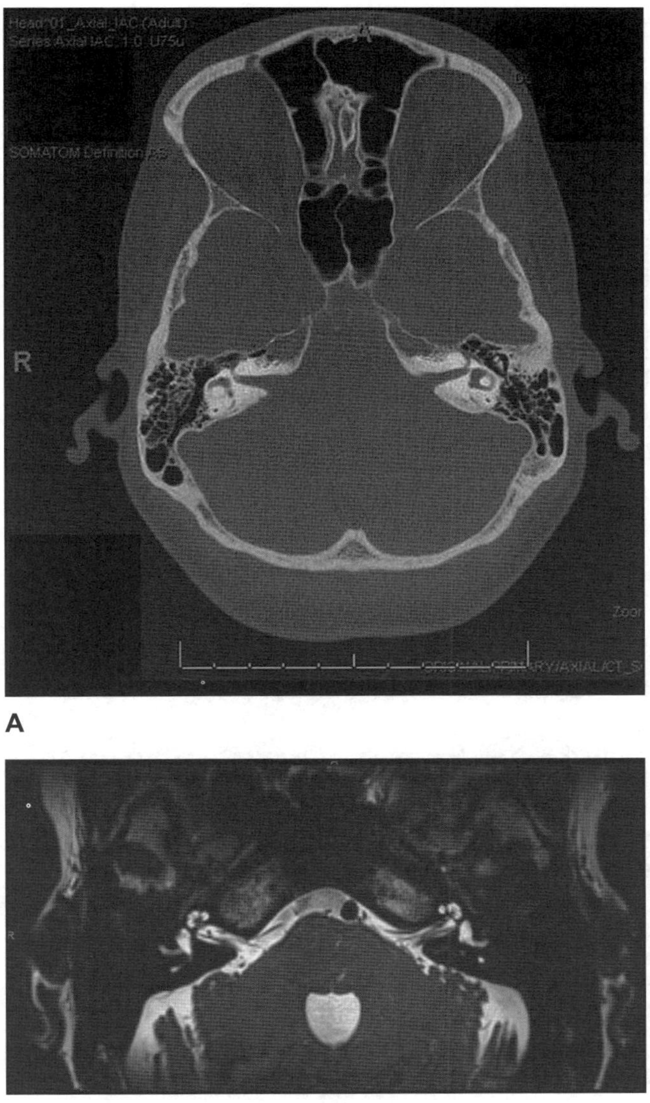

**FIGURE 8–4. A.** Computerized-tomography scan of the internal auditory canal. **B.** Magnetic resonance imaging scan of the internal auditory canal.

Family counseling is also important during the cochlear implant evaluation process. Ideally, this family counseling component is led by any member of the cochlear implant team with some training or background in family counseling. In many cases, however, the counseling role is the audiologist's responsibility. The purpose of the counseling is threefold: to help with the decision-making process of which cochlear implant device to choose, to evaluate the family's level of commitment to the aural rehabilitation process, and to ensure that the family has realistic expectations of what the cochlear implant can do, before proceeding with surgery. It is necessary that caregivers recognize that a cochlear implant will not "cure" the child's deafness. Caregivers should also be cognizant of the follow-up protocol after the surgery takes place. The surgery is only the first step in the implantation process. In order for children to receive benefit from a cochlear implant, the caregivers must be diligent in returning for programming appointments and following through with intervention.

## The Audiologic Evaluation

The audiologist is obviously central in the audiologic evaluation, which will determine whether or not the candidate meets the audiometric criteria. If the child meets the criteria, the audiologist's evaluation will also help in formulating a plan for aural habilitation after the surgery. In the case of children, unaided air- and bone-conduction threshold testing is completed to verify that the hearing loss is sensorineural in nature, as opposed to conductive or mixed. Otoacoustic emissions should also be performed, to rule out auditory neuropathy spectrum disorder (ANSD). While an ANSD diagnosis does not preclude cochlear implantation, it does affect the prognosis with the device and aural habilitation process (Roush, Frymark, Venediktov, & Wang, 2011). Audiologists will also assess aided speech perception skills, depending on the patient's age, linguistic, and cognitive levels. For children who are old enough to participate in speech perception testing, common measures include the Lexical Neighborhood Test or Multisyllabic Lexical Neighborhood Test

(Kirk, Pisoni, & Osberger, 1995), Early Speech Perception Test (Moog & Geers, 1990), Glendonald Auditory Screening Procedure (Erber, 1982), or the Phonetically-Balanced Kindergarten Lists (Haskins, 1949). There is no standardized battery for pediatric cochlear implant candidates, and audiologists report great variability in the speech perception tests that are utilized (Uhler & Gifford, 2014). The lack of a standardized test battery makes it even more important to integrate other audiologic results (e.g., audiogram, parent report questionnaires, aided audibility measures) when determining cochlear implant candidacy. The chapters on diagnostics (Chapter 2), verification (Chapter 4), and outcome measures (Chapter 6) describe these assessments in more detail. It is also typical clinical practice for audiologists to conduct aided sound-field testing with warble tones and speech as part of the evaluation procedure.

All prospective cochlear implant candidates should experience a hearing aid trial prior to implantation, to determine if they are receiving benefit from hearing aids. An exception to this rule is in cases of meningitis, where there is a concern for ossification of the cochlea that is a complication of that specific disease process. In nonmeningitic cases, the length of the hearing aid trial varies depending on the cochlear implant center, but is typically around 3 to 6 months. This is a critical step in the preimplantation process, because hearing aids are a less-invasive intervention approach than cochlear implants. If a patient shows benefit from hearing aids and is able to access sound, cochlear implantation may not be warranted. Benefit may be assessed through parent-report questionnaires or Aided Ling-6 sounds (see Chapter 6 for more information). Thus, as part of the evaluation process, audiologists should also perform real-ear or simulated real-ear hearing aid verification, to establish that the hearing aids are appropriately fit to prescriptive targets. As described earlier in this textbook, audiologists cannot effectively conclude that hearing aids are fit appropriately based on aided sound field testing (i.e., functional gain) alone.

## WHAT ARE THE CURRENT GUIDELINES FOR PEDIATRIC COCHLEAR IMPLANT CANDIDACY?

Table 8–1 shows the most recent criteria for pediatric cochlear implantation in the United States (Gifford, 2011). The table displays the criteria based on

**Table 8–1.** Audiometric and Speech Perception Criteria for Children, Based on Cochlear Implant Device Manufacturers' Labeled Indications (Gifford, 2011)

| | *Manufacturer* | | |
|---|---|---|---|
| | ***Advanced Bionics*** | ***Cochlear*** | ***MED-EL*** |
| Hearing Loss | Profound bilateral SNHL (>90 dB HL) | <2 years: Profound bilateral SNHL (>90 dB HL)<br>2+ years: severe-to profound bilateral SNHL | Profound, bilateral SNHL (90+ dB HL at 1000 Hz) |
| Speech Recognition (older children) | <4 years: <20% correct simple open-set words (e.g., Multisyllabic Lexical Neighborhood Test)<br>>4 years: <12% on difficult open-set words (i.e., PB-K) or <30% on open-set sentences (e.g., HINT-C) | ≤30% correct word recognition Multisyllabic Lexical Neighborhood Test or Lexical Neighborhood Test | <20% correct word recognition for Multisyllabic Lexical Neighborhood Test or Lexical Neighborhood Test |

the three cochlear implant manufacturers' indications, which are the specified criteria by which the manufacturers market their products. The three implant companies work independently of one another, which is why the labeled indications differ slightly. To summarize, the current FDA guidelines state that children must be at least 12 months of age at the time of surgery. The audiologic criteria for 12- to 24-month-olds are profound bilateral hearing loss (pure-tone average greater than 90 dB HL). For children older than 24 months, the audiologic criteria are less strict; the FDA approves candidacy for children with severe-to-profound hearing loss (pure-tone average greater than 70 dB HL). Regardless of age, children must demonstrate limited benefit from hearing aids, which is defined as making little to no progress in terms of auditory development. In children older than 2 years, auditory development may be assessed using speech perception measures. In children 2 years or younger, auditory development is often assessed using parent questionnaires. Typically, the Infant-Toddler Meaningful Auditory Scale (IT-MAIS), the Meaningful Auditory Integration Scale (MAIS) (Zimmerman-Phillips & Osberger, 1997), or the LittlEARS® (May-Mederake et al., 2010) are utilized (Uhler & Gifford, 2014).

## Unilateral Versus Bilateral Cochlear Implants

One decision that parents face if their child meets the audiometric criteria for cochlear implantation is whether to implant one ear (unilateral) or both ears (bilateral). In the 1990s, when the treatment effectiveness of cochlear implants was still being debated, unilateral cochlear implants were the standard approach to habilitation. Starting in the 2000s, increasing numbers of children began receiving two cochlear implants, either sequentially (the surgeries for each ear take place at different times, therefore, devices are activated months or years apart) or simultaneously (both ears are implanted at the same time). The rationale behind bilateral implantation is that binaural hearing (i.e., hearing from both ears) results in better speech understanding in quiet and noise, as well as better sound localization skills (Peters et al., 2007). Bilateral cochlear implants have become an accepted treatment approach for children with bilateral severe-to-profound hearing loss in recent years (Papsin & Gordon, 2008). The clinical recommendation to implant both ears is supported by evidence that children generally performed better on speech-in-noise and localization tasks in bilateral compared to unilateral conditions (Kühn-Inacker, Shehata-Dieler, Müller, & Helms, 2004; Litovsky et al., 2006). Studies have also shown between-group differences, with children with bilateral cochlear implants outperforming children with unilateral implants on spatial hearing skills, even as young as 2 to 3 years of age (Grieco-Calub & Litovsky, 2012).

## Expanding Candidacy for Pediatric Cochlear Implantation: Children with Residual Hearing

As Roland and Waltzman (2015) noted, the FDA guidelines are just that—guidelines for who should be a candidate for a cochlear implant. The guidelines are not rules that are set in stone. One aspect of the guidelines that has evolved over time is the trend to offer cochlear implantation for children with increasing amounts of residual hearing. When cochlear implants were first approved for children in 1990, they were intended for children with profound hearing loss and no open-set word recognition. Early on, researchers and clinicians observed that children with cochlear implants performed better than children with hearing aids who had hearing loss in the profound range on speech perception and language measures (Eisenberg, Kirk, Martinez, Ying, & Miyamoto, 2004; Spencer, Tye-Murray, & Tomblin, 1998; Tomblin, Spencer, Flock, Tyler, & Gantz, 1999). Studies published in the late 1990s and early 2000s offered evidence that children with preoperative open-set speech perception scores could make substantial improvements in word recognition following implantation (Cowan et al., 1997; Dettman et al., 2004; Eisenberg, Martinez, Sennaroglu, & Osberger, 2000; Gantz et al., 2000; Mondain et al., 2002; Zwolan et al., 1997). The adult cochlear implant literature provided further evidence that the candidacy criteria was overly restrictive, as it became evident that preoperative residual hearing was a significant positive predictor of postimplantation speech perception outcomes (Blamey et al., 1996; Gantz, Woodworth, Knutson, Abbas, & Tyler, 1993; Gomaa, Rubinstein, Lowder, Tyler, & Gantz, 2003; Rubinstein, Parkinson, Tyler, & Gantz, 1999). In 2003, candidacy was expanded to include children with some open-set word recognition abilities. The open-set criteria varies depending on the cochlear implant manufacturer indications (Gifford, 2011), as shown in Table 8–1.

There is growing recognition among many cochlear implant centers that the FDA guidelines may be too conservative with respect to degree of hearing loss. Specifically, there are children with hearing aids who do not meet all of the FDA criteria for cochlear implantation, but who might arguably have better perception and developmental outcomes with cochlear implants than they can achieve with hearing aids. As a result, it is now common practice to consider children with greater residual hearing for cochlear implants, both in the United States and internationally (Fitzpatrick, McCrae, & Schramm, 2006; Russell, Pine, & Young, 2013). The rationale for this expansion of candidacy is motivated by the expectation that children with more hearing will experience better outcomes if they avoid lengthy trials with hearing aids, because hearing aids cannot provide the same amount of auditory access as cochlear implants for children with severe-to-profound loss. There is also a strong argument to be made against pursuing an aggressive surgical approach via cochlear implantation, however. For children with significant usable hearing, the surgery may damage the structures of the inner ear, resulting in complete loss of residual hearing and natural acoustic perception.

Carlson et al. (2015) describes several different pediatric populations that may be considered with the expansion of cochlear implant candidacy. The first of these groups are children with asymmetric hearing loss, with the poorer ear in the severe-to-profound range and the better ear in the moderately-severe range or better. The most extreme example of these cases would be children with single-sided deafness: severe-to-profound hearing loss in one ear and normal-to-near normal hearing in the opposite ear. Considering cochlear implants as an option for children with single-sided deafness is a recent development and is discussed later in this chapter.

In the less extreme case of children with bilateral hearing loss that is asymmetric, one of the primary concerns is that they will have little access to binaural listening cues, because the poorer ear will have little to no auditory access due to the limits of acoustic amplification (Cadieux, Firszt, & Reeder, 2013). Binaural listening is critical for understanding speech in noise and sound localization. Thus, the argument is that these children may be good candidates for bimodal device use, in that they would receive electrical stimulation from the cochlear implant in the poorer ear and acoustic stimulation from the hearing aid in the better ear.

Another group that Carlson and colleagues describe are children with better than severe hearing loss in both ears who are showing lack of progress in auditory development, despite having well-fit hearing aids, full-time device use, and consistent aural habilitation services. These children are the group that should be considered with utmost caution, given the possibility of damaging the anatomical structures and eliminating whatever acoustic hearing still remains. Hearing preservation approaches are particularly important to this group; these techniques are described later in this chapter.

Despite the consensus that these two populations of children (asymmetric hearing loss and moderate-severe flat hearing loss) might benefit from cochlear implants, there is a dearth of high-quality research studies examining the effects of cochlear implants on outcomes of nontraditional pediatric candidates. Carlson et al. (2015) conducted a retrospective review of 51 pediatric patients who received cochlear implants at two different cochlear implant centers. They specifically examined patients based on the following criteria: (1) less than 70 dB HL PTA in the implanted or nonimplanted ear for children between 2 and 17 years, or less than 90 dB HL for children less than 2 years of age, and (2) speech perception scores greater than 30% in the best aided condition. At an average follow-up of 17 months postimplantation, patients showed significant gains in speech perception and language skills; on average, children showed a 63% improvement in speech perception scores postimplantation and 40% improvement in the bimodal condition. Carlson and his colleagues interpreted this as evidence for expansion of pediatric cochlear implant guidelines to include children who are demonstrating poor progress with hearing aids.

In another report of nontraditional pediatric candidates, Cadieux, Firszt, and Reeder (2013) described a within-subject case study of five adolescents with asymmetric hearing loss, ranging in age from 10 to 19 years. For all five children, one ear met the audiometric criteria for cochlear implantation, while the other ear did not. After implantation, the patients all wore hearing aids in the opposite ear. Hearing aids were fit to Desired Sensation Level prescriptive targets for soft, conversational, and loud speech, using real-ear verification procedures. Results were mixed, with three patients showing good postimplantation outcomes and two patients not demonstrating significant benefit from their cochlear implants compared to preimplant scores. The three patients with better outcomes demonstrated open-set speech recognition when they were tested with only their cochlear implant. They also demonstrated benefit on speech perception tests and sound localization in the bimodal condition, suggesting positive effects of using a cochlear implant and hearing aid in combination. These three patients had favorable case histories, specifically progressive hearing loss and consistent bilateral hearing aid use since early childhood. The other two patients did not show as much benefit postimplantation. Neither demonstrated open-set speech recognition with their cochlear implant following initial stimulation. They also did not show bimodal benefit in speech recognition or sound localization testing, although they reported experiencing bimodal benefit in daily life. The latter two participants both had profound hearing loss since birth in the poorer ear and had never worn a hearing aid in that ear. The lengthy period of auditory deprivation likely reduced the ability of the auditory nerve to respond to electrical stimulation in these two cases, which may be taken as evidence for a need to consider implantation at younger ages for children with these audiometric profiles. Interestingly, despite the lack of evidence that the latter two patients received objective benefit from their cochlear implants, both reported receiving subjective bimodal benefit. The results support the need for early, consistent hearing aid use for children with asymmetric hearing loss, even in cases where the poorer ear has a severe-to-profound hearing loss and is unlikely to demonstrate any clear benefit from acoustic amplification. The early stimulation of the auditory pathways may prime the poorer ear for later electric stimulation, if the family decides to pursue cochlear implantation at a later age (Gordon, Jiwani, & Papsin, 2011).

One of the major limitations of these studies is that they did not directly compare the performance of children with severe hearing loss who continued to use hearing aids to children with comparable degrees of hearing loss who received cochlear implants. There are only a few examples of direct comparisons in the research literature. Blamey et al. (2001) compared pediatric hearing aid users with severe hearing loss (average PTA = 78 dB HL) to pediatric cochlear implant users with profound hearing loss (average preoperative PTA = 106 dB HL). They found no significant differences between the two groups on measures of speech recognition, articulation, and language, but the cochlear implant group fit the more traditional profile of implant candidates and nearly all would have fit under current FDA guidelines, in that children had profound bilateral hearing loss. Fitzpatrick et al. (2012) tested 20 hearing aid users (average age = 12.5 years; average PTA = 68.7 dB HL) and 21 cochlear implant users (average age = 9.9 years; average preoperative PTA = 100.5 dB HL). Like the participants in the Blamey et al. study, the cochlear implant users fit the traditional guidelines for implantation. They found no significant differences between groups on speech perception measures in quiet or in noise, articulation, spelling, and word reading. The hearing aid users did perform significantly better on higher level language measures, including receptive vocabulary, global expressive and receptive language skills, nonword repetition, and reading comprehension. These results highlight the importance of evaluating both speech perception and language skills for children in the borderline cochlear implant candidacy range. If speech perception scores or speech production are the only factors considered, many children with cochlear implants appear to perform as well as children with hearing aids, which could be interpreted as evidence that cochlear implants are justified in borderline scenarios. When higher level language skills are taken into account, at least some children with moderately-severe or severe hearing loss appear to show benefits from conventional hearing aids over cochlear implants. Such evidence would suggest that the need for more aggressive surgical interventions is unnecessary for all children in the borderline candidacy range.

### Conclusions on Expanding Candidacy for Children with Residual Hearing

In this section, we emphasize the point that language, reading, and academic performance should be considered in combination with speech perception scores. Often, traditional audiological speech discrimination and word recognition measures are the focus of cochlear implant candidacy criteria and investigations of device efficacy (Fitzpatrick et al., 2012; Pisoni, 2000). Reliance on speech perception measures to determine candidacy becomes a challenge when clinicians encounter children who have substantial residual hearing and open-set speech perception scores with hearing aids (Eisenberg et al., 2004). Poor auditory access influences language skills, and language skills are associated with functional outcomes, including literacy and academic achievement. However, the associations between these factors is not always a direct, one-to-one relationship: Fitzpatrick et al. (2012) did not find a difference in speech perception scores between children with severe hearing loss who used hearing aids and children with cochlear implants, but did show an advantage for the hearing aid users on receptive vocabulary, grammar, and phonological memory. Therefore, the best approach to take when evaluating a child who is a borderline cochlear implant candidate is to conduct a comprehensive, multidisciplinary assessment, including assessments in the child's educational setting. This will allow the cochlear implant team to obtain a complete picture of the child's current level of functioning and make an informed decision of whether he or she would receive greater benefit from a cochlear implant than hearing aids.

It is also important to recognize the limitations of the current literature on cochlear implants in children with residual hearing. We are still lacking research designs with controlled trials, comparing children with cochlear implants and children with hearing aids who are in the borderline candidacy range. High quality research studies are greatly needed and will provide more guidance in the decision-making process for cochlear implants.

## WHEN IT IS TIME TO CONSIDER TRANSITIONING FROM A HEARING AID TO A COCHLEAR IMPLANT?

Researchers have maintained that children who are "nontraditional" cochlear implant candidates often struggle making progress with appropriately fit hearing aids and are likely the ones who will do the best with cochlear implants (Cadieux et al., 2013; Carlson et al., 2015). Unfortunately, infants and toddlers often cannot participate in speech perception tasks and may have limited evidence of language abilities, which leads to a difficult decision for families and audiologists. What do we do for so-called borderline candidates? These would include infants or toddlers with thresholds in the moderate-to-severe range, who show speech understanding with hearing aids and make some progress in terms of speech and spoken language acquisition, but less than what we would expect based on their audiometric thresholds. Should the child still be considered for cochlear implantation? By *not* considering cochlear implants as a treatment option, families and audiologists are put in the awkward position of essentially waiting for the child to fall further behind in developmental milestones before proceeding with cochlear implantation. To avoid such pitfalls, it is critical for audiologists to recognize the numerous factors that should be considered when deciding when to send a child for a cochlear implant evaluation.

The dilemma is further compounded by the fact that by waiting for the child to demonstrate developmental delays, we might be missing out on a window of brain plasticity for auditory development. We have a preponderance of evidence that "younger is better"—in other words, children benefit from early provision of cochlear implants. So how should parents and audiologists determine when it is appropriate to consider cochlear implantation? The consensus among researchers and clinicians is that the decision should not be based on audiometric thresholds alone (Fitzpatrick et al., 2009). We advocate for audiologists to consider several different factors when deciding whether it is time to refer a pediatric patient for a cochlear implant evaluation. These factors include auditory development questionnaires, aided audibility measures, and standardized language measures.

## Auditory Development Questionnaires

For younger children who cannot participate in speech perception testing and may have limited evidence of language use, auditory development questionnaires provide information that can be helpful in monitoring progress (Carlson et al., 2015). These questionnaires include parent-report measures such as the IT-MAIS, the MAIS, the LittlEARS Auditory Questionnaire (May-Mederake et al., 2010), and the Parents' Evaluation of Aural/Oral Performance of Children (PEACH) (Ching & Hill, 2007). Although the IT-MAIS and MAIS are often used in the clinical setting, the LittlEARS and PEACH have additional benefits that are useful in the decision-making process. One of these benefits is the inclusion of normative data, to allow for comparison to typically developing children (Bagatto, Brown, Moodie, & Scollie, 2011; Coninx et al., 2009). Figure 8–5 shows the mean and 95% confidence intervals for English-speaking children with the LittlEARS. By administering the LittlEARS at every audiology appointment, audiologists can identify children who are consistently outside of the normative range. These observations should encourage conversations with parents about the need to consider a cochlear implant. A second benefit is that the LittlEARS and PEACH have been translated into multiple languages (Geal-Dor, Jbarah, Meilijson, Adelman, & Levi, 2011; Kosaner, Sonuguler, Olgun, &

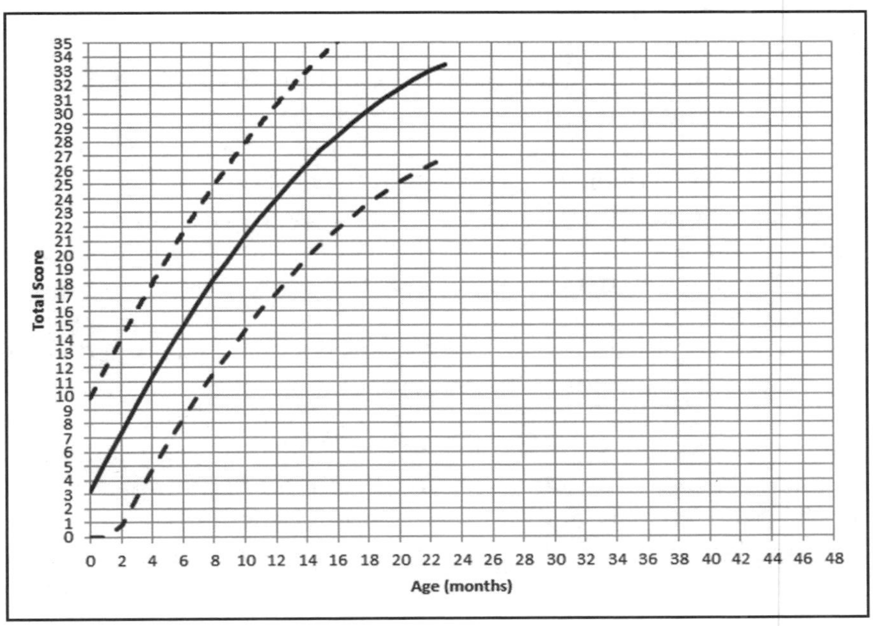


**FIGURE 8–5.** English-speaking normative curve and the minimum 95% confidence intervals from the Canadian-derived norms of the *LittlEARS®* parent-report questionnaire (Image courtesy of Marlene Bagatto, AuD, PhD).

Amann, 2013; Negro, García, & Quevedo, 2016; Rauhamäki, Lonka, Lipsanen, & Laakso, 2014; Spitzer & Zavala, 2011; Wang, Sun, Liang, Chen, & Zheng, 2013), making them feasible for use with culturally and linguistically diverse populations. Further discussion about auditory development questionnaires that have been used with pediatric cochlear implant candidates, as well as information regarding developmental "red flags" that audiologists should be aware of, can be found in Chapter 6 (Monitoring Outcomes).

## Moving Beyond Pure-Tone Average: Aided Audibility Measures

In a survey with Canadian audiologists, Fitzpatrick et al. (2009) found general agreement among practitioners that pure-tone average is insufficient to indicate whether a child is a candidate for a cochlear implant. The main limitation of using pure-tone average is that it does not take configuration of hearing loss into account. By definition, it is an average of thresholds at low, middle, and higher frequencies, and weights each region equally in its calculation. Also, there is not a valid way to estimate the pure-tone average when a child is wearing their hearing aid, as discussed in the section on the limitations of functional gain testing in Chapter 4. In the Fitzpatrick et al. (2009) study, audiologists indicated that they placed greater weight on thresholds in the high frequency region than the low frequency region when describing children as being in the borderline hearing range for candidacy. Thus, it seems important for audiologists to have evidence-based metrics for measuring auditory access, other than pure-tone average.

One strategy for measuring auditory access while still taking configuration into account is through audibility measures. As we discussed in Chapter 4, audibility is a measure of the amount of access to the speech spectrum. The audibility for speech can be quantified using metrics like the Speech Intelligibility Index (SII; ANSI S3.5:1997 R2007). The SII is a number between 0 and 1, where higher numbers mean that more of the speech spectrum is audible to the listener. The SII, by design, weights high-frequency sounds more heavily in the calculation because this region contributes more information to speech clarity than low frequency sounds. A major benefit of aided audibility measures is that they allow the audiologist to evaluate the configuration of the hearing loss, as well as determine how much access the individual has to speech with and without hearing aids.

We know that better aided audibility promotes language growth in children who are hard of hearing (Tomblin et al., 2015; Tomblin, Oleson, Ambrose, Walker, & Moeller, 2014). Unfortunately, we do not know how much access is *enough*. How much aided audibility does a child need to successfully acquire spoken language? Stiles, Bentler, and McGregor (2012) looked at aided SII as a predictor of vocabulary in children with mild to severe hearing loss. Results suggested that children with an aided SII of less than .65 are at risk for delays in receptive vocabulary. Figure 8–6 shows the relationship between aided SII and receptive vocabulary for the participants in Stiles et al.'s study.

It should be noted that vocabulary tends to be a relatively robust aspect of language for children with hearing loss (Geers & Nicholas, 2013; Moeller, Tomblin, & the OCHL Collaboration, 2015). Children who are hard of hearing tend to have more difficulty in the language domain of morphology and syntax (Delage & Tuller, 2007; McGuckian & Henry, 2007; Tomblin et al., 2015). Specifically, high-frequency, low-intensity s/z morphological markers appear to be vulnerable to the effects of hearing loss because they are difficult to hear, even with amplification. These morphological markers include third person singular -s ("He walk<u>s</u> to the store"), plural -s ("many cat<u>s</u>"), and possessive -s ("The girl'<u>s</u> hat"). To date, no researchers have examined whether there is a cutoff point based on the aided SII, at which children are at risk for morphosyntactic delays. Koehlinger, Owen Van Horne, Oleson, McCreery, and Moeller (2015) found that aided access to high-frequency sounds, particularly at 4000 Hz, supports grammatical development of s/z morphemes. Additional research, looking at children's aided access to high-frequency information (i.e., 4000 to 8000 Hz), is needed in this area. As researchers learn more about the relationship between audibility and language acquisition, the aided SII may

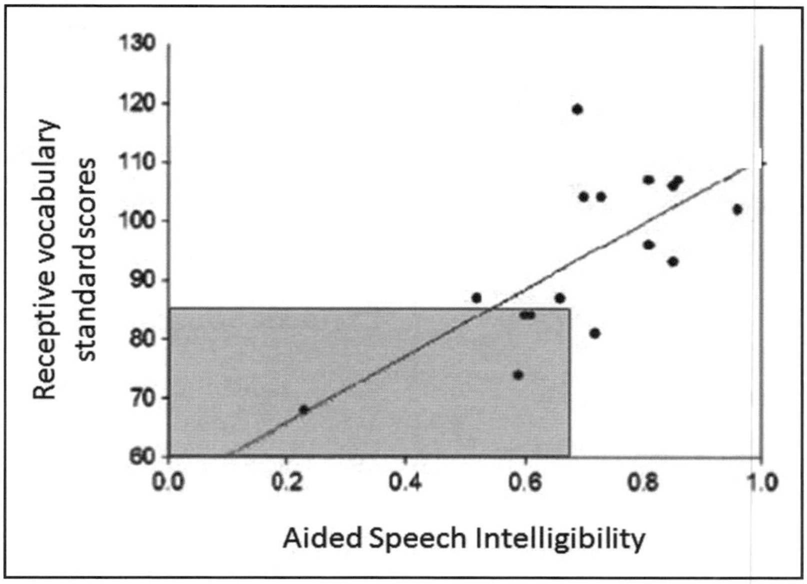


**FIGURE 8–6.** Association between aided Speech Intelligibility Index and receptive vocabulary in children with mild to severe hearing loss (Stiles, Bentler, & McGregor, 2012).

become a useful benchmark for determining cochlear implant candidacy for children in the borderline range.

Stiles et al. (2012) brings up another point regarding aided audibility, which relates to cochlear implant candidacy. One participant in his study, "Casey," had a severe-to-profound hearing loss and the lowest aided SII (0.23) of the 16 participants with hearing loss. Casey's hearing aids were appropriately fit to prescriptive targets, but even then, the aided SII was very low. Audiologists who are fitting hearing aids have likely encountered this situation. For children whose hearing loss is in the severe range (i.e., borderline cochlear implant candidates), aided audibility might be poor even when the hearing aids are matched to prescriptive targets. The output level required to provide sufficient audibility results in a simultaneous increase in the distortion of the hearing aid, which negates any improvement in the aided SII. In Casey's case, Stiles notes that his family was considering cochlear implantation, after audiologists and parents took into account the reduced access Casey could get from his hearing aids, as well as the struggles he was facing in terms of academic and language development.

## Standardized Measures for Older Children

One of the main reasons for considering cochlear implants for children with residual hearing and open-set speech perception skills is because they are falling behind their same-age, hearing classmates academically and/or socially. Therefore, it makes sense that multiple developmental domains should be considered when deciding whether it is time for a child to transition to a cochlear implant. These domains should include the three aspects of language, as described by Bloom and Lahey (1978) (Figure 8–7).

Each aspect of language should be evaluated as part of a comprehensive assessment of functioning when deciding if child should transition from hearing aids to a cochlear implant. Standardized, norm-referenced measures are available to assess each of these areas, and speech-language pathologists are trained to administer these measures. Although audiologists would not conduct these measures, taking a collaborative approach and expressing concerns to parents and other professionals when children are under-performing relative to their degree of hearing loss can initiate

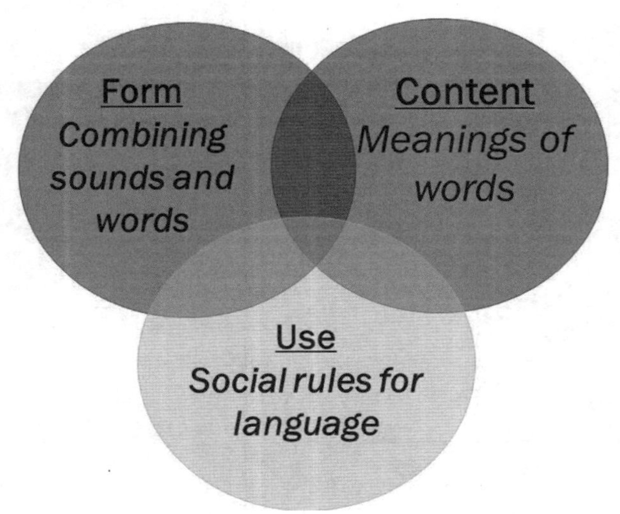


**FIGURE 8–7.** Bloom and Lahey's model of language (Bloom & Lahey, 1978).

a process of evaluation. In addition to evaluating language skills in older school-age children, literacy and academic assessments are also warranted. These literacy and academic assessments, such as the *Gray Oral Reading Test* (Wiederholt & Bryant, 2001), the *Oral and Written Language Scales* (Carrow-Woolfolk, 2011), or the *Woodcock-Johnson Tests of Achievement* (Schrank, Mather, & McGrew, 2014) will allow for comparisons to age- or grade-matched children with normal hearing and will give a sense of how delayed the child is compared to average performance. Educational specialists may be best qualified to administer these types of assessments, although speech-language pathologists are appropriate as well. The child's own educational service providers, particularly his or her regular education teacher and itinerant teacher of the deaf/hard of hearing, are also a good source of information.

## NEW DIRECTIONS IN COCHLEAR IMPLANTS

Cochlear implant technology and issues related to candidacy continue to evolve over time. Typically, these new technologies or strategies undergo trials with adults first. Once it is deemed safe in the adult, postlingually deaf population and benefits are clearly demonstrated, researchers will initiate clinical trials with the pediatric population. The following section will highlight two new applications of cochlear implants that are just starting to be used with children.

### Electroacoustic Stimulation

When considering the transition from hearing aids to cochlear implants, parents and audiologists express one major concern: irreversible loss of residual hearing during and after the implant surgery. This is a valid concern given the intracochlear trauma that occurs to the osseous spiral lamina, basilar membrane, and adjacent structures during the course of inserting the electrode array into the cochlea. In recent years, there has been a move toward designing electrode arrays that will cause less damage to the intracochlear structures. These electrode arrays are both thinner and shorter. Surgeons are also adjusting surgical techniques in an attempt to preserve cochlear anatomy and residual hearing (Gantz, Turner, Gfeller, & Lowder, 2005). The hope is that the combination of modified electrode designs and *soft surgical techniques* will result in expansion of cochlear implant candidacy, to include children with moderately-severe and severe hearing loss, particularly with significant low-frequency residual hearing.

> Soft-surgery cochlear implant techniques are a surgical approach designed to reduce trauma to the intracochlear structures and preserve residual hearing. Some of the procedures involve avoiding blood entry into the scala tympani, bone dust in the cochlea, and applying steroids at the cochleostomy site. For a review on the techniques and efficacy of soft surgery approaches, see Friedland and Runge-Samuelson (2009).

One motivation for reducing the trauma by using shorter, thinner electrode arrays is that low-frequency residual hearing will be preserved.

Patients with significant amounts of low-frequency hearing can then take advantage of technology that combines electric and acoustic stimulation into one device in the same ear. These strategies are known as electroacoustic stimulation (EAS) or Hybrid technology (Gantz & Turner, 2004; Turner, Gantz, & Reiss, 2008). The concept for a Hybrid electric/acoustic device first began in 1995, not long after standard-length cochlear implants were approved by the FDA. Dr. Bruce Gantz at the University of Iowa approached Cochlear Corporation, one of the major cochlear implant manufacturers, about designing a shorter-length electrode that would be implanted in the base of the cochlear, preserving the anatomy of the apical end (Gantz et al., 2016). The FDA began clinical trials in the US in 1999. The Nucleus® Hybrid™ L24 Cochlear Implant System was approved for use in individuals who are 18 years or older by the FDA in 2014.

The goal of Hybrid devices is to provide electrical stimulation in the mid- and high-frequency range and acoustic stimulation to the low frequencies. Hybrid candidates may have low-frequency residual hearing of less than or equal to 60 dB HL at 500 Hz and profound hearing loss (greater than 90 dB HL) at 1500 Hz and above. The darkened region in Figure 8–8 shows the audiometric range at which adult patients may be considered for a Hybrid device. Figure 8–9 compares the length of the two currently used electrode arrays in the internal Hybrid device, as well as the standard length array which can be placed 20 to 25 mm into the cochlea, while Figure 8–10 shows the insertion depth of these arrays.

These Hybrid devices appear to provide improved frequency resolution in adults, which has resulted in better speech perception in quiet and in noise compared to adults with standard length electrode arrays (Gantz, Turner, & Gfeller, 2006). Individuals using Hybrid devices and hearing aids in the opposite ear also show improved localization abilities (identifying where a sound is coming from) compared to listening with the short-electrode cochlear implant in one ear and hearing aid in the other ear (Dunn, Perreau, Gantz, & Tyler, 2010). A third demonstrated benefit of Hybrids in adults is music appreciation, which is typically described as sounding poor to listeners with electric-only hearing (Gfeller, Olszewski, Turner, Gantz, & Oleson, 2006).

The majority of Hybrid users demonstrate some preservation of residual hearing following

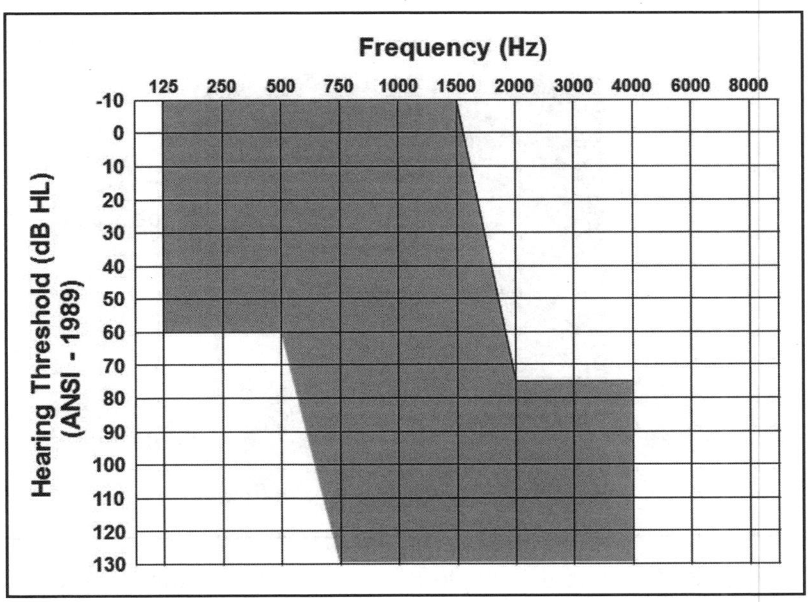


**FIGURE 8–8.** Audiometric range for candidacy of a Hybrid device, shown in gray. Image courtesy of Cochlear Americas, © 2017.

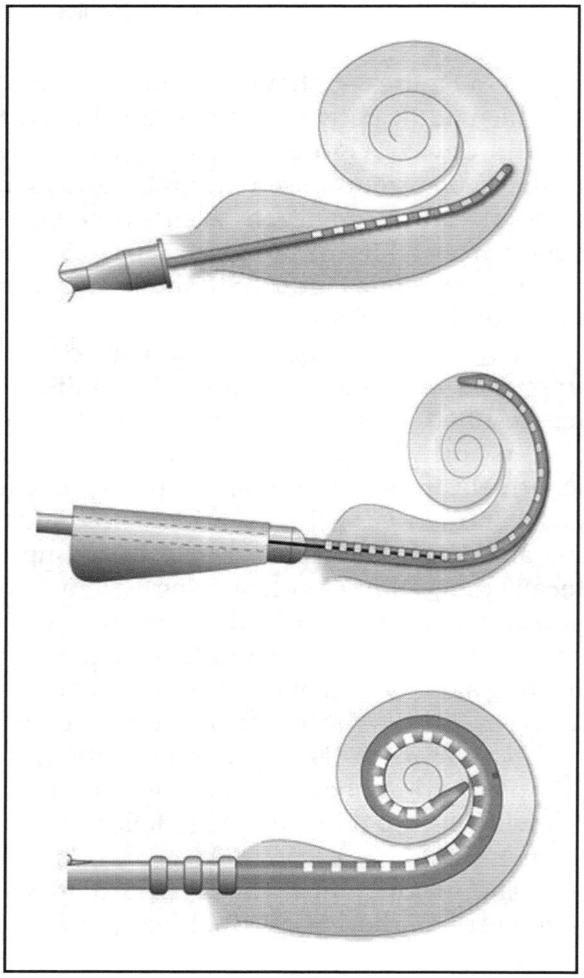

**FIGURE 8–9.** Schematic of the length of the two currently used electrode arrays in the internal Hybrid device, as well as the standard length array. The top image depicts the Hybrid S12 array, the middle image depicts the Hybrid L24 array, and the bottom image depicts the standard length array (22 to 25 mm). Image courtesy of Cochlear Americas, ©2017.

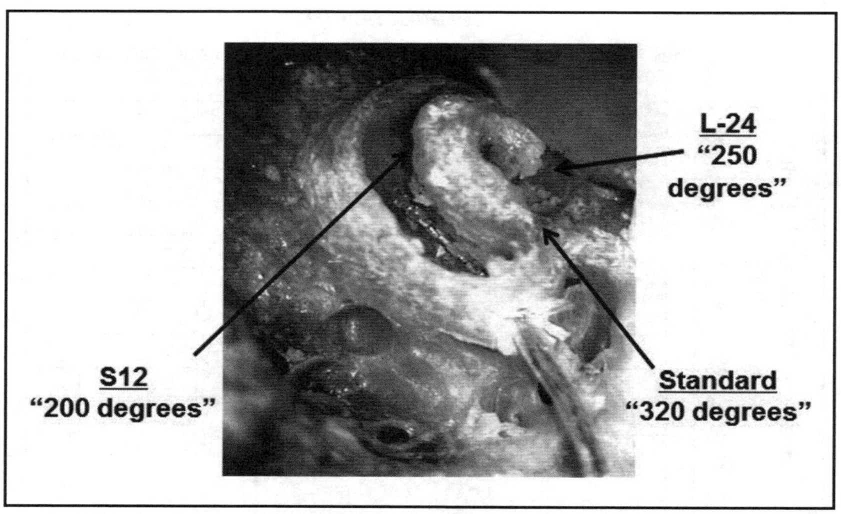


**FIGURE 8–10.** Insertion depth into the cochlea of the Hybrid S12, L24, and standard length arrays. Image courtesy of Cochlear Americas, © 2017.

the implantation surgery. In a recent study by Dedhia, Worman, Meredith, and Rubinstein (2016), 94% of adult Hybrid patients achieved some long-term hearing preservation. As previously stated, Hybrids were recently approved for use by the FDA in adults. Clinical FDA trials (known as Investigational Device Exemptions or IDEs) for children ages 5 to 15 years are currently underway. At the University of Iowa, five children have received Hybrid devices since 2011. These children did not meet the FDA-approved audiometric indications for adult Hybrid candidates (shown earlier in Figure 8–7), as they had poorer low-frequency hearing. Specifically, the children who have participated in the Hybrid IDE had a PTA between 60 and 90 dB HL from 125 to 1500 Hz and profound hearing loss above 1500 Hz (Gantz, Dunn, Walker, Van Voorst, Gogel, & Hansen, 2016). At initial activation, the average PTA loss was 5.6 dB HL. At the 24 months postoperative visit for four children and the 12 months postoperative visit for one child, all five had preserved functional hearing (defined as low-frequency pure-tone average of 125 to 1000 Hz that is better than 85 dB HL). Hearing thresholds below 1500 Hz were stable from the preoperative visit compared to the most recent visit for three of the participants. Two participants showed a decrease in thresholds following the surgery, although both maintained functional hearing. The children demonstrated significant improvements in speech perception in quiet by 8 months postimplantation compared to their preimplant word recognition scores. Localization skills also improved from preimplant to postimplant. Articulation, reading, and language skills were monitored across the five patients. Two patients showed stable performance over time, one patient showed a significant decrease in articulation (but was stable in language and reading scores), and one patient showed significant improvement in articulation and language (Gantz et al., 2016).

Performance with the Hybrid device in adolescents can also be compared between-groups, to children who use a standard-length electrode array in one ear and a hearing aid in the other ear. Figure 8–11 displays open-set speech perception scores on the Consonant-Nucleus-Consonant (CNC) test for adolescents with the L24 Hybrid device compared and adolescents with a standard length array. Both groups of children wore hearing aids in their opposite ears (i.e., bimodal configuration), but the children with standard arrays had poorer preimplant residual hearing, particularly in the low frequencies. Although these data indicate that the average speech perception scores for the Hybrid users were slightly lower compared to the bimodal users (bars on the far right of the figure), the results should be interpreted with caution, given the small number of patients and variability in individual results. When the individual data are examined, it appears that four out of the five Hybrid users achieved open-set speech perception scores that were similar to the children with the standard-length array. These preliminary data suggest that adolescents with low-frequency residual hearing may benefit from combined acoustic and electric hearing. Further longitudinal research is needed to fully establish the efficacy of this device.

## Single-Sided Deafness

Individuals with single-sided deafness or unilateral hearing loss (i.e., profound hearing loss in one ear, normal hearing in the opposite ear) experience difficulties with localization and speech perception in noise. These difficulties are due to the listener's inability to take advantage of binaural listening cues, which help with telling where sounds are coming from and listening in noisy environments. These problems have cascading effects on children with single-sided deafness, some of whom show delays in language, psychosocial, and academic outcomes (Bess & Tharpe, 1984; Lieu, Tye-Murray, Karzon, & Piccirillo, 2010). The traditional rehabilitative options for children and adults with unilateral hearing loss are contralateral routing of sound (CROS) hearing aids or bone-anchored hearing aids (BAHA). These treatment approaches are limited, in that they do not restore binaural auditory processing because the device is only improving detectability of sound originating from the side of the deaf ear. Therefore, the CROS and the BAHA provide

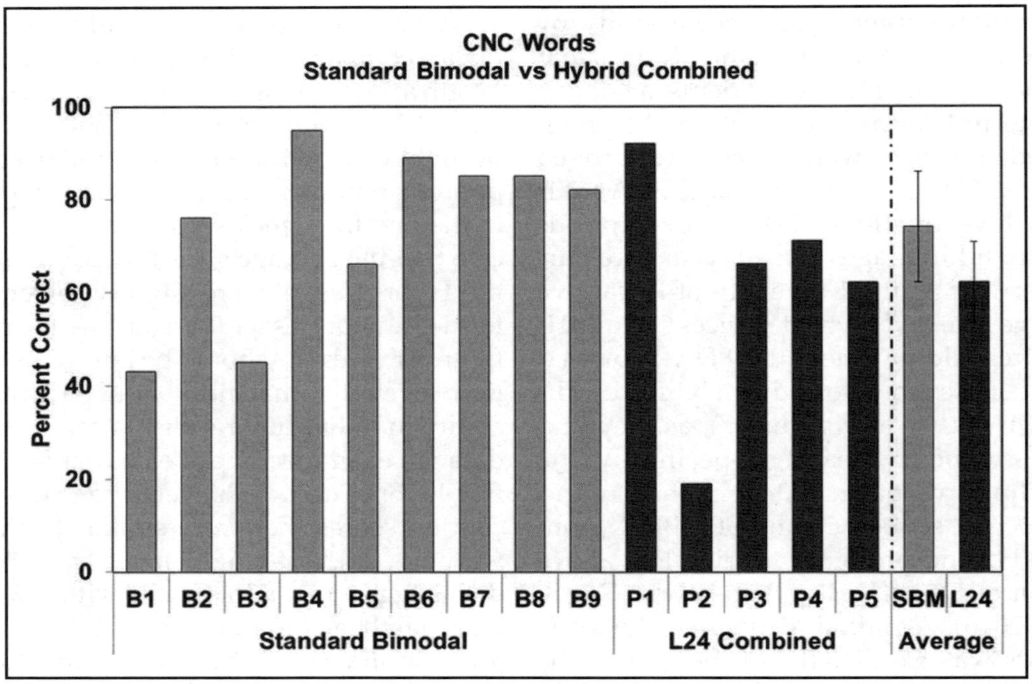


**FIGURE 8–11.** Individual results on the Consonant-Nucleus-Consonant word recognition measure for adolescents with a standard-length electrode in one ear and hearing aid in the other ear (standard bimodal, shown in light gray bars) and adolescents with the L24 Hybrid in one ear and hearing in the other ear (L24 Combined, shown in dark gray bars). Averaged results are shown to the right of the dotted line.

minimal improvement in sound localization for individuals with sensorineural hearing loss (Battista et al., 2013; Grantham et al., 2012) and only modest improvements in listening in noise (Desmet, Wouters, De Bodt, & Van de Heyning, 2014). In recent years, cochlear implants have been proposed as a method to restore auditory perception to the deaf ear. Preliminary results with adults are promising, in that adult patients showed improved speech perception and sound localization compared with CROS, BAHA, and unaided conditions preoperatively (Arndt et al., 2011). Several literature reviews on treatment efficacy for cochlear implants in single-sided deafness support the earlier positive results (Kamal, Robinson, & Diaz, 2012; Vlastarakos, Nazos, Tavoulari, & Nikolopoulos, 2014).

Providing cochlear implants to children with single-sided deafness is still rare, as surgeons are hesitant to provide this technology to children until the benefits for adults are more firmly established. Only a handful of studies have been published on the pediatric population. Plontke et al. (2013) published a case study of an 8-year-old boy with postlingual, acute deafness in one ear, following a skull fracture. MRI results indicated signs of fibrosis in the deaf ear, which would preclude the opportunity for cochlear implantation at later ages. Therefore, surgeons provided the child with a cochlear implant. Results showed improvements in speech perception in noise, localization, and subjective reports of satisfaction with the device. Because this report only documents results for an individual child with single-sided deafness, results cannot be generalized to other children with unilateral hearing loss. This is particularly true for children with congenital losses, who may have difficulty integrating binaural signals. Another case series by Távora-Vieira and Rajan (2015) supports this point. They examined cochlear implantation in four children with unilateral deafness, one of whom had a postlingual hearing loss. The child with postlingual hearing loss showed the most rapid improvement in localization and speech perception in noise of the four children. Two of the children with congenital hearing loss (ages 4.5 and 6.8 years at the time of implantation) did not show benefit from the device, and one of those became a nonuser after 7 weeks postimplantation. The fourth child, who was implanted at 17 months of age, was too young to participate in speech perception testing, but reportedly wore the device full-time. Based on this small number of case studies, it appears that professionals should be cautious about providing cochlear implants to children with congenital single-sided deafness who have experienced long periods of auditory deprivation in their deaf ear. Children with postlingual, sudden onset of deafness in one ear may derive binaural benefit from a cochlear implant. It is still too soon to tell if younger children, who are implanted during a sensitive period of binaural auditory development, could obtain more benefit from a cochlear implant compared to no treatment, BAHAs, or CROS hearing aids. Further high-quality research studies are needed before we can conclusively state that cochlear implants are a viable option for children with single-sided deafness.

## CONCLUSIONS

The decision on when to transition a child from hearing aids to a cochlear implant can be a difficult and emotional choice for parents. Important factors have to be weighed in the decision-making process; these factors include what might be lost for the child (e.g., residual acoustic hearing, a less drastic intervention approach), versus what might be gained (e.g., increased auditory access and localization, decreased listening effort). The process of documenting outcomes for children who wear hearing aids can provide clinical data to help to support decisions about when to transition from a hearing aid to a cochlear implant. Obtaining the right clinical information and having a willingness to share information about all possible treatment options are critical to this process. For children who are in the gray area for cochlear implant candidacy, audiologists can be a great support in helping family members make informed decisions. High-quality research is still needed to determine which treatment options are the most effective for individual children.

## REFERENCES


ANSI. (1997). S3. 5-1997 R-2007, American National Standards methods for the calculation of the Articulation Index. New York, NY: American National Standards Institute.

Arndt, S., Aschendorff, A., Laszig, R., Beck, R., Schild, C., Kroeger, S., . . . Wesarg, T. (2011). Comparison of pseudobinaural hearing to real binaural hearing rehabilitation after cochlear implantation in patients with unilateral deafness and tinnitus. *Otology & Neurotology, 32*(1), 39–47.

Bagatto, M. P., Brown, C. L., Moodie, S. T., & Scollie, S. D. (2011). External validation of the LittlEARS® Auditory Questionnaire with English-speaking families of Canadian children with normal hearing. *International Journal of Pediatric Otorhinolaryngology, 75*(6), 815–817.

Battista, R. A., Mullins, K., Wiet, R. M., Sabin, A., Kim, J., & Rauch, V. (2013). Sound localization in unilateral deafness with the Baha or TransEar device. *JAMA Otolaryngology-Head & Neck Surgery, 139*(1), 64–70.

Bess, F. H., & Tharpe, A. M. (1984). Unilateral hearing impairment in children. *Pediatrics, 74*(2), 206–216.

Blamey, P., Arndt, P., Bergeron, F., Bredberg, G., Brimacombe, J., Facer, G., . . . Peterson, A. (1996). Factors affecting auditory performance of postlinguistically deaf adults using cochlear implants. *Audiology and Neurotology, 1*(5), 293–306.

Blamey, P. J., Sarant, J. Z., Paatsch, L. E., Barry, J. G., Bow, C. P., Wales, R. J., . . . Tooher, R. (2001). Relationships among speech perception, production, language, hearing loss, and age in children with impaired hearing. *Journal of Speech, Language, and Hearing Research, 44*(2), 264–285.

Bloom, L. & Lahey, M. (1978). *Language development and disorders.* New York, NY: John Wiley.

Cadieux, J. H., Firszt, J. B., & Reeder, R. M. (2013). Cochlear implantation in nontraditional candidates: Preliminary results in adolescents with asymmetric hearing loss. *Otology & Neurotology, 34*(3), 408–415.

Carlson, M. L., Sladen, D. P., Haynes, D. S., Driscoll, C. L., DeJong, M. D., Erickson, H. C., . . . Davis, T. J. (2015). Evidence for the expansion of pediatric cochlear implant candidacy. *Otology & Neurotology, 36*(1), 43–50.

Carrow-Woolfolk, E. (2011). *Oral and Written Language Scales.* Minneapolis, MN: Pearson.

Ching, T. Y., & Hill, M. (2007). The Parents' Evaluation of Aural/Oral Performance of Children (PEACH) scale: Normative data. *Journal of the American Academy of Audiology, 18*(3), 220–235.

Coninx, F., Weichbold, V., Tsiakpini, L., Autrique, E., Bescond, G., Tamas, L., . . . Le Maner-Idrissi, G. (2009). Validation of the LittlEARS® Auditory Questionnaire in children with normal hearing. *International Journal of Pediatric Otorhinolaryngology, 73*(12), 1761–1768.

Cowan, R. S., DelDot, J., Barker, J., Barker, E. J., Sarant, J. Z., Pegg, P., . . . Hollow, R. (1997). Speech perception results for children with implants with different levels of preoperative residual hearing. *American Journal of Otology, 18,* S125–S126.

Dedhia, K., Worman, T., Meredith, M. A., & Rubinstein, J. T. (2016). Patterns of long-term hearing loss in hearing preservation cochlear implant surgery. *Otology & Neurotology, 37*(5), 478–486.

Delage, H., & Tuller, L. (2007). Language development and mild-to-moderate hearing loss: Does language normalize with age? *Journal of Speech, Language, and Hearing Research, 50*(5), 1300–1313.

Desmet, J., Wouters, K., De Bodt, M., & Van de Heyning, P. (2014). Long-term subjective benefit with a bone-conduction implant sound processor in 44 patients with single-sided deafness. *Otology & Neurotology, 35*(6), 1017–1025.

Dettman, S. J., D'Costa, W. A., Dowell, R. C., Winton, E. J., Hill, K. L., & Williams, S. S. (2004). Cochlear implants for children with significant residual hearing. *Archives of Otolaryngology–Head & Neck Surgery, 130*(5), 612–618.

Djourno, A., & Eyries, C. (1957). Auditory prosthesis by means of a distant electrical stimulation of the sensory nerve with the use of an indwelt coiling. *La Presse Médicale, 65*(63), 1417–1417.

Djourno, A., Eyries, C., & Vallancien, B. (1957). Electric excitation of the cochlear nerve in man by induction at a distance with the aid of micro-coil included in the fixture. *Comptes Rendus des Séances de la Société de Biologie et de ses Filiales, 151*(3), 423–425.

Dunn, C. C., Perreau, A., Gantz, B., & Tyler, R. (2010). Benefits of localization and speech perception with multiple noise sources in listeners with a short-electrode cochlear implant. *Journal of the American Academy of Audiology, 21*(1), 44–51.

Edelman, R. R., & Warach, S. (1993). Magnetic resonance imaging. *New England Journal of Medicine, 328*(10), 708–716.

Eisenberg, L. S., Kirk, K. I., Martinez, A. S., Ying, E. A., & Miyamoto, R. T. (2004). Communication abilities of children with aided residual hearing: Comparison with cochlear implant users. *Archives of Otolaryngology-Head & Neck Surgery, 130*(5), 563–569.

Eisenberg, L. S., Martinez, A. S., Sennaroglu, G., & Osberger, M. J. (2000). Establishing new criteria in selecting children for a cochlear implant: Performance of "platinum" hearing aid users. *Annals of Otology, Rhinology & Laryngology. Supplement, 185,* 30–33.

Erber, N. (1982). *Auditory training.* Washington, D.C.: Alexander Graham Bell Association for the Deaf.

Fitzpatrick, E., McCrae, R., & Schramm, D. (2006). A retrospective study of cochlear implant outcomes in children with residual hearing. *BMC Ear, Nose and Throat Disorders, 6*(1), 1–6.

Fitzpatrick, E., Olds, J., Durieux-Smith, A., McCrae, R., Schramm, D., & Gaboury, I. (2009). Pediatric cochlear implantation: How much hearing is too much? *International Journal of Audiology, 48*(2), 91–97.

Fitzpatrick, E. M., Olds, J., Gaboury, I., McCrae, R., Schramm, D., & Durieux-Smith, A. (2012). Comparison of outcomes in children with hearing aids and cochlear implants. *Cochlear Implants International, 13*(1), 5–15.

Friedland, D. R., & Runge-Samuelson, C. (2009). Soft cochlear implantation: Rationale for the surgical approach. *Trends in Amplification, 13*(2), 124–138.

Gantz, B. J., Dunn, C., Oleson, J., Hansen, M., Parkinson, A., & Turner, C. (2016). Multicenter clinical trial of the Nucleus Hybrid S8 cochlear implant: Final outcomes. *Laryngoscope, 126,* 962–973.

Gantz, B. J., Dunn, C., Walker, E., Van Voorst, T., Gogel, S., & Hansen, M. (2016). Outcomes of adolescents with a short electrode cochlear implant with preserved residual hearing. *Otology & Neurotology, 37*(2), e118–e125.

Gantz, B. J., Rubinstein, J. T., Tyler, R. S., Teagle, H., Cohen, N. L., Waltzman, S. B., . . . Kirk, K. I. (2000). Long-term results of cochlear implants in children with residual hearing. *Annals of Otology, Rhinology & Laryngology. Supplement, 185,* 33–36.

Gantz, B. J., & Turner, C. (2004). Combining acoustic and electrical speech processing: Iowa/Nucleus Hybrid implant. *Acta Oto-Laryngologica, 124*(4), 344–347.

Gantz, B. J., Turner, C., & Gfeller, K. E. (2006). Acoustic plus electric speech processing: Preliminary results of a multicenter clinical trial of the Iowa/

Nucleus Hybrid implant. *Audiology and Neurotology, 11*(Suppl. 1), 63–68.

Gantz, B. J., Turner, C., Gfeller, K. E., & Lowder, M. W. (2005). Preservation of hearing in cochlear implant surgery: Advantages of combined electrical and acoustical speech processing. *Laryngoscope, 115*(5), 796–802.

Gantz, B. J., Woodworth, G. G., Knutson, J. F., Abbas, P. J., & Tyler, R. S. (1993). Multivariate predictors of audiological success with multichannel cochlear implants. *Annals of Otology, Rhinology & Laryngology, 102*(12), 909–916.

Geal-Dor, M., Jbarah, R., Meilijson, S., Adelman, C., & Levi, H. (2011). The Hebrew and the Arabic version of the LittlEARS® Auditory Questionnaire for the assessment of auditory development: Results in normal hearing children and children with cochlear implants. *International Journal of Pediatric Otorhinolaryngology, 75*(10), 1327–1332.

Geers, A. E., & Nicholas, J. G. (2013). Enduring advantages of early cochlear implantation for spoken language development. *Journal of Speech, Language, and Hearing Research, 56*(2), 643–655.

Gfeller, K. E., Olszewski, C., Turner, C., Gantz, B., & Oleson, J. (2006). Music perception with cochlear implants and residual hearing. *Audiology and Neurotology, 11*(Suppl. 1), 12–15.

Gifford, R. H. (2011). Who is a cochlear implant candidate? *Hearing Journal*, *64*(6), 16–18.

Gomaa, N. A., Rubinstein, J. T., Lowder, M. W., Tyler, R. S., & Gantz, B. J. (2003). Residual speech perception and cochlear implant performance in postlingually deafened adults. *Ear and Hearing, 24*(6), 539–544.

Gordon, K., Jiwani, S., & Papsin, B. (2011). What is the optimal timing for bilateral cochlear implantation in children? *Cochlear Implants International, 12*(Suppl. 2), S14–S18.

Grantham, D. W., Ashmead, D. H., Haynes, D. S., Hornsby, B. W., Labadie, R. F., & Ricketts, T. A. (2012). Horizontal plane localization in single-sided deaf adults fitted with a bone-anchored hearing aid (Baha). *Ear and Hearing, 33*(5), 595–603.

Grieco-Calub, T. M., & Litovsky, R. Y. (2012). Spatial acuity in two-to-three-year-old children with normal acoustic hearing, unilateral cochlear implants and bilateral cochlear implants. *Ear and Hearing, 33*(5), 561–572.

Haskins, H. L. (1949). *A phonetically balanced test of speech discrimination skills for children* (Unpublished master's thesis). Northwestern University, Evanston, IL.

Heman-Ackah, S. E., Roland, J. T., Haynes, D. S., & Waltzman, S. B. (2012). Pediatric cochlear implantation: Candidacy evaluation, medical and surgical considerations, and expanding criteria. *Otolaryngologic Clinics of North America, 45*(1), 41–67.

Herman, G. T. (2009). *Fundamentals of computerized tomograph: Image reconstruction from projections.* London, UK: Springer Science & Business Media.

Hyde, M., Punch, R., & Komesaroff, L. (2010). Coming to a decision about cochlear implantation: Parents making choices for their deaf children. *Journal of Deaf Studies and Deaf Education, 15*(2), 162–178.

Kamal, S. M., Robinson, A. D., & Diaz, R. C. (2012). Cochlear implantation in single-sided deafness for enhancement of sound localization and speech perception. *Current Opinion in Otolaryngology & Head and Neck Surgery, 20*(5), 393–397.

Kirk, K. I., Pisoni, D. B., & Osberger, M. J. (1995). Lexical effects on spoken word recognition by pediatric cochlear implant users. *Ear and Hearing, 16*(5), 470–481.

Koehlinger, K., Van Horne, A. O., Oleson, J., McCreery, R., & Moeller, M. P. (2015). The role of sentence position, allomorph, and morpheme type on accurate use of s-related morphemes by children who are hard of hearing. *Journal of Speech, Language, and Hearing Research, 58*(2), 396–409.

Kosaner, J., Sonuguler, S., Olgun, L., & Amann, E. (2013). Young cochlear implant users' auditory development as measured and monitored by the LittlEARS® Auditory Questionnaire: A Turkish experience. *International Journal of Pediatric Otorhinolaryngology, 77*(8), 1359–1363.

Kühn-Inacker, H., Shehata-Dieler, W., Müller, J., & Helms, J. (2004). Bilateral cochlear implants: A way to optimize auditory perception abilities in deaf children? *International Journal of Pediatric Otorhinolaryngology, 68*(10), 1257–1266.

Lieu, J. E., Tye-Murray, N., Karzon, R. K., & Piccirillo, J. F. (2010). Unilateral hearing loss is associated with worse speech-language scores in children. *Pediatrics, 125*(6), e1348–e1355.

Litovsky, R. Y., Johnstone, P. M., Godar, S., Agrawal, S., Parkinson, A., Peters, R., & Lake, J. (2006). Bilateral cochlear implants in children: Localization acuity measured with minimum audible angle. *Ear and Hearing, 27*(1), 43–59.

May-Mederake, B., Kuehn, H., Vogel, A., Keilmann, A., Bohnert, A., Mueller, S., . . . Stroele, A. (2010). Evaluation of auditory development in infants and toddlers who received cochlear implants under the age of 24 months with the LittlEARS® Auditory Questionnaire. *International Journal of Pediatric Otorhinolaryngology, 74*(10), 1149–1155.

McGuckian, M., & Henry, A. (2007). The grammatical morpheme deficit in moderate hearing impairment.

*International Journal of Language & Communication Disorders*, *42* (suppl. 1), 17–36.

Moeller, M. P., Tomblin, J. B., & the OCHL Collaboration. (2015). Epilogue: Conclusions and implications for research and practice. *Ear and Hearing*, *36*, 92S–98S.

Mondain, M., Sillon, M., Vieu, A., Levi, A., Reuillard-Artieres, F., Deguine, O., . . . Uziel, A. (2002). Cochlear implantation in prelingually deafened children with residual hearing. *International Journal of Pediatric Otorhinolaryngology*, *63*(2), 91–97.

Moog, J. S., & Geers, A. E. (1990). *Early speech perception test*. St. Louis, MO: Central Institute for the Deaf.

Negro, A.-S. G., García, J.-L. P., & Quevedo, M. S. (2016). Production and evaluation of a Spanish version of the LittlEARS® Auditory Questionnaire for the assessment of auditory development in children. *International journal of Pediatric Otorhinolaryngology*, *83*, 99–103.

Papsin, B. C., & Gordon, K. A. (2008). Bilateral cochlear implants should be the standard for children with bilateral sensorineural deafness. *Current Opinion in Otolaryngology & Head and Neck Surgery*, *16*(1), 69–74.

Peters, B. R., Litovsky, R., Parkinson, A., & Lake, J. (2007). Importance of age and postimplantation experience on speech perception measures in children with sequential bilateral cochlear implants. *Otology & Neurotology*, *28*(5), 649–657.

Pisoni, D. B. (2000). Cognitive factors and cochlear implants: Some thoughts on perception, learning, and memory in speech perception. *Ear and Hearing*, *21*(1), 70–78.

Plontke, S. K., Heider, C., Koesling, S., Hess, S., Bieseke, L., Goetze, G., & Rahne, T. (2013). Cochlear implantation in a child with posttraumatic single-sided deafness. *European Archives of Oto-Rhino-Laryngology*, *270*(5), 1757–1761.

Rauhamäki, T., Lonka, E., Lipsanen, J., & Laakso, M. (2014). Assessment of early auditory development of very young Finnish children with LittlEARS® Auditory Questionnaire and McArthur Communicative Developmental Inventories. *International Journal of pediatric otorhinolaryngology*, *78*(12), 2089–2096.

Roland, J. T., & Waltzman, S. B. (2015). Expanded pediatric cochlear implant candidacy. *Otolaryngology-Head and Neck Surgery*, *152*(4), 592–593.

Roush, P., Frymark, T., Venediktov, R., & Wang, B. (2011). Audiologic management of auditory neuropathy spectrum disorder in children: A systematic review of the literature. *American Journal of Audiology*, *20*(2), 159–170.

Rubinstein, J., Parkinson, W., Tyler, R., & Gantz, B. (1999). Residual speech recognition and cochlear implant performance: Effects of implantation criteria. *Otology & Neurotology*, *20*(4), 445–452.

Russell, J. L., Pine, H. S., & Young, D. L. (2013). Pediatric cochlear implantation: Expanding applications and outcomes. *Pediatric Clinics of North America*, *60*(4), 841–863.

Schrank, F. A., Mather, N., & McGrew, K. S. (2014). *Woodcock-Johnson IV Tests of Achievement*. Rolling Meadows, IL: Riverside.

Spencer, L. J., Tye-Murray, N., & Tomblin, J. B. (1998). The production of English inflectional morphology, speech production and listening performance in children with cochlear implants. *Ear and Hearing*, *19*(4), 310–318.

Spitzer, J. B., & Zavala, J. S. (2011). Development of Spanish version of the LittlEARS® parental questionnaire for use in the United States and Latin America. *Audiology Research*, *1*(2), 23–29.

Stiles, D. J., Bentler, R. A., & McGregor, K. K. (2012). The speech intelligibility index and the pure-tone average as predictors of lexical ability in children fit with hearing aids. *Journal of Speech, Language, and Hearing Research*, *55*(3), 764–778.

Távora-Vieira, D., & Rajan, G. P. (2015). Cochlear implantation in children with congenital and noncongenital unilateral deafness: A case series. *Otology & Neurotology*, *36*(2), 235–239.

Tomblin, J. B., Harrison, M., Ambrose, S. E., Walker, E. A., Oleson, J. J., & Moeller, M. P. (2015). Language outcomes in young children with mild to severe hearing loss. *Ear and Hearing*, *36*, 76S–91S.

Tomblin, J. B., Oleson, J. J., Ambrose, S. E., Walker, E., & Moeller, M. P. (2014). The influence of hearing aids on the speech and language development of children with hearing loss. *JAMA Otolaryngology-Head & Neck Surgery*, *140*, 403–409. http://dx.doi:10.1001/jamaoto.2014.267

Tomblin, J. B., Spencer, L., Flock, S., Tyler, R., & Gantz, B. (1999). A comparison of language achievement in children with cochlear implants and children using hearing aids. *Journal of Speech, Language, and Hearing Research*, *42*(2), 497–511.

Turner, C., Gantz, B. J., & Reiss, L. (2008). Integration of acoustic and electrical hearing. *Journal of Rehabilitation Research and Development*, *45*(5), 769–778.

Uhler, K., & Gifford, R. H. (2014). Current trends in pediatric cochlear implant candidate selection and postoperative follow-up. *American Journal of Audiology*, *23*(3), 309–325.

Vlastarakos, P. V., Nazos, K., Tavoulari, E.-F., & Nikolopoulos, T. P. (2014). Cochlear implantation for single-sided deafness: The outcomes. An evidence-based approach. *European Archives of Oto-Rhino-Laryngology*, *271*(8), 2119–2126.

Volta, A., & Banks, J. (1800). I. On the electricity excited by the mere contact of conducting substances of different kinds. *The Philosophical Magazine: Comprehending the Various Branches of Science, the Liberal and Fine Arts, Agriculture, Manufactures, and Commerce, 7*(28), 289–311.

Wang, L., Sun, X., Liang, W., Chen, J., & Zheng, W. (2013). Validation of the Mandarin version of the LittlEARS® Auditory Questionnaire. *International Journal of Pediatric Otorhinolaryngology, 77*(8), 1350–1354.

Wiederholt, J.L., & Bryant, B.R. (2001). *Gray Oral Reading Tests, Fourth Edition*, Austin, TX: Pro-Ed.

Wilson, B. S., & Dorman, M. F. (2008). Cochlear implants: A remarkable past and a brilliant future. *Hearing Research, 242*(1), 3–21.

Zimmerman-Phillips, S., & Osberger, M. (1997). *Meaningful Auditory Integration Scale (IT-MAIS) for Infants and Toddlers*. Sylmar, CA: Advanced Bionics Corporation.

Zwolan, T. A., Zimmerman-Phillips, S., Ashbaugh, C. J., Hieber, S. J., Kileny, P. R., & Telian, S. A. (1997). Cochlear implantation of children with minimal open-set speech recognition skills. *Ear and Hearing, 18*(3), 240–251.

# 9

# Special Populations in Pediatric Amplification

*Elizabeth A. Walker and Ryan W. McCreery*

## INTRODUCTION

To this point, this textbook has focused primarily on the amplification process for children with bilateral sensorineural hearing loss. However, there are other types of hearing loss where amplification may be beneficial, as emerging evidence suggests that these types of hearing loss can impact a child's development and ability to function in daily life. The process of providing amplification to children who fall into the categories of special populations will meet the same standards and use the same processes as children with bilateral sensorineural hearing loss. Some approaches need to be adapted or alternative tools will be used to meet those goals, but the guiding principles are always providing amplification at the earliest possible age and maximizing audibility, which will permit access to the child's auditory environment.

Several types of hearing loss or comorbid conditions require special considerations during the amplification process. Minimal hearing loss is a term that has been used to describe children with either hearing loss in only one ear, known as unilateral hearing loss, or hearing loss that is bilateral, but mild in degree. The provision of amplification for children with minimal hearing loss has been inconsistent, with estimates suggesting that amplification is recommended in the majority of cases. At the same time, more than 50% of children experience substantial delays between identification and fitting of amplification (Fitzpatrick, Whittingham, & Durieux-Smith, 2014). This pattern persists despite the fact that children with minimal hearing loss may be at risk for delays in speech, language and academic domains. The topic of children with auditory neuropathy spectrum disorder (ANSD) and how this relates to diagnostic considerations was discussed in Chapter 2. This population also requires unique considerations in the fitting and verification of amplification. Specific amplification considerations for children with additional disabilities also are discussed. Alternative management strategies are highlighted to allow audiologists to meet the goals of promoting consistent hearing aid use and aided audibility, while monitoring auditory development outcomes in these special populations.

## MINIMAL HEARING LOSS

Minimal hearing loss is an umbrella term that is used to describe children with mild bilateral hearing loss or unilateral hearing loss. Over the years, there has been further specification of the audiometric criteria for minimal hearing loss. In 2005, the National Workshop on Mild and Unilateral Hearing Loss convened and set forth a working definition. Mild bilateral hearing loss was defined as a pure-tone average (PTA) at 500, 1000, and 2000 Hz between 20 and 40 dB; high-frequency hearing loss was defined as pure-tone thresholds greater than 25 dB HL at two or more frequencies above 2000 Hz *in both ears*; and unilateral hearing loss was defined as a PTA at 500, 1000, and 2000 Hz greater than or equal to 20 dB HL, or thresholds greater than 25 dB HL at two or more frequencies above 2000 Hz in the poorer ear, and a PTA in the better ear less than or equal to 15 dB. Children with mild hearing loss in the better ear (i.e., asymmetric hearing loss) also fall into this minimal hearing loss category in some reports (Fitzpatrick, Whittingham et al., 2014; Wake et al., 2006; Walker, Spratford, Ambrose, Holte, & Oleson, 2017).

In the past, children with minimal hearing loss were underrepresented in the research literature and underserved clinically, based on the rationale that these children had sufficient access to speech, and therefore, would experience little negative impact on development (Tharpe, 2007). Contrary evidence emerged starting in the 1980s and 1990s, which demonstrated that children with mild or unilateral hearing loss are at risk for delays in language, psychosocial, and academic outcomes (Bess, Dodd-Murphy, & Parker, 1998; Bess, Tharpe, & Gibler, 1986; Davis, Elfenbein, Schum, & Bentler, 1986). Despite the fact that research suggests that without early identification and intervention, children with minimal hearing loss may struggle, both academically and socially, there is a situation of *clinical equipoise* surrounding this population. In other words, there is a lack of clear guidelines regarding clinical management with this population. This uncertainty results in a variety of treatment approaches, ranging from (1) a failure-based approach of waiting to see developmental delays occur to (2) a front-loading approach of providing amplification and speech-language services soon after confirmation of hearing loss (Fitzpatrick, Whittingham et al., 2014; Winiger, Alexander, & Diefendorf, 2016).

> Clinical equipoise is uncertainty or ambiguity in the expert clinical community regarding the benefits of a specific treatment approach (Freedman, 1987).

### Prevalence

*Prevalence* rates answer the question of how many people have this condition right now. Prevalence estimates of minimal hearing loss vary depending on the age group examined and the audiometric definitions used. It is difficult to determine the prevalence of mild bilateral hearing loss in newborns because newborn hearing screening programs are often set up to target moderate or greater hearing loss (Gravel et al., 2005). The best estimates of prevalence for minimal hearing loss at birth range from 0.4 to 1.3 per 1000 newborns (Johnson et al., 2005; Watkin & Baldwin, 1999). The prevalence rate increases as children get older, due to acquired hearing loss or because of congenital cases that were false negatives on the newborn hearing screen. Bess et al. (1998) reported that the prevalence of minimal hearing loss in school-age children was 54 per 1000 children. In Bess et al.'s population-based sample, unilateral hearing loss occurred the most often (30 per 1000), followed by high-frequency hearing loss (14 per 1000) and mild bilateral hearing loss (10 per 1000).

> Prevalence is the number of individuals with an identified condition at a specific time period.

## Etiology

Minimal hearing loss shares many of the same etiologies as bilateral hearing loss or hearing loss of a greater degree. Tharpe and Sladen (2008) provided an overview of the possible causes of minimal hearing loss. Some common etiologies include genetic causes, such as the Connexin (GJB2) gene (Liu et al., 2005; Wake et al., 2006), enlarged vestibular aqueduct syndrome (Callison & Horn, 1998), and mitochondrial gene mutations (Jacobs et al., 2005). Viral or bacterial infections, such as congenital cytomegalovirus or meningitis (Fortnum & Davis, 1993; Fowler & Boppana, 2006), may also result in minimal hearing loss. Additional etiologies include noise induced hearing loss, prematurity, sudden idiopathic hearing loss, and ANSD (to be discussed later in this chapter).

## Outcomes

Children with minimal hearing loss are at risk for delays in multiple developmental domains, including language, psychosocial, and academic achievement (Blair, Peterson, & Viehwig, 1985; Davis et al., 1986). Winiger et al. (2016) recently conducted a literature review on outcomes and treatment approaches for children with minimal hearing loss. They reviewed 102 articles and reported that research on children with minimal hearing loss has been reported on for over 50 years, but studies separating these children into respective categories of unilateral hearing loss and mild hearing loss are more recent. Although the challenges children with mild hearing loss and unilateral hearing loss face often overlap, there are important distinctions that make it advantageous to review their outcomes separately. Differences between unilateral and mild hearing loss are important for clinicians to consider, despite the fact that these two conditions are often combined under the umbrella of minimal hearing loss. A child with unilateral hearing loss is likely to experience difficulties in listening situations where binaural hearing is beneficial, including listening in background noise or locating talkers in noisy environments. Bilateral mild hearing loss creates deficits in terms of access to soft sounds or sounds originating from a distance. These differences should be considered when examining different treatment approaches for the two groups, which can have an effect on outcomes. The following review discusses research related to outcomes for these children and presents results based on studies in which children with minimal hearing loss are categorized as one group, studies focusing on children with mild hearing loss, and studies focusing on children with unilateral hearing loss.

### *Minimal Hearing Loss*

Several studies have combined children with unilateral and mild hearing losses in a single study. Porter, Sladen, Ampah, Rothpletz, and Bess (2013) explored group differences between 26 children with normal hearing and 27 children with minimal hearing loss. Participants were between the ages of 4 to 9 years, and were evaluated on language, literacy, memory, psychosocial, and academic achievement. The minimal hearing loss group included children with bilateral mild hearing loss, bilateral high-frequency hearing loss, or unilateral hearing loss. Porter et al. found no significant differences between the children with normal hearing and the children with minimal hearing loss on any of the language, memory, or academic measures. Attention-related difficulties were the only area in which there was a significant group difference, with teachers rating children with hearing loss as having significantly more problems than children with normal hearing. Whether the attention-related difficulties were a behavioral manifestation of minimal hearing loss or related to a separate behavioral problem can be difficult to resolve, because many children with minimal hearing loss have listening difficulties that can appear to be the result of off-task or inattentive behavior.

Other researchers have suggested that language and psychosocial development are vulnerable in the early school years for children with minimal hearing loss, but this gap may close by adolescence. Factors, such as grade-level retention, must be taken into account when interpreting group differences, however. In a seminal paper by Bess et al. (1998), third graders with minimal hearing loss (i.e., unilateral, slight or mild) scored lower than children with normal hearing on academic achievement tests. In contrast to the third graders, there were no significant differences in a separate cohort of sixth and ninth graders. It is worth noting that this closing of the achievement gap may have been illusory. More than one third of the sixth graders and almost half of the ninth graders with minimal hearing loss were retained for one or more years in school. The normal-hearing control group consisted of grade-mates, not age-mates; therefore, many of the children with minimal HL who achieved grade-level performance in middle school and high school were older than their hearing peers and had more educational experience due to retention. Practical considerations related to grade-level retention make interpretation of the difficulties experienced by children with minimal hearing loss challenging to generalize from research to practice.

### Mild Hearing Loss

As in studies of children with minimal hearing loss, research that specifically examines children with mild hearing loss has suggested somewhat mixed outcomes. Some studies indicate that these children are likely to experience delays relative to same-age peers with normal hearing and other studies indicate that they are performing within the average range on different outcome measures. Prior to the 1980s, there was little research on outcomes in children with mild hearing loss because it was commonly assumed that they had sufficient residual hearing to achieve similar levels of performance compared to children with normal hearing. Several studies in the 1980s refuted that claim. Davis et al. (1986) examined school-age children who were hard of hearing (mild ranging to severe hearing loss) on language, academic, and psychosocial measures. Degree of hearing loss did not appear to influence performance on outcome measures, and children with mild hearing loss in the sample showed significant delays in receptive vocabulary compared to test norms on a standardized receptive vocabulary test. Another study by Blair et al. (1985) focused exclusively on children with mild hearing loss (20 to 45 dB HL in the better ear) in early elementary grades. This study demonstrated the differences in results when comparing children to normative data from standardized tests versus a matched group of children with normal hearing from the same local community. The children with mild hearing loss performed within the average range on academic achievement measures when they were compared to the normative sample of standardized tests. When they were compared to same-age hearing children from their school district, they achieved lower scores on those same tests. Thus, even though they were within normal limits for academics based on standardized test measures, evidence suggests that they performed significantly below their classmates, and the gap increased compared to grade-mates at higher grade levels.

More recent results are consistent with Blair and his colleagues' findings from 30 years ago. Đoković et al. (2014) compared 144 children with mild bilateral hearing loss (pure-tone average between 20 and 40 dB HL in both ears) to 160 children with normal hearing. The children with mild hearing loss had not received intervention (i.e., hearing aids). They performed significantly worse compared to the children with normal hearing on morphosyntactic and phonological short-term memory tasks. There were no significant differences between groups on measures of vocabulary knowledge. Similar to Blair et al. (1985), the children with mild hearing loss were within the average range on standardized tests. Walker et al. (2015) examined children with mild hearing loss in the better ear (mild hearing loss or worse in the poorer ear). Children with mild hearing loss who were full-time hearing aid users were compared to children with mild hearing loss who did not use hearing aids. The groups were matched on socioeconomic status, but the full-time hearing aid users had significantly worse better-ear pure-tone averages compared to the nonusers, even though both groups had mild hearing loss. Results showed that the full-time hearing aid users had significantly higher scores on vocabulary and morphosyntax measures than the nonusers. Both groups were within the average range for vocabulary skills, but the nonusers were outside of the average range, on average, for morphosyntactic skills (Figure 9–1). These results suggest that children with mild hearing loss may be especially vulnerable in aspects of language related to form (i.e., morphology, syntax, phonology).

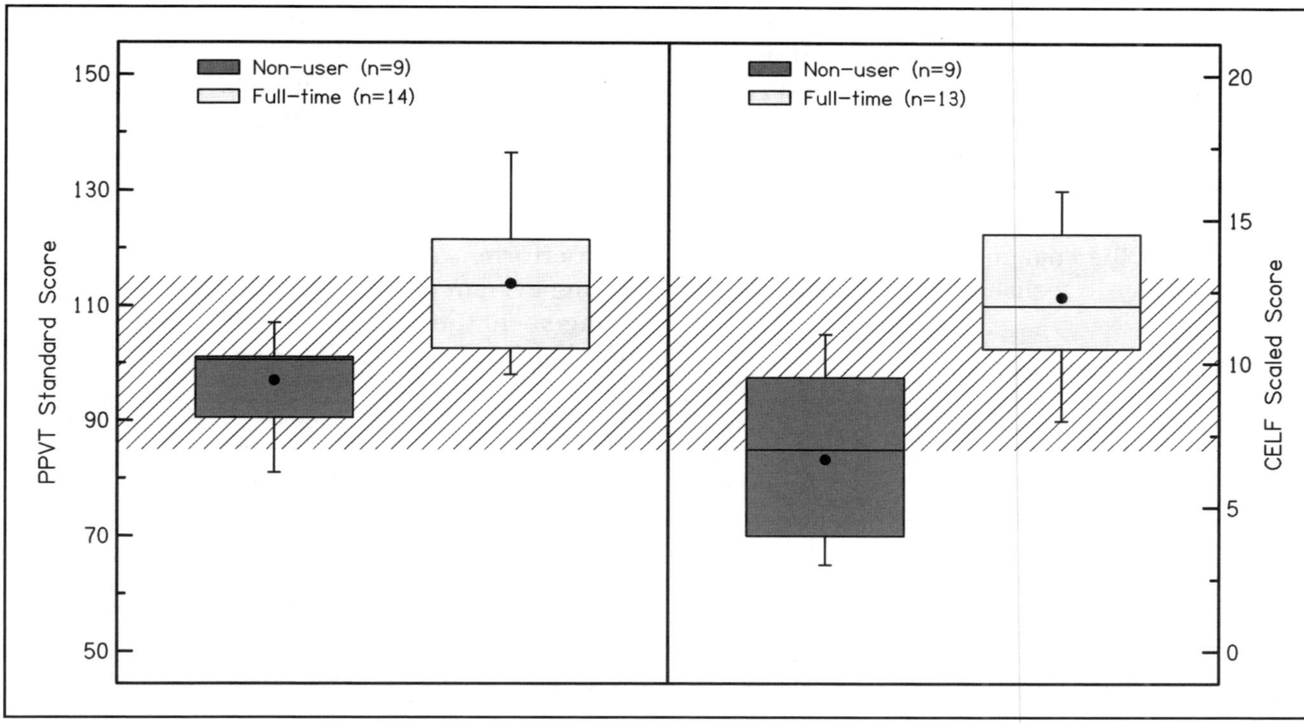


**FIGURE 9–1.** Box plots of Peabody Picture Vocabulary Test-Fourth Edition scores (*left panel*) and Clinical Evaluation of Language Fundamentals-Fourth Edition Word Structure subtest scores (*right panel*) as a function of hearing aid use group (full-time users, part-time users, and nonusers). The central lines represent the median values, the filled circles represent the mean values, and the box limits are the 25th and 75th percentiles. The lower and upper fences are the minimum and maximum, respectively. The hatched lines display the average range for the normative samples of both tests. Adapted from Walker et al. (2015).

In contrast to the research studies that found a negative impact of minimal hearing loss, a number of studies suggest that children with mild hearing loss are not at risk for language delays (Briscoe, Bishop, & Norbury, 2001; Kiese-Himmel & Ohlwein, 2003; Norbury, Bishop, & Briscoe, 2001; Wake et al., 2006; Wolgemuth, Kamhi, & Lee, 1998). Wake and colleagues (2006) investigated differences between children with normal hearing and 48 children with slight/mild hearing loss (pure-tone average between 16 and 40 dB HL in the better ear) in first or fifth grade on language measures and phonological short-term memory. Like Đoković et al. (2014), the children with mild hearing loss had not received any intervention in the form of amplification. Phonological short-term memory was the only measure in which children with slight/mild hearing loss performed significantly worse than children with normal hearing, results that are consistent with Đoković et al. (2014). Based on the lack of group differences on language measures, Wake et al. concluded that children with mild hearing loss do not require intervention to achieve grade-level performance.

The lack of coherence in research findings for children with mild hearing loss has contributed to clinical equipoise regarding the provision of hearing aids and early intervention for children with this degree of hearing loss. While children with mild hearing loss are clearly at risk for delays in some areas of language development, other areas may appear to be within the normal range. This discrepancy highlights the need for approaches to monitoring auditory development outcomes by audiologists and language assessment by speech-language pathologists that examine a wide range of speech and language skills, instead of more general measures. Red flags for children with mild hearing loss could include greater difficulty in listening situations with noise and reverberation, difficulty understanding speech from a distance, or concerns for inattentive behavior. Audiologists may also assess speech recognition in noise or at lower sensation levels instead of testing in quiet or at average conversational levels, as these conditions will highlight the challenges children with mild hearing loss face in realistic listening conditions.

### *Unilateral Hearing Loss*

Audiology students often hear in their classes and in clinic that "two ears are better than one." This maxim reflects the notion that binaural listening is superior to monaural listening. There is substantial research evidence in the adult and pediatric literature to support the benefits of binaural hearing, both in terms of sound localization (i.e., identifying what direction a sound is coming from) and listening in background noise.

Children with unilateral hearing loss face specific difficulties with localizing sounds, including speech. The ability to locate the location of a talker in listening situations with noise and reverberation can be an important support strategy for accessing visual cues. Bess et al. (1986) examined horizontal sound localization in 25 school-age children with unilateral hearing loss. Compared to the normal-hearing comparison group, children with unilateral hearing loss showed significantly poorer localization to 500 and 3000 Hz tones. Within the unilateral group, localization skills were associated with degree of hearing loss in the impaired ear; children with more severe hearing loss made more localization errors. Speech perception in background noise is also challenging in cases of unilateral hearing loss. A number of studies have shown poorer performance while listening in noise (Bess & Tharpe, 1984; Bess et al., 1986; Ruscetta, Arjmand, & Pratt, 2005). Ruscetta and colleagues found that children with unilateral hearing loss need a significantly more favorable signal-to-noise ratio to repeat back sentences and nonsense syllables compared to children with normal hearing. The direction of the signal makes a difference in speech perception performance for this population (Winiger et al., 2016). Due to the head shadow effect, speech perception is significantly more difficult when the signal is directed toward the poorer ear (Ruscetta et al., 2005). In general, speech perception performance improves within the unilateral group when the signal is directed toward the ear with normal thresholds. However, some children with unilateral hearing loss perform worse than children with normal hearing even in this more advantageous listening arrangement (Bess & Tharpe, 1984; Bovo, Martini, Agnoletto, & Beghi, 1988).

> Head shadow effect is the physical effect of the head and shoulders acting as a barrier, which reduces the amplitude of incoming sound. When a signal is directed toward the ear with poorer hearing, sounds (particularly high-frequency information) get attenuated, creating challenges with audibility and speech recognition (Schleich, Nopp, & D'Haese, 2004; Tyler, Dunn, Witt, & Preece, 2003; Van Wanrooij & Van Opstal, 2004).

In addition to the auditory challenges that accompany unilateral hearing loss, this population has also demonstrated difficulties with academic achievement and language acquisition. While normal hearing in one ear might be considered sufficient to support access to the cues needed to develop speech and language, the high prevalence of delays in these skills in children with unilateral hearing loss support the idea that language acquisition occurs in noisy listening environments that require binaural hearing. Kiese-Himmel (2002) reported that children with unilateral hearing loss were delayed in producing two-word combinations (but not delayed in first word productions). These data were collected through retrospective parent interviews, rather than direct testing; therefore, these results should be interpreted with some caution. Culbertson and Gilbert (1986) compared 25 children with unilateral hearing loss to 25 children with normal hearing and found significantly lower performance on reading and written language measures in the unilateral group. Furthermore, children with unilateral hearing loss were more likely to be retained and had increased behavioral problems. Consistent with the Culbertson and Gilbert study, Klee and Davis-Dansky (1986) found that children with unilateral hearing loss were significantly more likely to be retained in school compared to hearing peers matched on age, I.Q., sex, race, and socioeconomic status. However, they did not find significant differences between groups on standardized language tests.

More recently, Lieu, Tye-Murray, Karzon, and Piccirillo (2010) conducted a case-control study, comparing children with unilateral hearing loss to their siblings with normal hearing. Including siblings as the hearing comparison group allowed the authors to control for family-specific effects, such as socioeconomic status. Results indicated that the children with unilateral hearing loss had significantly lower language comprehension and production scores than their siblings. They were also more likely to receive additional services in school (i.e., Individualized Education Programs or 504 plans). The latter finding highlights a change in how the U.S. educational system manages children who are experiencing difficulty in school. Between the 1980s and the 2000s, grade retention has been gradually replaced by a focus on increasing special education or additional support services (Winiger et al., 2016). Children with unilateral hearing loss may need additional supports listening in a classroom with noise and reverberation, including hearing assistance technology, if the hearing loss appears to have an adverse effect on academic, functional, or language outcomes.

> Individualized Education Programs (IEPs) are a legal document that outlines special education service delivery plans, as described in Part B of the Individuals with Disabilities Education Act (IDEA, 2004). All children who qualify for special education within the public school setting are mandated to have an IEP.
>
> 504 Plans are services in the general education setting that provide accessibility to instruction and accommodations, as described in Section 504 of the Rehabilitation Act of 1973. 504 plans are intended for children who have a documented disability that is not severe enough to qualify for special education services.

### *Summary of Outcomes for Children with Minimal Hearing Loss*

Children with minimal hearing loss demonstrate a wide range of performance, with some studies showing significant delays relative to hearing peers and other studies showing no difference between groups. As Wininger et al. (2016) point out, however, children with minimal hearing loss who perform within normal limits on standardized tests may not be achieving their full potential. In particular, children with minimal hearing loss display vulnerabilities in the areas of speech recognition, receptive and expressive language, academic achievement, and psychosocial outcomes, listening effort and localization. Audiologists need to be aware of the potential for these deficits and select appropriate tools to monitor outcomes in children with minimal hearing loss, even if the child does not use hearing aids.

## Intervention Options for Minimal Hearing Loss

The Joint Committee on Infant Hearing and the American Academy of Pediatricians recommend that children with minimal hearing loss receive early identification and intervention (JCIH, 2007); however, the appropriate path for audiological management after identification and referral to early intervention is not always clear (Fitzpatrick et al., 2016; Walker et al., 2015). Specifically, audiologists and parents may be cautious about pursuing amplification once the hearing loss has been confirmed as mild or unilateral. The American Academy of Audiology (AAA) Pediatric Amplification guidelines recommend that children with mild hearing loss receive hearing aids (AAA, 2013). Bagatto and Tharpe (2014) have expanded on these recommendations. They described an individualized, case-by-case method for considering amplification for children with mild hearing loss. For the purposes of this discussion, audiological intervention options for children with mild hearing loss will be distinguished from children with unilateral hearing loss.

### *Intervention Options for Children with Mild Hearing Loss*

There are three main intervention options that are often considered for children with mild hearing loss: (1) hearing aids, (2) hearing assistance technology, such as a remote-microphone system, and (3) no amplification with monitoring of auditory and communication development. Hearing aids and hearing assistance technology may be considered together or as separate options for intervention.

The study by Walker and colleagues (2015) highlights the potential benefits of amplification for children with mild hearing losses. As noted earlier in this chapter, they included children with mild hearing loss who received amplification and children with mild hearing loss who did not. Among the group of children with hearing aids, some children wore their hearing aids nearly all day, whereas others were part-time hearing aids users according to either hearing aid data logging or parent report. The children with mild hearing loss who were full-time hearing aid users had significantly higher scores on measures of vocabulary and grammar than children who did not wear hearing aids. There were no differences between groups on speech recognition in noise or speech production scores. The children with mild hearing loss in this study were not randomly assigned to these groups, and the children who received hearing aids were more likely than the children without hearing aids to have received early intervention. These factors make it difficult to establish a causal link between hearing aid use and outcomes in children with mild hearing loss. However, from a practical standpoint, these limitations have limited implications for intervention, because current best practices dictate that children should receive both amplification and intervention, and the combination of the two factors appear to provide some benefit to children with mild hearing loss. Further research is needed, but the potential risk for developmental concerns combined with the potential benefits of early intervention and amplification for this population support the recommendation that hearing aids should be provided to children with mild hearing loss.

There are potential challenges to establishing hearing aid use in children with mild hearing loss that audiologists must anticipate. Parents of children with mild bilateral hearing loss often do not report significant concerns for hearing, as these children have good audibility for average speech in quiet listening situations. In one-on-one listening situations, it can be nearly impossible to determine whether or not a child has mild hearing loss. Reassurance of the parents' perspectives can help them to understand that their child does hear well in specific listening conditions, but may not have access to incidental learning or speech spoken from a distance. The use of tools like the Situational Hearing Aid Response Profile (SHARP), as discussed in Chapter 4, can be useful in cases of mild bilateral hearing loss for showing the effects of distance on unaided audibility, as well as the positive effects of amplification in those situations. Parents of children with mild hearing loss may be more willing to consider a trial period with a loaner hearing aid than to consider purchasing hearing aids for their child. A trial with a loaner hearing aid can demonstrate the benefits of amplification for parents with appropriate counseling about the situations where hearing aids are most likely to help.

As outlined in Chapter 7, a wide range of hearing assistance technologies is available. These technologies can provide support in some specific listening situations for children with mild hearing loss. Hearing assistance technologies can be used with or without hearing aids. Remote microphone hearing assistance technologies, including frequency- and digital-modulation systems (FM and DM, respectively) can be particularly helpful for situations with a single talker of interest (such as a parent, caregiver, or teacher) and background noise. One disadvantage to remote-microphone systems is that there is typically only a single microphone that can be arduous to pass around to multiple conversational partners. A companion microphone that can be more easily passed around or a hand-held beamforming microphone array, such as the Phonak Roger pen, can provide benefit in listening situations with multiple talkers in background noise. Importantly, hearing assistance technologies alone provide limited, if any, amplification to the signal, so audibility may not be optimized for these devices. Additionally, a hearing assistance technology device that occludes the ear canal can reduce situational awareness for children with mild bilateral hearing loss. The degree of occlusion of the ear canal should be minimized to the greatest extent possible to avoid creating greater loss of audibility than the child would have without using a device.

The third option for children with mild hearing loss is monitoring of auditory and developmental outcomes without hearing aids or hearing assistance technology. Some families may elect not to pursue amplification or may feel that amplification provides a limited benefit for their child. In those cases, the child should continue to be monitored through the early intervention program in their area, if the program serves children with mild hearing loss. The child's audiological status should continue to be monitored on an annual basis to reevaluate any progression or fluctuation in hearing, as well as to monitor the impact of changes in middle ear status on the child's hearing. Importantly, if a family decides not to pursue amplification, the child should continue to receive audiological care and monitoring or developmental surveillance through the early intervention program. As children get older and their listening needs change, particularly as education transitions from small group activities to didactic listening in large groups, children with mild hearing loss may need greater support than they have previously received.

### *Intervention Options for Children with Unilateral Hearing Loss*

Unlike children with mild bilateral hearing loss, children with unilateral hearing loss have unbalanced or absent binaural cues that will create specific listening challenges in terms of localization of sound and background noise. The magnitude of difficulty experienced by children with unilateral hearing loss and the appropriate audiological intervention will be dictated by the degree of hearing loss in their impaired ear. For the purposes of discussing intervention, a distinction will be made between children with unilateral hearing loss who have aidable hearing in their impaired ear and children with unilateral hearing loss who do not have aidable hearing in their impaired ear. The definition of aidable hearing is debatable, but in general, children with unilateral hearing loss who have pure-tone averages in their impaired ear above 70 dB HL are not considered to have aidable hearing. Children with bilateral hearing loss with thresholds above 70 dB HL are routinely considered to have aidable hearing. However, in the case of children with one normal ear, there have been some case reports of complaints of poor sound quality and even poorer overall performance with amplification in the impaired ear than without, a phenomenon known as binaural interference (Jerger, Silman, Lew, & Chmiel, 1993). Therefore, a distinction will be made based on the presence of aidable hearing that will guide audiological intervention decisions for children with unilateral hearing loss. Clinicians may determine that a child with a pure-tone average greater than 70 dB HL may be a candidate for amplification based on the aided audibility that can be achieved with a hearing aid or an older child's preference to use a hearing aid. Speech recognition outcomes and questionnaires may be particularly important to demonstrate that the provision of amplification is beneficial in children with normal hearing in one ear and severe-to-profound hearing loss in the other ear.

**Intervention Options for Children with Aidable Unilateral Hearing Loss.** For children with unilateral hearing loss who have aidable hearing in their impaired ear, the provision of amplification is the preferred audiological intervention. With aidable hearing, the use of amplification creates the potential for at least partial restoration of binaural cues. Further, there is evidence that delaying the provision of amplification to an ear with hearing loss can increase the likelihood of auditory deprivation and poorer perception in the impaired ear over time (Gelfand & Silman, 1993). The mechanisms for these changes in the auditory system have not been definitively identified, and it is unclear whether or not auditory stimulation from hearing aids would have avoided the changes that have been documented in those studies. Nonetheless, many children with aidable unilateral hearing loss receive both objective and subjective improvements with amplification (Briggs, Davidson & Lieu, 2011). There is some evidence to suggest that children with unilateral hearing loss may use their hearing aids less consistently than children with bilateral hearing loss (McKay, Knightly, Marsh, Amann, & Gravel, 2007). Studies of hearing aid use in children with unilateral hearing loss have often included children with severe or profound unilateral hearing losses, a group that may have limited potential to benefit from amplification. The amplification fitting process for children with aidable unilateral hearing loss should follow the same selection and verification procedures as children with bilateral hearing loss. Some outcome measures designed for children with bilateral hearing loss may not be sensitive to the specific challenges of children with unilateral hearing loss, but alternative tools have not been developed and validated for this purpose.

**Intervention Options for Children with Severe to Profound Unilateral Hearing Loss**. Children with severe to profound unilateral hearing loss are not considered to have aidable hearing, as discussed in the previous section. For this reason, amplification for the impaired ear may not be effective or accepted by the child (Kiese-Himmel, Ohlwein, & Kruse, 2000). As an alternative to amplifying the impaired ear, there are four audiological intervention options: (1) contralateral routing of sound, (2) hearing assistance technology, (3) cochlear implant, or (4) monitoring of audiological status and development. Each of the options has potential advantages and drawbacks for providing auditory access to children with severe to profound unilateral hearing loss.

Contralateral Routing of Sound (CROS) devices transmit sound from the impaired ear to the normal-hearing ear so that it can be perceived. The transmission of sound can be achieved using a wire or wireless radio-frequency transmission from a transmitter with a microphone on the impaired ear to a receiver that is worn on the ear with normal hearing. Alternatively, bone conduction devices, including bone conduction hearing aids or osseointegrated auditory devices, can be used as CROS devices that send the signal from the impaired ear to the normal-hearing ear via bone conduction. In both cases, the sound from both ears is received in the normal-hearing ear, which means that CROS devices do not restore access to binaural cues. Instead, the CROS minimizes the head shadow effect by transmitting sounds from the impaired side of the head that would otherwise be inaudible because of transmission around the head. This is primarily limited to frequencies above 2 kHz, where the wavelength of sound is shorter than the distance between the two ears. It is important for clinicians to temper patient expectations in light of the minimal amount of auditory information that is being made audible by CROS devices. The situations where CROS devices are most beneficial tend to be in situations where there is a diffuse noise source or noise directed at the good ear and a target talker or speech on the impaired side.

A study by Lin and colleagues (2006) evaluated subjective preference and speech recognition in noise for a group of adults with unilateral hearing loss, comparing a wireless CROS hearing aid and a osseointegrated bone conduction device. The study found positive benefits for speech perception in noise where the target talker was directed toward the poorer ear and subjective benefits in terms of patient preference. Similar comparative studies have not been conducted in children, to date. A review of outcomes from CROS studies conducted with children who have unilateral hearing loss highlighted minimal situational improvements and potential for negative results if the child could not appropriately orient the CROS device toward a talker of interest and away from background noise (McKay et al., 2008). For these reasons, audiologists have been reluctant to provide CROS devices to young children before they can orient toward talkers of interest. There are currently no guidelines and limited evidence to suggest an appropriate age where CROS devices might be beneficial to children. Further research is needed to determine the extent to which CROS devices may be beneficial for children with severe-to-profound unilateral hearing loss.

Another potential future option for severe-to-profound unilateral hearing loss in children is cochlear implantation. Cochlear implantation for adults with unilateral hearing loss started as a potential treatment for debilitating tinnitus, but improvements in hearing were noted as a potential side benefit (Vermeire & Van de Heyning, 2008). Unlike CROS devices, cochlear implants may be able to restore access to binaural hearing in children with unilateral hearing loss, although there are some important caveats. The only evidence for cochlear implantation for children with unilateral hearing loss has been case studies, which have indicated that speech recognition and localization outcomes are highly variable. Additional information regarding outcomes for children with unilateral hearing loss who receive cochlear implants is provided in Chapter 8 of this textbook (see also Peters, Ramakers, Smit, & Grolman, 2015, for a review of the literature). It is worth noting that a large proportion of children with unilateral hearing loss are likely to have structural anomalies to the cochlea or auditory nerve that preclude cochlear implantation. In the future, cochlear implantation may become a viable option for some children with unilateral severe or profound hearing loss, but further research is needed before this practice gains clinical acceptance among audiologists.

## AUDITORY NEUROPATHY SPECTRUM DISORDER

ANSD is a type of hearing loss that involves an abnormal or absent neural response at the site of the auditory nerve or auditory brainstem. In addition, outer hair cell function is intact, as shown by preneural cochlear responses including otoacoustic emissions and/or cochlear microphonic (Roush, Frymark, Venediktov, & Wang, 2011). ANSD was first described in the 1990s by Starr, Picton, Sininger, Hood, and Berlin (1996). It has been referred to by a number of different terms, including auditory neuropathy, auditory dysynchrony, auditory synaptopathy, or inner hair cell pathology (Vlastarakos, Nikolopoulos, Tavoulari, Papacharalambous, & Korres, 2008). More recently, the term ANSD has been utilized to reflect the growing awareness that this is not a single disorder, but rather a spectrum of pathologies along the auditory pathway. Because ANSD is so heterogeneous, there is wide variation in outcomes, making audiological management a challenge.

### Prevalence and Incidence

ANSD is relatively rare, with Vlastarakos et al. (2008) reporting a prevalence rate between 0.23 and 2% in infants who are considered to be "at risk" for hearing loss (e.g., neonatal intensive care unit graduates). This prevalence rate increases in children who have been diagnosed with a permanent hearing loss, with estimates between 2 and 15% (Rance, 2005; Sininger, 2002). ANSD makes up approximately 8% of newly identified cases of hearing loss per year, reflecting the incidence rate of the disorder (Madden, Hilbert, Rutter, Greinwald, & Choo, 2002).

> Incidence rate is the number of newly identified cases of a specific disorder, in a given time period.

### Etiology

As previously stated, ANSD is a multifaceted spectrum of disorders. A variety of possible causes have been identified, including prematurity and hyperbilirubinemia. Ototoxic medications, such as furosemide and aminoglycosides, have also been implicated as causal factors (Coenraad, Goedegebure, van Goudoever, & Hoeve, 2011; Lobarinas, Salvi, & Ding, 2013). ANSD may also be due to syndromic or nonsyndromic genetic conditions (Roush et al., 2011). Examples of syndromic conditions include hereditary sensorimotor neuropathy (also referred to as Charcot-Marie-Tooth disease) and Friedreich's ataxia. Nonsyndromic genetic forms include the Otoferlin (OTOF) gene, a recessive gene mutation (Varga et al., 2003).

#### *Outcomes*

Children with ANSD may present with pure-tone averages in the normal to profound range (Rance

& Starr, 2011). Some children may have progressive or fluctuating hearing loss (Madden et al., 2002). Therefore, it is not surprising that outcomes for children with ANSD can vary widely. In particular, children with ANSD demonstrate large individual differences in speech perception outcomes. Speech perception skills in ANSD are characterized by several hallmark features. One feature is that there is not a linear relationship between speech perception abilities and audibility (Rance, 2005). In other words, individuals with better audibility will not necessarily have better speech understanding compared to individuals with poorer audibility, as we typically see in cases of sensorineural hearing loss. Temporal resolution appears to be associated with speech perception skills in ANSD, as children with ANSD who have greater temporal processing deficits tend to have poorer speech recognition in quiet, unaided conditions (Rance, McKay, & Grayden, 2004). A second characteristic of ANSD is that speech perception in noise is particularly difficult (Kraus et al., 2000; Rance & Barker, 2008). Research suggests that the underlying cause of speech perception challenges is related to a reduced ability to integrate cues coming from both ears. As a result, individuals with ANSD have poor localization skills, and localization supports speech perception in noise (Zeng, Kong, Michalewski, & Starr, 2005).

Temporal resolution is the ability to detect differences in sound duration.

We know less about speech production and language outcomes for children with ANSD compared to speech perception outcomes. One of the major questions in the ANSD literature is whether children with ANSD perform similarly to hearing peers, but also how they compare to children with sensorineural hearing loss. This question is critical to determining appropriate audiological management of children with ANSD because it informs us on whether children with ANSD should receive intervention that is similar to children with sensorineural hearing loss or if alternative approaches are warranted. Research on this topic is often hampered by small numbers of participants and challenges with controlling for factors that may influence outcomes, such as degree of hearing loss, aided audibility, chronological age, and socioeconomic status. Recent studies have begun to shed light on expected outcomes for ANSD, however.

Two studies from Australia compared children with ANSD to children with sensorineural hearing loss. Rance, Barker, Sarant, and Ching (2007) examined vocabulary comprehension and speech production skills in 12 school-age children with ANSD. On average, the children scored below the average range relative to the standardized tests norms, suggesting that they had delays compared to their same-age peers with normal hearing. The children with ANSD were also matched with a group of children who had sensorineural hearing loss, which allowed the researchers to control for chronological age and degree of hearing loss. Results indicated that there were no significant differences between the children with ANSD and the children with sensorineural hearing loss. This suggests that children with ANSD can develop spoken language skills that are commensurate with the level of performance expected for children with sensorineural hearing loss.

The second study from Australia included children with mild-to-profound hearing loss who participated in a population-based longitudinal study (Longitudinal Outcomes of Children with Hearing Impairment; LOCHI). Ching et al. (2013) compared 47 preschool-age children with ANSD to a group of children with sensorineural hearing loss. They found no differences between the ANSD group and the group with sensorineural hearing loss on a variety of measures (i.e., speech production, receptive and expressive language). A limitation of this study was that they did not examine the influence of audiological management within the ANSD group; in other words, children with hearing aids and cochlear implants were combined into one group. This makes it difficult to determine whether a specific treatment approach (hearing aids versus cochlear implant) was associated with more difficulties in speech and language outcomes.

Finally, researchers with the OCHL study, a longitudinal study in the United States, compared the speech production, speech perception, and language outcomes of 12 children with

ANSD and children with similar degrees of mild-to-moderately-severe sensorineural hearing loss (Walker, McCreery, Spratford, & Roush, 2016). All of the participants wore bilateral hearing aids that were verified based on the American Academy of Audiology (AAA) pediatric amplification guidelines. Children in the two groups were matched on a number of factors, including better-ear pure-tone average, better-ear aided audibility, gender, socioeconomic status, and newborn hearing screening result (i.e., pass or refer). Consistent with the findings of Rance and Barker (2008) and Ching et al. (2013), there were no significant differences between groups on any of the language measures. Although the literature on spoken language outcomes in children with ANSD is sparse, these three studies (Rance & Barker, 2008; Ching et al., 2013; Walker et al., 2016) suggest that children with ANSD benefit from audiological intervention, similar to children with sensorineural hearing loss. Given the varying presentations of ANSD in children, pediatric audiologists who encounter this population need to have a clear understanding regarding appropriate clinical interventions for this population, which will be discussed in the next section.

### *Intervention Options for ANSD*

There has been a great deal of debate about best practices for audiological management of children with ANSD. This debate arises from a general uncertainty regarding the treatment effectiveness of hearing aids versus cochlear implants. When ANSD was first being described, there were some recommendations for minimizing hearing aid usage (Berlin, 1999) or providing hearing aids with low gain, relative to prescriptive targets based on hearing thresholds and real-ear-to-coupler difference (Hood, 1998). Some of this early research indicated that children with ANSD had poor outcomes with hearing aids (Berlin, 1999; Berlin et al., 2003; Raveh, Buller, Badrana, & Attais, 2007). This research should be interpreted with some caution, however, because the studies did not report on outcomes of children with mild-to-moderately-severe hearing loss, who were fit with hearing aids set to prescriptive targets (either Desired Sensation Level or National Acoustics Laboratory).

Currently, the American Academy of Audiology (AAA) Pediatric Amplification guidelines recommend that children with ANSD undergo a trial with hearing aids if hearing sensitivity is so poor that it limits the audibility of speech. Hearing aids should be fit according to the AAA Pediatric Amplification best-practice guidelines (AAA, 2013), using prescriptive gain targets for soft and conversational speech levels and MPO targets for pure-tones via real-ear probe microphone measurements or simulated real-ear measurements, depending on the developmental level of the child (Bagatto et al., 2005; Scollie et al., 2005). Recent evidence supports the use of appropriately fit hearing aids for children with ANSD who have auditory thresholds in the hard of hearing range (Walker et al., 2016).

Cochlear implants have been closely examined as an intervention approach for ANSD (Breneman, Gifford, & DeJong, 2012; Buss et al., 2002; Rance & Barker, 2008; Raveh, Buller, Badrana, & Attias, 2007; Shallop, Peterson, Facer, Fabry, & Driscoll, 2001; Teagle et al., 2010). In 2008, an international working group convened in Como, Italy, to discuss guidelines for clinical management of ANSD. The group consensus was that cochlear implantation should be considered a viable treatment option for children with ANSD. Unlike children with sensorineural hearing loss, children with ANSD may be considered candidates for cochlear implants regardless of audiometric thresholds, if they show limited progress in speech recognition and language acquisition with hearing aids.

Several reasons have been proposed to explain why cochlear implants may benefit some patients with ANSD, including cases of milder hearing loss. One proposed reason is that the cochlear implant electrode array effectively bypasses damaged inner hair cells, which hearing aids cannot do. This electrical signal directly stimulates the spiral ganglion and increases the number of firing neural elements. The second proposed reason is that the electrical stimulation increases synchronized neural firing along the auditory nerve (Rance, 2014). This increase in synchronization benefits individuals with ANSD who have difficulty with temporal resolution.

Many of the studies looking at the treatment effectiveness of cochlear implants for

ANSD focused on children with hearing loss in the severe-to-profound range (Jeong, Kim, Kim, Bae, & Kim, 2007; Miyamoto, Kirk, Renshaw, & Hussain, 1999; Trautwein, Sininger, & Nelson, 2000; Vermeire, Brokx, Van de Heyning, Cochet, & Carpentier, 2003). Some of these studies showed improvements in speech recognition skills following implantation (Madden et al., 2002; Mason, De Michele, Stevens, Ruth, & Hashisaki, 2003). Breneman et al. (2012) demonstrated that children with ANSD who used cochlear implants performed similarly to children with sensorineural hearing loss on speech perception tests, when the two groups were matched on age at initial stimulation and length of cochlear implant experience. The authors point out, however, that children should first have a hearing aid trial with hearing aids that have been fit using best practice techniques, to determine if auditory progress can be made with acoustic amplification.

Hearing assistance technologies, including remote microphone FM and DM systems, are also often noted as a solution in noise for children with ANSD (Rance, 2013). However, research supporting this recommendation has largely been based on some studies that suggest that children with ANSD have greater difficulty in background noise than peers with sensorineural hearing loss of comparable degree, but not on evidence suggesting that these systems can overcome the dysfunction of the auditory system that many children with ANSD experience even in quiet listening conditions. Given the limited evidence for benefit from hearing assistance technologies in children with ANSD, these systems should be recommended on a case-by-case basis for children with documented difficulty listening in background noise based on a functional listening evaluation or aided measures of speech recognition.

## HEARING LOSS AND ADDITIONAL DISABILITIES

Up to 40% of children with hearing loss have additional disabilities, based on the Gallaudet Research Institute (GRI) annual survey (2011). In children with severe-to-profound hearing loss, estimates of comorbidity range as high as 48% (Chilosi et al., 2010). Most of these comorbid conditions consist of intellectual, behavioral, or motor disabilities. As discussed in Chapter 6 (Monitoring Outcomes), identifying these additional disabilities is important for determining appropriate clinical management. The following sections will describe two disabilities that can co-occur with hearing loss and may require different clinical management approaches, specifically Autism Spectrum Disorder and Down syndrome.

### Autism Spectrum Disorder (ASD)

The term ASD is used to describe a neurodevelopmental disorder that is characterized by impaired social and communicative interactions with others. Prior to 2013, ASD was divided into subgroups, including Autism, Asperger Disorder, Rett syndrome, childhood disintegrative disorder (CDD), and pervasive developmental delay— not otherwise specified (PDD-NOS). In 2013, the fifth edition of the *Diagnostic and Statistical Manual of Mental Disorders* (DSM-V; American Psychiatric Association, 2013) revised the description of ASD, collapsing the categories of Autism, Asperger, CDD, and PDD-NOS into a single condition. Rett syndrome was given its own diagnostic category due to its genetic basis. Individuals with ASD are diagnosed in two domains: (1) social communication/interactions, and (2) repetitive and restricted behaviors. Recent estimates by the Centers for Disease Control (CDC) indicate the prevalence of ASD is 1 in 68 children, with boys being more likely to be diagnosed than girls (Baio, 2014).

There are inconsistencies in the research literature regarding the prevalence of hearing loss in children with ASD, as it can be challenging to obtain reliable behavioral thresholds in this population. Fitzpatrick, Lambert, Whittingham, and Leblanc (2014) examined the prevalence of ASD in children with hearing loss, including children from Canada who had been seen for audiological services over an 8-year period. Out of 785 children with hearing loss, 2.2% ($n = 17$) had also received a diagnosis of ASD. Beers, McBoyle, Kakande, Santos, and Kozak (2014) conducted a systematic review of the literature on autism and hearing loss, and reported that there is no indication that children with ASD are more likely to have hearing loss than the general population of children.

> *Diagnostic and Statistical Manual of Mental Disorders:* classifications of mental disorders used by psychologists, psychiatrists, and related professionals to diagnose mental health issues.

Traditional methods of pediatric audiological assessment for children with ASD may not be feasible because they may be uninterested (or overly interested) in conditioned play techniques such as dropping blocks, or they may be unresponsive to auditory stimuli (Beers et al., 2014). Children with ASD may also be resistant to wearing headphones, insert earphones, bone oscillators, or probes for tympanometry or otoacoustic emissions due to tactile sensitivity. For children with confirmed hearing loss, fitting hearing aids using probe-tube measurements can also be a challenge due to tactile issues. Collaborating with parents and speech-language pathologists prior to testing can be highly beneficial in preparing children for an audiological appointment. Children with ASD have difficulty transitioning to new surroundings, and novel people, situations, and stimuli can cause anxiety. Parents and speech-language pathologists (or any service provider who knows the child well) can help familiarize the child with the situation through picture schedules or online videos (Davis & Stiegler, 2005). Another evidence-based strategy for working with children with ASD are Social Stories, which are individually tailored stories designed to promote appropriate behavior (Gray & Garand, 1993). For children with ASD who have diagnosed hearing loss, Social Stories may be an effective approach for eliciting compliance during audiological assessment or hearing aid fittings. The audiologist may work with the child's service provider to develop Social Stories related to visiting the audiology clinic.

Best practices for audiological intervention in children with ASD and hearing loss are consistent with intervention for children without ASD. If the hearing loss is diagnosed and deemed to be aidable, hearing aids should be selected, fit, and verified using prescriptive targets and real-ear or simulated real-ear measures. One important point related to children with ASD is that they may be hypersensitive to sound. In these cases, it may be beneficial to reduce the MPO levels at the initial fitting and gradually increase it at follow-up appointments. This procedure may facilitate acceptance of the hearing aids by the child (Beers et al., 2014). To the best of our knowledge, only one study has been published regarding uptake of amplification in children with ASD. Fitzpatrick, Lambert and colleagues (2014) examined 17 children with ASD and hearing loss, and found that 13 out of the 17 were fit with hearing aids after diagnosis (one child did not receive amplification, one received a cochlear implant, and two received an FM system). Further research is needed regarding the acceptance and effectiveness of hearing aids in this population.

Cochlear implants are another habilitation option for children with ASD and hearing loss in the severe-to-profound range. Although research on treatment effectiveness with cochlear implants and ASD is limited, one study indicated improvements in social communication, awareness of sound, vocalizations, and eye contact following implantation (Donaldson, Heavner, & Zwolan, 2004). Another study by Daneshi and Hassanzadeh (2007) reported that children with ASD showed slower gains in auditory perception skills following implantation, compared to other children with cochlear implants and multiple disabilities. Daneshi and Hassanzadeh recommend a multidisciplinary approach, utilizing service providers with experience working with the ASD population, to facilitate optimal outcomes in these children.

## Down Syndrome

Down syndrome is a genetic disorder that is the result of a third copy of chromosome 21 (hence, Down syndrome may also be referred to as Trisomy 21). An estimated 5400 infants are born with Down syndrome each year in the United States, making it the most common chromosomal disorder and a leading cause of intellectual disabilities (Sherman, Allen, Bean, & Freeman, 2007). Prevalence is approximately 1 in 700 births (Raut et al., 2011), with prevalence being five times higher in older mothers than younger mothers (Shin et al., 2009). The overexpression of additional genetic material on chromosome 21 has a cascading effect on physical and cognitive development. Individuals with Down syndrome have characteristic facial and physical features, including microcephaly (small head circumference), macroglossia (proportionally large tongue), hypotonia (low muscle tone), and short stature (Korenberg et al., 1994). Down syndrome is often associated with congenital heart defects, metabolic problems (usually in the form of hypothyroidism), and increased risk of leukemia (Fong & Brodeur, 1987; Roizen & Patterson, 2003). Life expectancy has greatly improved for adults with Down syndrome due to medical advances in the treatment of cardiac and thyroid anomalies, as well as leukemia. In the 1960s, average life expectancy was in the 30s. Currently, it is in the 50s to 60s (Mégarbané et al., 2009).

Hearing loss identification and intervention is critical in the clinical management of this population, from birth through adulthood (Roizen & Patterson, 2003). The incidence of hearing loss during infancy occurs more often than in healthy infants or babies with other developmental delays (Raut et al., 2011). Hearing loss may present as conductive, sensorineural, or mixed, although conductive hearing loss is most common. Children with Down syndrome show a higher incidence of chronic otitis media, due in part to anatomical differences in the eustachian tube as well as slower development of the immune system, resulting in more frequent upper respiratory infections. Further, stenotic ear canals occur in approximately 40% of children with Down syndrome (Shott, Joseph, & Heithaus, 2001). Recent evidence suggests that close monitoring and aggressive treatment of otitis media results in improved hearing and subsequent improvements in quality of life (Labby, Mace, Buncke, & MacArthur, 2016).

Given the high likelihood of language and cognitive delays, improving auditory access for children with Down syndrome is of paramount importance. Once hearing loss has been confirmed, early intervention in the form of amplification will help children with Down syndrome maximize their communication outcomes. Real-ear or simulated real-ear measures should always be used to fit hearing aids, as with any population of children. In particular, it is critical that the real-ear-to-coupler difference (RECD) is measured, rather than using the average values, because children with Down syndrome will likely have smaller-than-average ear canals and/or PE tubes (thus, the RECD will probably be far off from the average values for a given age). Due to the chronic middle ear problems that are associated with Down syndrome, bone-anchored hearing aids (BAHAs) are also a viable option in cases of permanent conductive hearing loss that cannot be improved through medical or surgical interventions (Porter & Tharpe, 2010).

## SUMMARY AND CONCLUSIONS

The process of diagnosing hearing loss and fitting hearing aids on children with bilateral, permanent hearing loss is complex. The complexity can increase significantly for children who have other types of hearing loss or other comorbid developmental conditions that complicate the picture. The overall framework of diagnosis of hearing loss, hearing aid candidacy, feature selection, verification, and outcomes assessment that we have outlined in this textbook is an effective starting point for children with more complicated hearing loss or associated conditions. This chapter provides important alternative considerations in terms of adapting candidacy, timelines for amplification, intervention, and the type of amplification that might be effective for these subgroups. Although it may have appeared repetitive at times during this chapter, the need for further research in all of these areas is essential. The need for further research into strategies for managing children with multiple disabilities is increasing and could be one of the next scientific leaps in the area of pediatric amplification. Children with hearing loss are already a small subpopulation, and the special populations of children with hearing loss are even more difficult to study because of their small numbers and large heterogeneity. Clinicians can serve a vital role in the research process with these patients by publishing findings and case series to help the scientific community generalize and develop alternative audiological interventions to help these children.

## REFERENCES


American Academy of Audiology. (2013). *Clinical practice guidelines: Pediatric amplification*. Reston, VA: Author.

American Psychiatric Association. (2013). *Diagnostic and statistical manual of mental disorders* (5th ed.). Washington, DC: Author.

Bagatto, M. P., & Tharpe, A. M. T. (2014). Decision support guide for hearing aid use in infants and children with minimal/mild bilateral hearing loss. In J. Northern (Ed.), *A Sound Foundation through early amplification. Proceedings of 6th International Conference* (pp. 145–151). Chicago, IL: Phonak AG.

Bagatto, M., Moodie, S., Scollie, S., Seewald, R., Moodie, S., Pumford, J., & Liu, K. R. (2005). Clinical protocols for hearing instrument fitting in the Desired Sensation Level method. *Trends in Amplification, 9*(4), 199–226.

Baio, J. and the Autism and Developmental Disabilities Monitoring Network. (2014). Prevalence of autism spectrum disorder among children aged 8 years. *Morbidity and Mortality Weekly Report. Surveillance Summaries, 63*(2), 1–21.

Beers, A. N., McBoyle, M., Kakande, E., Santos, R. C. D., & Kozak, F. K. (2014). Autism and peripheral hearing loss: A systematic review. *International Journal of Pediatric Otorhinolaryngology, 78*(1), 96–101.

Berlin, C. I. (1999). Auditory neuropathy: Using OAEs and ABRs from screening to management. *Seminars in Hearing, 20*, 307–315.

Berlin, C. I., Hood, L., Morlet, T., Rose, K., & Brashears, S. (2003). Auditory neuropathy/dys-synchrony: Diagnosis and management. *Mental Retardation and Developmental Disabilities Research Reviews, 9*(4), 225–231.

Bess, F. H., Dodd-Murphy, J., & Parker, R. A. (1998). Children with minimal sensorineural hearing loss: Prevalence, educational performance, and functional status. *Ear and Hearing, 19*(5), 339–354.

Bess, F. H., & Tharpe, A. M. (1984). Unilateral hearing impairment in children. *Pediatrics, 74*(2), 206–216.

Bess, F. H., Tharpe, A. M., & Gibler, A. M. (1986). Auditory performance of children with unilateral sensorineural hearing loss. *Ear and Hearing, 7*(1), 20–26.

Blair, J. C., Peterson, M. E., & Viehweg, S. H. (1985). The effects of mild sensorineural hearing loss on academic performance of young school-age children. *Volta Review, 87*, 87–93.

Bovo, R., Martini, A., Agnoletto, M., & Beghi, A. (1988). Auditory and academic performance of children with unilateral hearing loss. *Scandinavian Audiology, Suppl 30*, 71–74.

Breneman, A. I., Gifford, R. H., & DeJong, M. D. (2012). Cochlear implantation in children with auditory neuropathy spectrum disorder: Long-term outcomes. *Journal of the American Academy of Audiology, 23*(1), 5–17.

Briggs, L., Davidson, L., & Lieu, J. E. (2011). Outcomes of conventional amplification for pediatric unilateral hearing loss. *Annals of Otology, Rhinology & Laryngology, 120*(7), 448–454.

Briscoe, J., Bishop, D. V., & Norbury, C. F. (2001). Phonological processing, language, and literacy: A comparison of children with mild-to-moderate sensorineural hearing loss and those with specific language impairment. *Journal of Child Psychology and Psychiatry, 42*(03), 329–340.

Buss, E., Labadie, R. F., Brown, C. J., Gross, A. J., Grose, J. H., & Pillsbury, H. C. (2002). Outcome of cochlear implantation in pediatric auditory neuropathy. *Otology & Neurotology, 23*(3), 328–332.

Callison, D. M., & Horn, K. L. (1998). Large vestibular aqueduct syndrome: An overlooked etiology for progressive childhood hearing loss. *Journal of the American Academy of Audiology, 9*, 285–291.

Chilosi, A. M., Comparini, A., Scusa, M. F., Berrettini, S., Forli, F., Battini, R., . . . Cioni, G. (2010). Neurodevelopmental disorders in children with severe to profound sensorineural hearing loss: A clinical study. *Developmental Medicine & Child Neurology, 52*(9), 856–862.

Ching, T. Y., Day, J., Dillon, H., Gardner-Berry, K., Hou, S., Seeto, M., . . . Zhang, V. (2013). Impact of the presence of auditory neuropathy spectrum disorder (ANSD) on outcomes of children at three years of age. *International Journal of Audiology, 52*(S2), S55–S64.

Coenraad, S., Goedegebure, A., van Goudoever, J. B., & Hoeve, L. J. (2011). Risk factors for auditory neuropathy spectrum disorder in NICU infants compared to normal-hearing NICU controls. *Laryngoscope, 121*(4), 852–855.

Culbertson, J. L., & Gilbert, L. E. (1986). Children with unilateral sensorineural hearing loss: Cognitive, academic, and social development. *Ear and Hearing, 7*(1), 38–42.

Daneshi, A., & Hassanzadeh, S. (2007). Cochlear implantation in prelingually deaf persons with additional disability. *Journal of Laryngology & Otology, 121*(07), 635–638.

Davis, J. M., Elfenbein, J., Schum, R., & Bentler, R. A. (1986). Effects of mild and moderate hearing impairments on language, educational, and psychosocial behavior of children. *Journal of Speech and Hearing Disorders, 51*(1), 53–62.

Davis, R., & Stiegler, L. N. (2005). Toward more effective audiological assessment of children with autism spectrum disorders. *Seminars in Hearing, 26*, 241–252.

Đoković, S., Gligorović, M., Ostojić, S., Dimić, N., Radić-Šestić, M., & Slavnić, S. (2014). Can mild bilateral sensorineural hearing loss affect developmental abilities in younger school-age children? *Journal of Deaf Studies and Deaf Education, 19*(4), 484–495.

Donaldson, A. I., Heavner, K. S., & Zwolan, T. A. (2004). Measuring progress in children with autism spectrum disorder who have cochlear implants. *Archives of Otolaryngology-Head & Neck Surgery, 130*(5), 666–671.

Fitzpatrick, E. M., Durieux-Smith, A., & Whittingham, J. (2010). Clinical practice for children with mild bilateral and unilateral hearing loss. *Ear and Hearing, 31*(3), 392–400.

Fitzpatrick, E., Grandpierre, V., Durieux-Smith, A., Gaboury, I., Coyle, D., Na, E., & Sallam, N. (2016). Children with mild bilateral and unilateral hearing loss: Parents' reflections on experiences and outcomes. *Journal of Deaf Studies and Deaf Education, 21*(1), 34–43.

Fitzpatrick, E. M., Lambert, L., Whittingham, J., & Leblanc, E. (2014). Examination of characteristics and management of children with hearing loss and autism spectrum disorders. *International Journal of Audiology, 53*(9), 577–586.

Fitzpatrick, E. M., Whittingham, J., & Durieux-Smith, A. (2014). Mild bilateral and unilateral hearing loss in childhood: A 20-year view of hearing characteristics, and audiologic practices before and after newborn hearing screening. *Ear and Hearing, 35*(1), 10–18.

Fong, C. T., & Brodeur, G. M. (1987). Down's syndrome and leukemia: Epidemiology, genetics, cytogenetics and mechanisms of leukemogenesis. *Cancer Genetics and Cytogenetics, 28*(1), 55–76.

Fortnum, H., & Davis, A. (1993). Hearing impairment in children after bacterial meningitis: Incidence and resource implications. *British Journal of Audiology, 27*(1), 43–52.

Fowler, K. B., & Boppana, S. B. (2006). Congenital cytomegalovirus (CMV) infection and hearing deficit. *Journal of Clinical Virology, 35*(2), 226–231.

Freedman, B. (1987). Equipoise and the ethics of clinical research. *New England Journal of Medicine, 317*(3), 141–145.

Gallaudet Research Institute. (2011). *Regional and National Summary Report of Data from the 2009–10 Annual Survey of Deaf and Hard of Hearing Children and Youth.* Washington, DC: Gallaudet University. Retrieved from http://research.gallaudet.edu/Demographics/2012_National_Summary.pdf

Gelfand, S. A., & Silman, S. (1993). Apparent auditory deprivation in children: Implications of monaural versus binaural amplification. *Journal of the American Academy of Audiology, 4*(5), 313–318.

Gravel, J. S., White, K. R., Johnson, J. L., Widen, J. E., Vohr, B. R., James, M., . . . Sullivan-Mahoney, M. (2005). A multisite study to examine the efficacy of the otoacoustic emission/automated auditory brainstem response newborn hearing screening protocol recommendations for policy, practice, and research. *American Journal of Audiology, 14*(2), S217–S228.

Gray, C. A., & Garand, J. D. (1993). Social stories: Improving responses of students with autism with accurate social information. *Focus on Autistic Behavior, 8*, 1–10.

Individuals with Disabilities Education Improvement Act of 2004, 20 U.S.C. § 1400 et seq. (2004).

Hood, L. J. (1998). Auditory neuropathy: What is it and what can we do about it? *Hearing Journal, 51*(8), 10–12.

Jacobs, H. T., Hutchin, T. P., Käppi, T., Gillies, G., Minkkinen, K., Walker, J., . . . Melchionda, S. (2005). Mitochondrial DNA mutations in patients with postlingual, nonsyndromic hearing impairment. *European Journal of Human Genetics, 13*(1), 26–33.

Jeong, S.-W., Kim, L.-S., Kim, B.-Y., Bae, W.-Y., & Kim, J.-R. (2007). Cochlear implantation in children with auditory neuropathy: Outcomes and rationale. *Acta Oto-Laryngologica, 127*(S558), 36–43.

Johnson, J. L., White, K. R., Widen, J. E., Gravel, J. S., James, M., Kennalley, T., . . . Vohr, B. R. (2005). A multicenter evaluation of how many infants with permanent hearing loss pass a two-stage otoacoustic emissions/automated auditory brainstem response newborn hearing screening protocol. *Pediatrics, 116*(3), 663–672.

Joint Committee on Infant Hearing (2007). Year 2007 position statement: Principles and guidelines for early hearing detection and intervention programs. *Pediatrics, 120*(4), 898–921.

Jerger, J., Silman, S., Lew, H. L., & Chmiel, R. (1993). Case studies in binaural interference: Converging evidence from behavioral and electrophysiologic measures. *Journal of the American Academy of Audiology, 4*(2), 122–131.

Kiese-Himmel, C. (2002). Unilateral sensorineural hearing impairment in childhood: Analysis of 31 consecutive cases. *International Journal of Audiology, 41*(1), 57–63.

Kiese-Himmel, C., & Ohlwein, S. (2003). Characteristics of children with permanent mild hearing impairment. *Folia Phoniatrica Et Logopaedica, 55*(2), 70–79.

Kiese-Himmel C, Ohlwein S, Kruse E. (2000). Acceptance of hearing aids for children: A longitudinal analysis. *Phoniatrie Und Padaudiolie, 48*, 758–764.

Klee, T. M., & Davis-Dansky, E. (1986). A comparison of unilaterally hearing-impaired children and normal-hearing children on a battery of standardized language tests. *Ear and Hearing, 7*(1), 27–37.

Korenberg, J. R., Chen, X. N., Schipper, R., Sun, Z., Gonsky, R., Gerwehr, S., . . . Disteche, C. (1994). Down syndrome phenotypes: The consequences of chromosomal imbalance. *Proceedings of the National Academy of Sciences, 91*(11), 4997–5001.

Kraus, N., Bradlow, A. R., Cheatham, M. A., Cunningham, J., King, C. D., Koch, D. B., . . . Wright, B. A. (2000). Consequences of neural asynchrony: A case of auditory neuropathy. *Journal of the Association for Research in Otolaryngology, 1*(1), 33–45.

Labby, A., Mace, J. C., Buncke, M., & MacArthur, C. J. (2016). Quality of life improvement after pressure equalization tube placement in Down syndrome: A prospective study. *International Journal of Pediatric Otorhinolaryngology, 88*, 168–172.

Lieu, J. E., Tye-Murray, N., Karzon, R. K., & Piccirillo, J. F. (2010). Unilateral hearing loss is associated with worse speech–language scores in children. *Pediatrics, 125*(6), e1348–e1355.

Lin, L. M., Bowditch, S., Anderson, M. J., May, B., Cox, K. M., & Niparko, J. K. (2006). Amplification in the rehabilitation of unilateral deafness: Speech in noise and directional hearing effects with bone-anchored hearing and contralateral routing of signal amplification. *Otology & Neurotology, 27*(2), 172–182.

Liu, X. Z., Pandya, A., Angeli, S., Telischi, F. F., Arnos, K. S., Nance, W. E., & Balkany, T. (2005). Audiological features of GJB2 (connexin 26) deafness. *Ear and Hearing, 26*(3), 361–369.

Lobarinas, E., Salvi, R., & Ding, D. (2013). Insensitivity of the audiogram to carboplatin induced inner hair cell loss in chinchillas. *Hearing Research, 302*, 113–120.

Madden, C., Hilbert, L., Rutter, M., Greinwald, J., & Choo, D. (2002). Pediatric cochlear implantation in auditory neuropathy. *Otology & Neurotology, 23*(2), 163–168.

Mason, J. C., De Michele, A., Stevens, C., Ruth, R. A., & Hashisaki, G. T. (2003). Cochlear implantation in patients with auditory neuropathy of varied etiologies. *Laryngoscope, 113*(1), 45–49.

Mégarbané, A., Ravel, A., Mircher, C., Sturtz, F., Grattau, Y., Rethoré, M. O., . . . Mobley, W. C. (2009). The 50th anniversary of the discovery of trisomy 21: The past, present, and future of research and treatment of Down syndrome. *Genetics in Medicine, 11*(9), 611–616.

McKay, S., Gravel, J. S., & Tharpe, A. M. (2008). Amplification considerations for children with minimal or mild bilateral hearing loss and unilateral hearing loss. *Trends in Amplification, 12*(1), 43–54.

McKay, S., Knightly, C., Marsh, R., Amann, C., Gravel, J. S. (2007, December). *Perceived listening difficulties in children with unilateral hearing loss.* Poster presented at A Sound Foundation Through Early Amplification—International Conference, Chicago, IL.

Miyamoto, R. T., Kirk, K. H., Renshaw, J., & Hussain, D. (1999). Cochlear implantation in auditory neuropathy. *Laryngoscope, 109*(2), 181–185.

Norbury, C. F., Bishop, D. V., & Briscoe, J. (2001). Production of English finite verb morphology: A comparison of SLI and mild-moderate hearing impairment. *Journal of Speech, Language, and Hearing Research, 44*(1), 165–178.

Peters, J. P., Ramakers, G. G., Smit, A. L., & Grolman, W. (2015). Cochlear implantation in children with unilateral hearing loss: A systematic review. *Laryngoscope, 126*(3), 713–721.

Porter, H., Sladen, D. P., Ampah, S. B., Rothpletz, A., & Bess, F. H. (2013). Developmental outcomes in early school-age children with minimal hearing loss. *American Journal of Audiology, 22*, 263–270.

Porter, H., & Tharpe, A. M. (2010). Hearing loss among persons with Down syndrome. *International Review of Research in Mental Retardation, 39*, 195–220.

Rance, G. (2005). Auditory neuropathy/dys-synchrony and its perceptual consequences. *Trends in Amplification, 9*(1),1–43.

Rance, G. (2013). Journal Club: In autism study, FM system enhances listening, attention, and behavior. *Hearing Journal, 66*(7), 4–5.

Rance, G. (2014). An update on auditory neuropathy spectrum disorder in children. In J. Northern (Ed.), *A Sound Foundation through early amplification: Proceedings of the 2013 International Conference* (pp. 137–144). Chicago, IL: Phonak AG.

Rance, G., & Barker, E. J. (2008). Speech perception in children with auditory neuropathy/dyssynchrony managed with either hearing aids or cochlear implants. *Otology & Neurotology, 29*(2), 179–182.

Rance, G., Barker, E. J., Sarant, J. Z., & Ching, T. Y. (2007). Receptive language and speech production in children with auditory neuropathy/dyssynchrony type hearing loss. *Ear and Hearing, 28*(5), 694–702.

Rance, G., McKay, C., & Grayden, D. (2004). Perceptual characterization of children with auditory neuropathy. *Ear and Hearing, 25*(1), 34–46.

Rance, G., & Starr, A. (2011). Auditory neuropathy/dys-synchrony type hearing loss. *Comprehensive Handbook of Pediatric Audiology*, 225–242.

Raut, P., Sriram, B., Yeoh, A., Hee, K. Y., Lim, S. B., & Daniel, M. L. (2011). High prevalence of hearing loss in Down syndrome at first year of life. *Annals of the Academy of Medicine–Singapore*, *40*(11), 493–498.

Raveh, E., Buller, N., Badrana, O., & Attias, J. (2007). Auditory neuropathy: Clinical characteristics and therapeutic approach. *American Journal of Otolaryngology*, *28*(5), 302–308.

Roizen, N. J., & Patterson, D. (2003). Down's syndrome. *Lancet*, *361*(9365), 1281–1289.

Roush, P., Frymark, T., Venediktov, R., & Wang, B. (2011). Audiologic management of auditory neuropathy spectrum disorder in children: A systematic review of the literature. *American Journal of Audiology*, *20*(2), 159–170.

Ruscetta, M. N., Arjmand, E. M., & Pratt, S. R. (2005). Speech recognition abilities in noise for children with severe-to-profound unilateral hearing impairment. *International Journal of Pediatric Otorhinolaryngology*, *69*(6), 771–779.

Schleich, P., Nopp, P., & D'Haese, P. (2004). Head shadow, squelch, and summation effects in bilateral users of the MED-EL COMBI 40/40+ cochlear implant. *Ear and Hearing*, *25*(3), 197–204.

Scollie, S., Seewald, R., Cornelisse, L., Moodie, S., Bagatto, M., Laurnagaray, D., . . . Pumford, J. (2005). The desired sensation level multistage input/output algorithm. *Trends in Amplification*, *9*(4), 159–197.

Shallop, J. K., Peterson, A., Facer, G. W., Fabry, L. B., & Driscoll, C. L. (2001). Cochlear implants in five cases of auditory neuropathy: Postoperative findings and progress. *Laryngoscope*, *111*(4), 555–562.

Sherman, S. L., Allen, E. G., Bean, L. H., & Freeman, S. B. (2007). Epidemiology of Down syndrome. *Mental Retardation and Developmental Disabilities Research Reviews*, *13*(3), 221–227.

Shin, M., Besser, L. M., Kucik, J. E., Lu, C., Siffel, C., & Correa, A. (2009). Prevalence of Down syndrome among children and adolescents in 10 regions of the United States. *Pediatrics*, *124*(6), 1565–1571.

Shott, S. R., Joseph, A., & Heithaus, D. (2001). Hearing loss in children with Down syndrome. *International Journal of Pediatric Otorhinolaryngology*, *61*(3), 199–205.

Sininger, Y. S. (2002). Identification of auditory neuropathy in infants and children. *Seminars in Hearing*, *23*, 193–200.

Starr, A., Picton, T. W., Sininger, Y., Hood, L. J., & Berlin, C. I. (1996). Auditory neuropathy. *Brain*, *119*(3), 741–753.

Teagle, H. F., Roush, P. A., Woodard, J. S., Hatch, D. R., Zdanski, C. J., Buss, E., & Buchman, C. A. (2010). Cochlear implantation in children with auditory neuropathy spectrum disorder. *Ear and Hearing*, *31*(3), 325–335.

Tharpe, A. M. (2007, December). Minimal hearing loss in children: The facts and the fiction. *Sound Foundation through early amplification. Proceedings from the 4th International Conference* (pp. 213-219). Chicago, IL: Phonak AG.

Tharpe, A. M., & Sladen, D. P. (2008). Causation of permanent unilateral and mild bilateral hearing loss in children. *Trends in Amplification*, *12*(1), 17–25.

Trautwein, P. G., Sininger, Y. S., & Nelson, R. (2000). Cochlear implantation of auditory neuropathy. *Journal of the American Academy of Audiology*, *11*(6), 309–315.

Tyler, R. S., Dunn, C. C., Witt, S. A., & Preece, J. P. (2003). Update on bilateral cochlear implantation. *Current Opinion in Otolaryngology & Head and Neck Surgery*, *11*(5), 388–393.

Van Wanrooij, M. M., & Van Opstal, A. J. (2004). Contribution of head shadow and pinna cues to chronic monaural sound localization. *Journal of Neuroscience*, *24*(17), 4163–4171.

Varga, R., Kelley, P. M., Keats, B. J., Starr, A., Leal, S. M., Cohn, E., & Kimberling, W. J. (2003). Nonsyndromic recessive auditory neuropathy is the result of mutations in the otoferlin (OTOF) gene. *Journal of Medical Genetics*, *40*(1), 45–50.

Vermeire, K., Brokx, J. P., Van de Heyning, P. H., Cochet, E., & Carpentier, H. (2003). Bilateral cochlear implantation in children. *International Journal of Pediatric Otorhinolaryngology*, *67*(1), 67–70.

Vermeire, K., & Van de Heyning, P. (2008). Binaural hearing after cochlear implantation in subjects with unilateral sensorineural deafness and tinnitus. *Audiology and Neurotology*, *14*(3), 163–171.

Vlastarakos, P. V., Nikolopoulos, T. P., Tavoulari, E., Papacharalambous, G., & Korres, S. (2008). Auditory neuropathy: Endocochlear lesion or temporal processing impairment? Implications for diagnosis and management. *International Journal of Pediatric Otorhinolaryngology*, *72*(8), 1135–1150.

Wake, M., Tobin, S., Cone-Wesson, B., Dahl, H.-H., Gillam, L., McCormick, L., . . . Ukoumunne, O. C. (2006). Slight/mild sensorineural hearing loss in children. *Pediatrics*, *118*(5), 1842–1851.

Walker, E., McCreery, R., Spratford, M., & Roush, P. (2016). Children with auditory neuropathy spectrum disorder fitted with hearing aids applying the American Academy of Audiology Pediatric Amplification Guideline: Current practice and outcomes. *Journal of the American Academy of Audiology*, *27*(3), 204–218.

Walker, E. A., Holte, L., McCreery, R. W., Spratford, M., Page, T., & Moeller, M. P. (2015). The influence of hearing aid use on outcomes of children with mild hearing loss. *Journal of Speech, Language, and Hearing Research, 58*(5), 1611–1625.

Walker, E. A., Spratford, M., Ambrose, S. E., Holte, L., & Oleson, J. (2017). Service delivery to children with mild hearing loss: current practice patterns and parent perceptions. *American Journal of Audiology, 28,* 38–52.

Watkin, P., & Baldwin, M. (1999). Confirmation of deafness in infancy. *Archives of Disease in Childhood, 81*(5), 380–389.

Winiger, A. M., Alexander, J. M., & Diefendorf, A. O. (2016). Minimal hearing loss: From a failure-based approach to evidence-based practice. *American Journal of Audiology, 25,* 1–14.

Wolgemuth, K. S., Kamhi, A. G., & Lee, R. F. (1998). Metaphor performance in children with hearing impairment. *Language, Speech, and Hearing Services in Schools, 29*(4), 216–231.

Zeng, F. G., Kong, Y. Y., Michalewski, H. J., & Starr, A. (2005). Perceptual consequences of disrupted auditory nerve activity. *Journal of Neurophysiology, 93*(6), 3050–3063.

# 10

# Case Studies in Pediatric Amplification

*Ryan W. McCreery and Elizabeth A. Walker*

## INTRODUCTION

The goal of this textbook is to provide a theoretical framework to support the provision of hearing aids to children. For clinicians and students, illustrative case examples can be helpful to bring the concepts described in the text into a realistic clinical context and to apply the fundamental concepts to their own patients. The case studies that follow were developed to illustrate key concepts presented in the preceding chapters. Some case studies illustrate multiple aspects of promoting cumulative auditory experience for children with hearing loss. Each case study includes a background section that describes relevant case history or demographic information. Clinical outcomes data are provided whenever possible to illustrate the application of concepts presented in the book. A summary of each case is provided to highlight the main points of each case, as well as unresolved questions and recommendations that might be provided in specific situations. None of the case studies presented in this chapter are representative of actual children. Names were invented to make the cases seem more realistic, but any resemblance to a real person is purely coincidental.

## CASE STUDY 1: CALEB

### Background

Caleb was first seen by an audiologist at 5 years of age after he failed a hearing screening as part of a kindergarten health check by his pediatrician. Caleb's parents did not have concerns about his hearing or speech and language development. His parents did note that he would often seem to ignore their requests or had difficulties listening, which they attributed to him being an active 5-year-old. Caleb passed his universal newborn hearing screening at birth with an automated auditory brainstem response (AABR) and did not have any history of chronic middle ear problems during early childhood.

## Clinical Data

### Diagnostic Data

Tympanometry was normal Type A in both ears using a 226 Hz probe tone. Ipsilateral acoustic reflexes were present in both ears at a screening level of 90 dB SPL at 1000 and 2000 Hz. Pure-tone audiometry was assessed using computer-assisted conditioned play audiometry (CPA). Results indicated a symmetrical mild hearing loss from 500 to 4000 Hz in both ears (Figure 10–1). Bone conduction assessment could not be completed, as Caleb lost interest in the play task before it could be completed. These findings are consistent with bilateral mild hearing loss. The absence of middle ear dysfunction and normal immittance suggests that the loss may be sensorineural, but bone conduction assessment was needed to verify the type of loss.

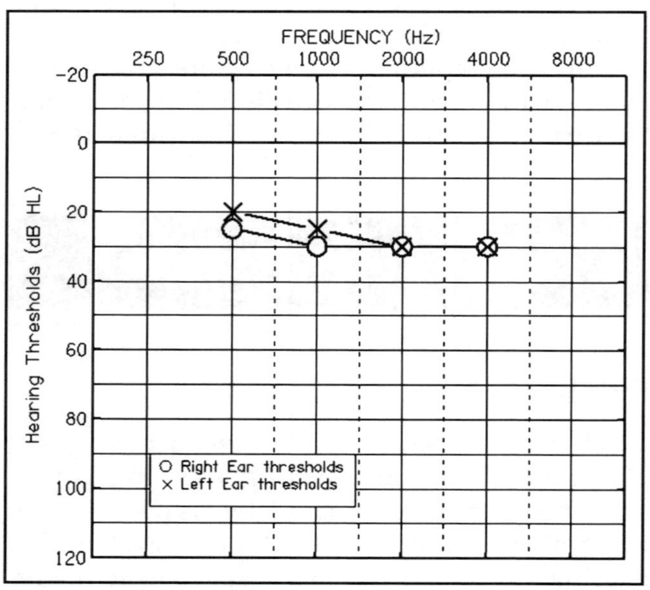


**FIGURE 10–1.** Caleb's first audiogram at 5 years of age, following a failed kindergarten hearing screening. These results are consistent with mild, bilateral hearing loss. The type of hearing loss cannot be definitively determined without bone-conduction thresholds.

The recommendations from the audiologist were to re-test Caleb's hearing in conjunction with evaluation by an Ear, Nose, and Throat (ENT) physician to confirm the type of hearing loss. Caleb was seen two weeks later by ENT and audiology. Air-conduction thresholds were consistent with the previous evaluation, and bone-conduction thresholds were obtained at levels within 5 dB of the air-conduction thresholds at each frequency, consistent with mild, bilateral sensorineural hearing loss. The ENT provided recommendations for genetic assessment and imaging, as well as providing medical clearance to proceed with hearing aids for both ears.

### Amplification Data

Caleb and his parents were counseled about the recommendation for bilateral hearing aids for children with mild hearing loss. Caleb's parents expressed concerns that the kindergarten screening was the first indication that there might be any problem with Caleb's hearing and that Caleb seemed to function quite well in a wide variety of listening situations without hearing aids. Caleb's parents also expressed concerns about the potential for bullying that might occur if Caleb wore hearing aids at school. Caleb's audiogram was converted to an SPL-o-gram to demonstrate how Caleb's hearing loss affects audibility for speech (Figure 10–2). Without hearing aids, Caleb has audibility of .51 for average speech and audibility of .39 for soft speech at 1 meter. At 4 meters, Caleb's unaided audibility drops to .19 for average speech. Based on those results, Caleb's parents agreed to a 3-month trial with loaner hearing aids to determine whether or not hearing aids were beneficial.

Caleb was fitted with bilateral hearing aids. The SPL-o-gram results from verification using real-ear measurements are shown in Figure 10–3. Note the improvements in audibility from the unaided results under the same conditions in Figure 10–2. Speech recognition assessment in background noise was completed using the Computer-Assisted Speech Perception Assessment (CASPA) (Boothroyd, 1999). Caleb was tested with and without his hearing aids. In the unaided condition, Caleb had 64% phonemes correct at a +5 dB signal-to-noise ratio (SNR) with a 60 dB speech-shaped noise masker and a 65 dB presentation level.

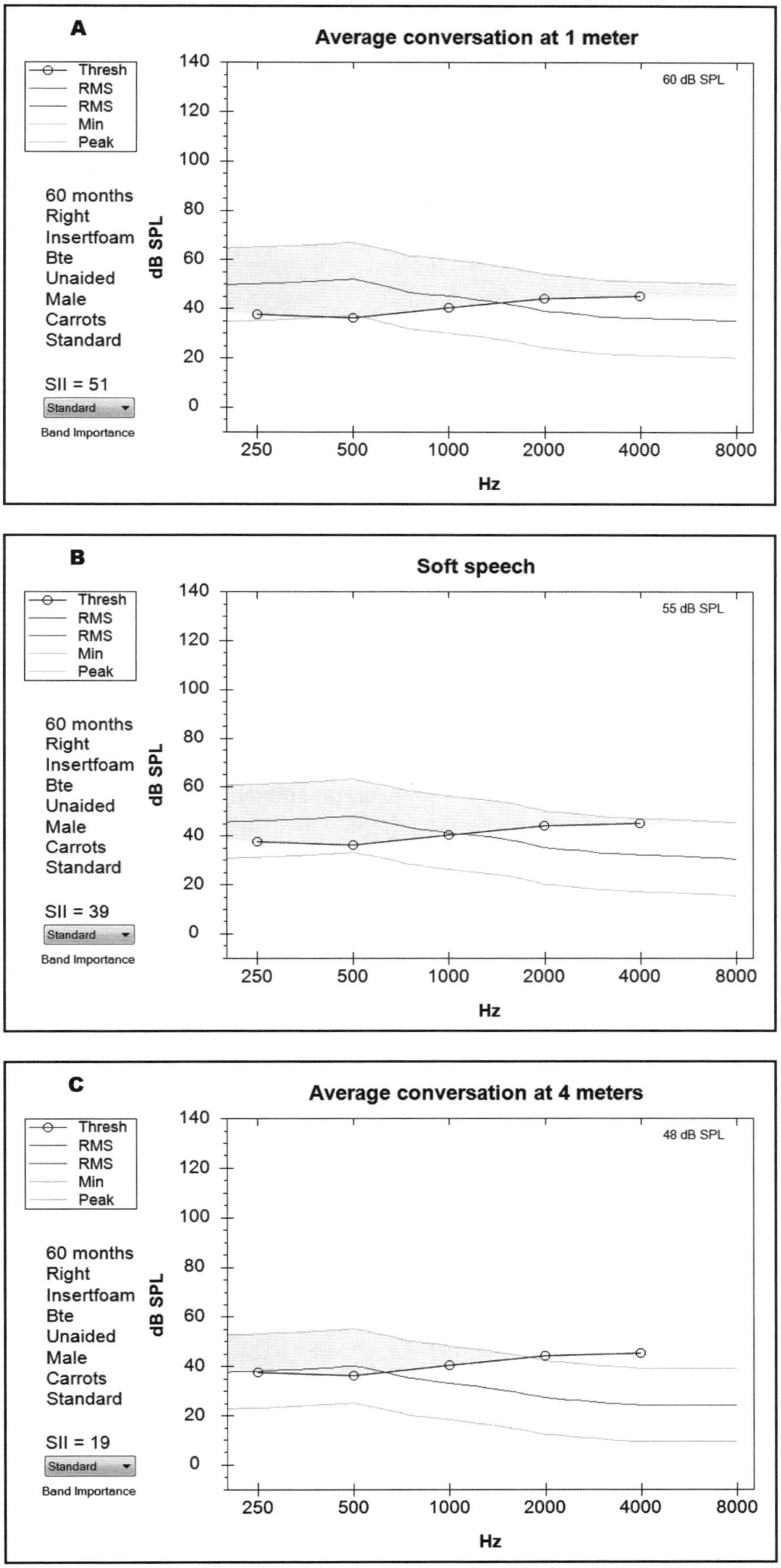


**FIGURE 10–2.** Unaided audibility as a function of frequency for Caleb's hearing loss in the right ear. Audibility for average speech at 1 meter (**A**), soft speech at 1 meter (**B**), and average speech at 4 meters (**C**). Both distance and input level have an impact on unaided audibility.

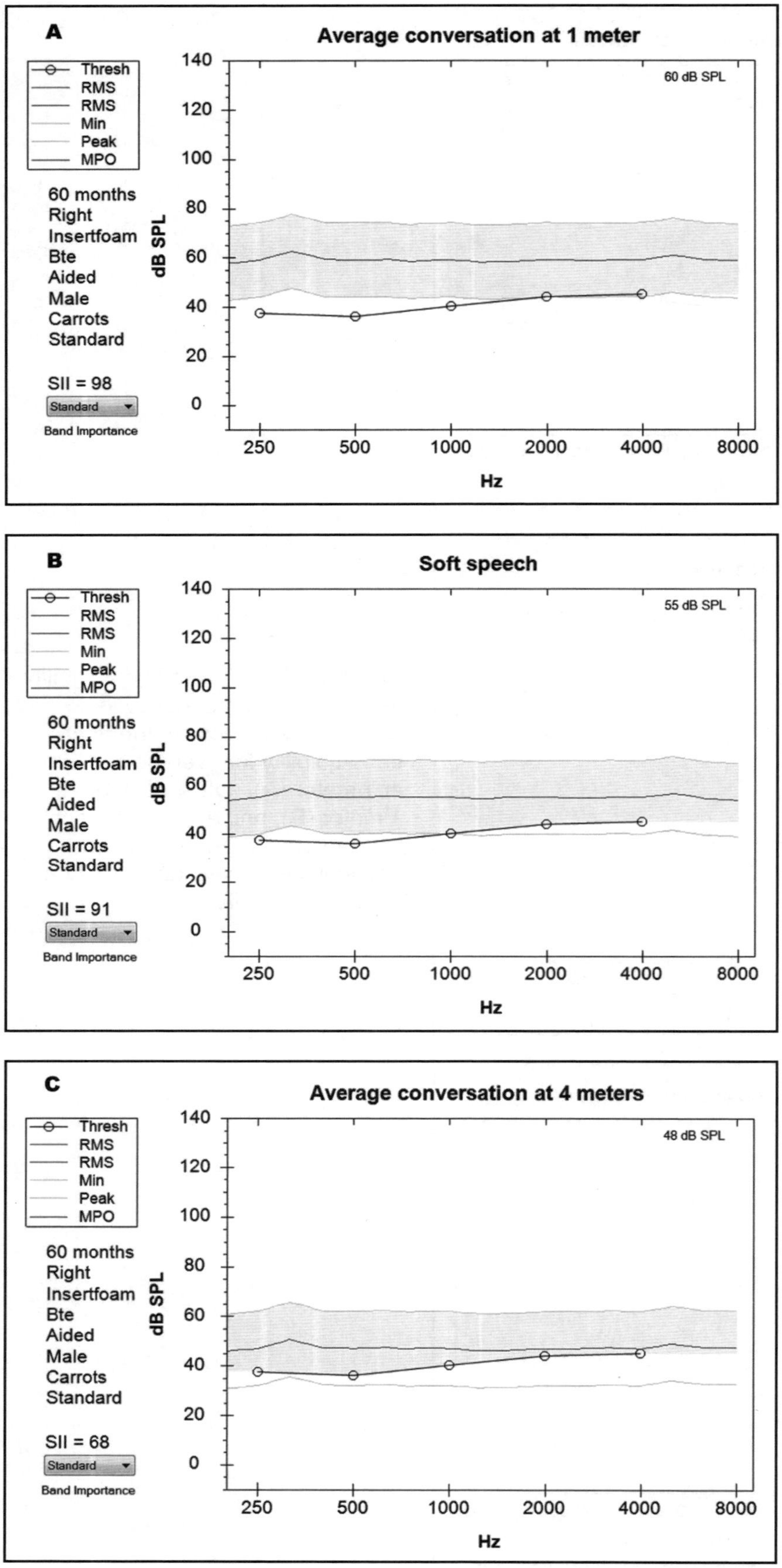


**FIGURE 10–3.** Aided audibility based on Caleb's fitting with loaner hearing aids. Aided audibility for average speech at 1 meter (**A**), soft speech at 1 meter (**B**), and average speech at 4 meters (**C**).

With hearing aids, Caleb's phoneme recognition in noise improved to 90% at the same SNR. Caleb and his parents were counseled about the results and sent home with the loaner hearing aids.

### *Follow-Up After the Hearing Aid Trial*

Caleb and his parents returned to the audiology clinic after two months of loaner hearing aid use. Caleb's parents reported several listening situations where Caleb seemed to hear better with the loaner hearing aids compared to his prior experience. Caleb's parents reported that he was using the hearing aids for approximately nine hours per day, which was consistent with the data logging recorded by the hearing aids of approximately eight hours per day of hearing aid use. Caleb's parents requested an extended period of time with the loaner hearing aids so that they could apply for private funding to purchase Caleb's own hearing aids.

## Case Summary

Caleb's case highlights several important considerations for fitting children with mild, bilateral hearing loss. First, mild bilateral hearing loss may occur with otitis media or other forms of middle ear dysfunction, which makes immittance and bone conduction results essential in differentiating these two conditions that require different types of management. Parents of children with mild hearing loss often do not report concerns about their child's hearing or development. If concerns are present, the concerns may be dismissed as typical behavior for the child's age or may be isolated to specific situations. Comparisons of unaided and aided audibility may help to quantify the limitations of audibility that occur with mild hearing loss, particularly if distances greater than one meter are simulated in a computer program, such as the Situational Hearing Aid Response Profile (SHARP). In this case, a difference between unaided and aided phoneme recognition was observed for Caleb. However, studies have suggested that speech recognition in noise may not be sensitive to differences in hearing aid performance for children with mild hearing loss, even when differences are observed in language abilities (Walker et al., 2015).

# CASE STUDY 2: KATIE

## Background

Katie is a 4-year-old seen in the audiology clinic for a post-operative evaluation following insertion of tympanostomy tubes by her ENT physician. An audiological evaluation at the ENT office indicated abnormal results, but the audiologist at the ENT clinic could not obtain consistent responses. Katie's parents had concerns for her hearing and her speech and language development. These concerns were assumed to be related to chronic middle ear problems since infancy. Katie did not pass her newborn hearing screening at birth, but her parents were told at the hospital that many babies fail the hearing screening so they should not be concerned. Katie had bilateral tympanostomy tubes placed at 18 months, but postoperative hearing evaluation could not be completed due to limited cooperation.

## Clinical Data

### *Diagnostic Data*

Katie had flat (Type B) tympanograms, with large equivalent ear canal volumes in both ears, consistent with patent bilateral tympanostomy tubes. Audiometric assessment using CPA was obtained using insert earphones. Air-conduction results revealed elevated thresholds in the mild-to-moderate range from 250 to 4000 Hz. Masked bone-conduction responses were measured within the normal range from 500 to 4000 Hz for both ears (Figure 10–4). These results indicated a mild-to-moderate conductive hearing loss in both ears despite patent tympanostomy tubes.

Katie was referred back to her ENT physician for medical evaluation of the origin of her conductive hearing loss. Katie's parents were counseled about the hearing loss. Amplification was recommended if further medical management of the conductive hearing loss was not determined to be possible by her ENT.

### ENT Evaluation

In a follow-up evaluation, Katie's ENT confirmed that the tympanostomy tubes were patent in both ears. Microscopic examination of the ear canal was reported to be grossly normal. The ENT ordered a high-resolution computerized tomography (CT) scan of Katie's temporal bones to evaluate the status of the middle ear. The results of the CT scan indicated that Katie had fixation of her stapes footplates in both ears. The ENT offered Katie's parents the option of surgical management of the middle ear problems or hearing aids. Given the potential risks associated with surgical management, including the potential need for amplification even if the surgery was successful, Katie's parents elected to get hearing aids for their daughter. The ENT provided medical clearance and recommended follow-up evaluation in six months to monitor the stability of Katie's audiometric thresholds.

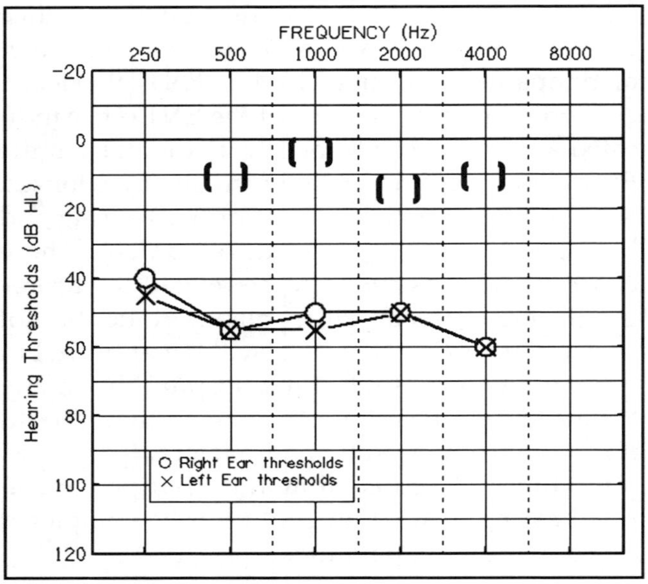


**FIGURE 10–4.** Katie's audiogram is consistent with a mild-to-moderate conductive hearing loss in both ears.

### Amplification Data

Katie was fitted with bilateral behind-the-ear (BTE) hearing aids. Verification was completed using a measured real-ear-to-coupler difference (RECD). Aided audibility for Katie's hearing aid fitting is shown in Figure 10–5.

Word recognition in quiet was completed in unaided and aided conditions in quiet using the Lexical Neighborhood Test (LNT; Kirk, Pisoni & Osburger, 1995) in sound field at 65 dB SPL.

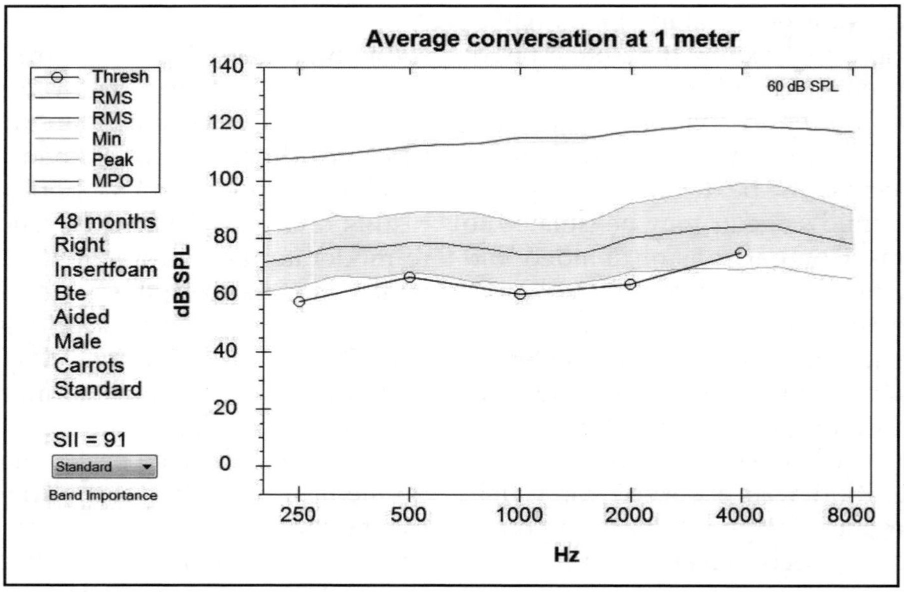


**FIGURE 10–5.** Katie's SPL-o-gram for her right ear for average speech (60 dB SPL).

Without her hearing aids, Katie correctly recognized 64% of the words averaged across two lists. With amplification, Katie correctly recognized 88% of the words averaged across two lists. The 24% improvement in performance with her hearing aids was a significant improvement based on the binomial theorem (Thornton & Raffin, 1978; see also Carney & Schlauch, 2007). Katie and her parents were oriented to the function of the hearing aids and provided with information about the types of changes in behavior that would be expected with amplification.

## Case Summary

Katie's case example highlights several important diagnostic issues that can occur with children with chronic middle ear problems. The presence of middle ear dysfunction related to fluid often is assumed to be the source of hearing loss, particularly if the loss is conductive. In many cases, that is a reasonable assumption, but one that should be verified after middle ear dysfunction is resolved, either spontaneously or through medical management. Acoustic reflexes can be useful in confirming the presence of conductive or mixed components to hearing loss in children, but only in cases where the child has a normal (Type A) tympanogram, which was not the case with Katie. Audiologists also often struggle with decision-making about when to provide amplification for children with persistent conductive hearing losses and when to rely on medical management from the ENT to resolve the hearing loss. The audiologist and ENT should work together to develop a treatment plan that includes periodic re-evaluation, even if the ENT decides not to manage the child's middle ear problem surgically. Some ENTs will take a less aggressive approach of monitoring the child's hearing status over time. There is currently limited guidance about the length of time that a conductive hearing loss must persist to warrant the use of hearing aids. In cases where conductive hearing losses persist for three months without a clear plan for medical management, the option of amplification should be discussed with the child's parents or caregivers and their managing physician. For conductive hearing losses that may be expected to resolve, loaner hearing aids may be provided so that families do not have to purchase permanent amplification for a temporary condition. If amplification is recommended, audiometric thresholds should be monitored regularly to ensure that thresholds are stable and that the hearing aids provide consistent audibility.

# CASE STUDY 3: CLAIRE

## Background

Claire is a 6-year-old who was being evaluated by a speech-language pathologist at her local education agency to determine if she qualified for an individualized education program (IEP). She failed her newborn hearing screen twice, but her family did not initially pursue follow-up. At age 3, her parents took her for an audiological evaluation with an ENT because of concerns about speech and language development.

## Clinical Data

### *Diagnostic Data*

Diagnostic testing took place at age 3 years, 2 months. Claire had normal (Type A) tympanograms in both ears. Audiometric assessment using CPA was obtained using insert earphones. Air-conduction results revealed elevated thresholds in the 70 to 80 dB range from 250 to 4000 Hz in both ears. Bone-conduction responses indicated no air-bone gap (Figure 10–6). These results indicated a bilateral, severe sensorineural hearing loss. Her better-ear pure-tone average was 66.25 dB HL.

### *Amplification Data*

Amplification was recommended for Claire, and she was fit with bilateral, behind-the-ear (BTE) hearing aids at age 3 years, 5 months. Verification was completed using sound-field aided thresholds. At age 7, when she was seen for her IEP evaluation, an educational audiologist completed

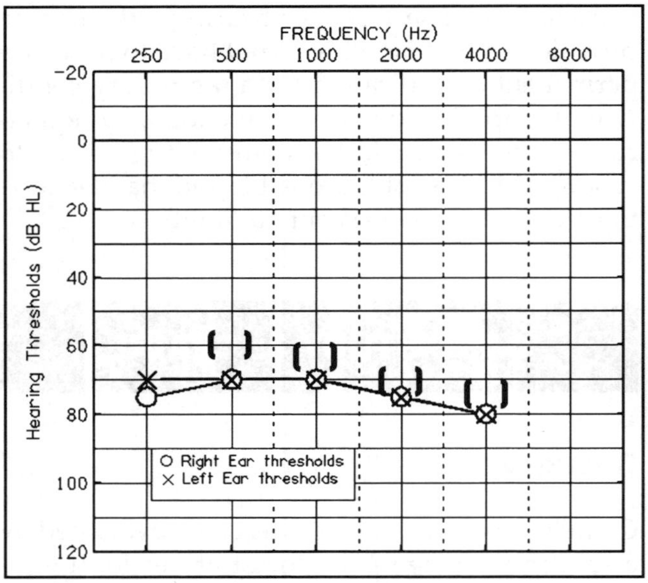


**FIGURE 10–6.** Claire's first audiogram at 3 years of age. These results are consistent with a severe, bilateral, sensorineural hearing loss.

real-ear testing with Claire's hearing aids. Claire's target SII, based on DSL prescriptive targets, was .68. Her measured SII was .39. This discrepancy indicates that Claire's hearing aids were not optimally fit relative to prescriptive targets, and she was substantially under-amplified. Data logging indicated that she was wearing her hearing aids 2.3 hours per day in the right ear and 2 hours per day in the left ear. Her parents reported experiencing resistance in getting Claire to wear her hearing aids on a regular basis. They did not notice any difference in Claire's listening behaviors with or without hearing aids.

### *Speech and Language Data*

Speech and language norm-referenced tests were administered as part of the IEP evaluation. Standard scores of 100 represent average performance on these measures, with a standard deviation equal to 15. For receptive vocabulary, Claire achieved a standard score of 48 (3.5 standard deviations below average), for expressive grammar, she achieved a standard score of 55 (3 standard deviations below average), and for articulation, she achieved a standard score of less than 40 (4 standard deviations below average). Based on these scores, she qualified for an IEP. The IEP specified that she would participate in the regular education classroom with pull-out services with a speech-language pathologist, itinerant teacher of the deaf/hard of hearing, and reading and math specialists. She would also have a full-time sign language interpreter in the regular-education classroom.

# CASE STUDY 4: JAMES

## Background

James is a 6-year-old being evaluated by a speech-language pathologist at his local education agency to determine if he qualified for an IEP. His parents reported that he passed his newborn hearing screen. His parents began to suspect a hearing loss around age 3 due to speech and language delays.

## Clinical Data

### *Diagnostic Data*

Diagnostic testing took place at age 3 years, 3 months. James had normal (Type A) tympanograms in both ears. Audiometric assessment using CPA was obtained using insert earphones. Air-conduction results revealed elevated thresholds in the 70 to 80 dB range from 250 to 4000 Hz in both ears. Bone-conduction responses indicated no air-bone gap (Figure 10–7). These results indicated a bilateral, severe sensorineural hearing loss. His better-ear pure-tone average was 66.25 dB HL. Based on family history, James' parents suspected that he may have had a mild hearing loss at birth that progressed to severe hearing loss over time.

### *Amplification Data*

Amplification was recommended for James, and he was fit with bilateral, behind-the-ear (BTE) hearing aids at age 3 years, 4 months. Verification was completed using simulated real-ear mea-

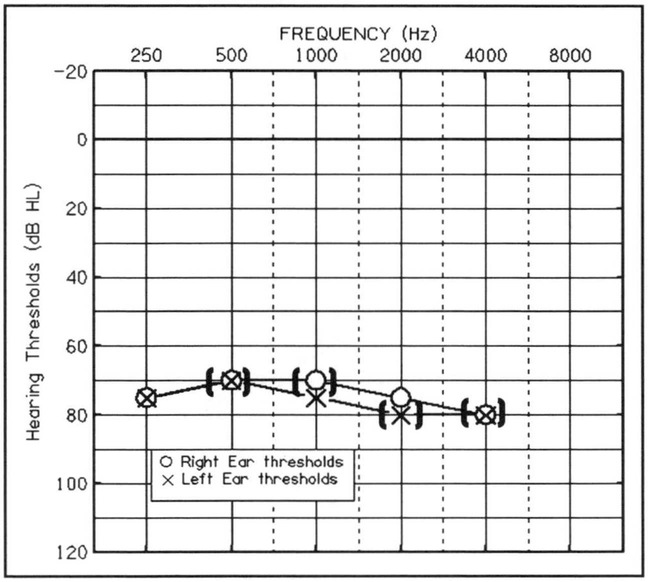


**FIGURE 10–7.** James' first audiogram at 3 years of age. These results are consistent with a severe, bilateral, sensorineural hearing loss.

sures. The audiologist measured James' real-ear-to-coupler difference in both ears. At age 6, when he was seen for his IEP evaluation, an educational audiologist completed real-ear testing with James' hearing aids. James' target SII based on DSL prescriptive targets was .70. His measured SII was .68, indicating that his hearing aids were well matched to prescriptive targets. Data logging indicated that he was wearing his hearing aids 12 hours per day in both ears.

### Speech and Language Data

Speech and language standardized, norm-referenced tests were administered as part of the IEP evaluation. Standard scores of 100 represent average performance on these measures, with one standard deviation equal to 15. For receptive vocabulary, he achieved a standard score of 85 (1 standard deviation below average), for expressive grammar, he achieved a standard score of 95 (within the average range), and for articulation, he achieved a standard score of 100 (within the average range). Based on these scores, James did not qualify for an IEP. His parents successfully advocated for a 504 plan. The 504 plan stated that he must receive accommodations in the regular-education classroom. These accommodations included preferential seating and a digital modulation system that connected to his hearing aids.

## CASE SUMMARY FOR CLAIRE AND JAMES

These two cases offer a clear demonstration of differences in developmental outcomes as the result of two malleable factors: aided audibility and hearing aid use. James and Claire's cases are very similar in several respects as both were identified with hearing loss as later ages and fit with hearing aids soon after confirmation of hearing loss. Their pure-tone averages were identical. From there, their cases diverge significantly. Claire's hearing aids were not optimally fit, and she likely would have benefitted from increased gain that met prescriptive targets at conversational and soft levels of speech. Claire was also at a disadvantage in that she did not wear her hearing aids on a consistent basis. Although this is speculative, it is possible that if she had received sufficient audibility from her hearing aids, she may have been more willing to wear them throughout the day. After a number of years of reduced cumulative auditory experience, Claire displayed significant delays in multiple domains of language acquisition, including vocabulary, grammar, and phonology, compared to same-age, hearing peers. James, on the other hand, had hearing aids that closely matched DSL prescriptive targets and wore his hearing aids during all waking hours. After three years of hearing aid experience, he achieved scores within the average range in terms of grammar and articulation, and slightly below average for vocabulary. Although degree of hearing loss may influence outcomes for children who are hard of hearing, these case studies illustrate that aided audibility and hearing aid use moderate that relationship. Ensuring that children have adequate audibility through real-ear verification methods can maximize perceived benefit from amplification. Audiologists and related service providers can also inform parents about data logging and encourage consistent use of hearing aids over time.

## CASE STUDY 5: BRANDON

### Background

Brandon is a 5-year-old boy with mild-to-severe sensorineural hearing loss in both ears. Brandon was diagnosed with hearing loss at 2 months of age after he did not pass his newborn hearing screening. Brandon was enrolled in an early intervention program through his local public school district within a few weeks of his diagnosis. Brandon was fitted with bilateral, BTE hearing aids in both ears at 3 months of age and received intervention once per week from an Early Childhood Special Educator until he was 3 years of age. At age 3, Brandon transitioned from home-based early intervention to a preschool program based at a nearby elementary school that includes both group and individualized therapy. When Brandon was fitted with hearing aids as an infant, his parents struggled to establish consistent hearing aid use. Brandon's parents reported that he would wear the hearing aids for about 2 hours per day at a follow-up appointment around his first birthday. His hearing aid use increased to only about 4 hours per day by 3 years of age. Data logging from Brandon's hearing aids were consistent with his parents' estimates of his hearing aid use. Brandon's parents and early intervention provider have consistently expressed concerns about his lack of responsiveness to sound and inconsistent hearing aid use.

### Clinical Data

Brandon returned to the clinic for his annual hearing evaluation and hearing aid check. Brandon's parents reported no new concerns for his hearing, although his mother reiterated her previous concerns about Brandon's lack of responsiveness with hearing aids. She reported that Brandon does sometimes respond well with hearing aids, but other times a device check is necessary because he does not seem to be responding. Brandon's

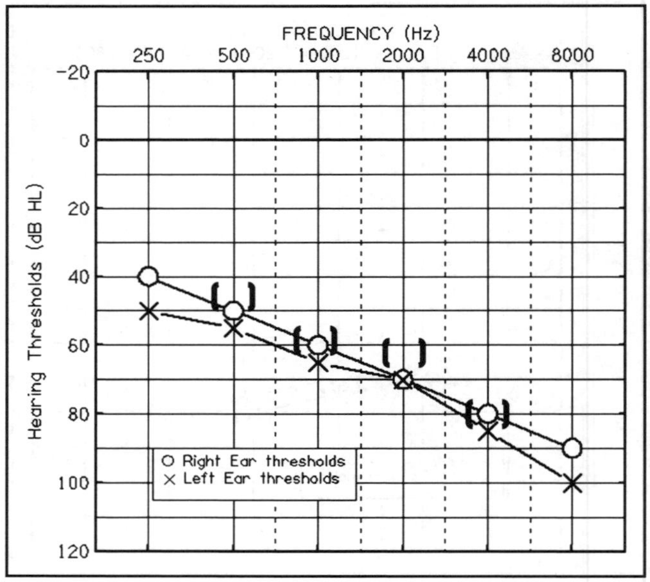


**FIGURE 10–8.** Brandon's audiogram at 5 years of age indicates bilateral moderate-to-severe hearing loss in both ears.

audiometric thresholds (Figure 10–8) were stable compared to his last hearing evaluation at 4 years of age, indicating mild, sloping to severe bilateral sensorineural hearing loss in both ears. Tympanometry was consistent with normal middle ear function in both ears.

Hearing aid verification using in situ real-ear measures suggested that Brandon had adequate audibility for his degree of hearing loss compared to normative data (Figure 10–9) for both average and soft speech input levels. Data logging from Brandon's hearing aid indicated an average daily hearing aid use of approximately 5 hours per day, roughly consistent with his mother's report that Brandon wears the hearing aids at school, but not regularly at home. Brandon's parents tried incentives and sticker charts to increase his hearing aid use at the suggestion of his early intervention provider, but the progress in increasing his hearing aid use had been minimal.

Speech recognition was assessed using the LNT monosyllabic word lists at a 65 dB SPL level in sound field with Brandon wearing his hearing aids. Brandon correctly identified 44% of the words, but several of his verbal responses were

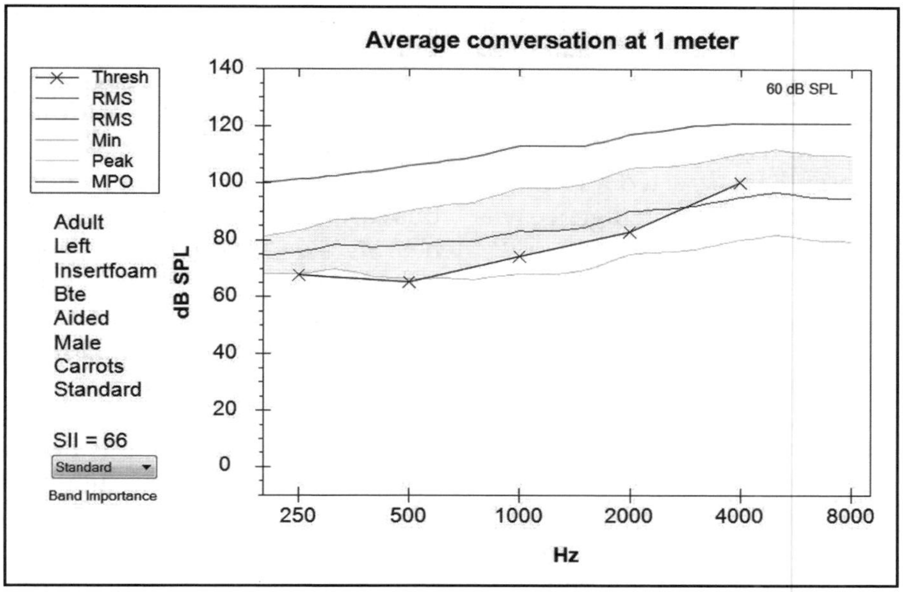


**FIGURE 10–9.** Brandon's SPL-o-gram for average speech (60 dB SPL).

unintelligible to the audiologist. The audiologist changed tasks to the Word Intelligibility by Picture Identification (WIPI) (Ross & Lerman, 1971) test, which allows the child to point to a picture instead of providing a verbal response. Brandon's correctly recognized 60% of the words on the WIPI using a point-to-picture response. Brandon's parents had completed the Parents' Evaluation of Aural/Oral Performance in Children (PEACH; Ching & Hill, 2007) at his previous evaluation at 4 years of age. Brandon's score on the PEACH based on his mother's rating of his auditory abilities was in the borderline at-risk range the previous year. At 5 years old, Brandon's PEACH score was identical to his score the year before, placing him again within the borderline at-risk range.

The results of the audiometric evaluation, the hearing aid verification, and the outcome measures were discussed with Brandon's parents. Several red flags were apparent based on Brandon's parents' concerns, as well as the outcome measures completed during the visit. The first potential problem area was Brandon's inconsistent hearing aid use, particularly at home. Brandon's parents shared the concerns of the audiologist regarding his limited hearing aid use, but were unsure about what can be done to address the problem beyond what had already been attempted. Brandon's speech recognition was poorer than would be expected for his degree of hearing loss in quiet, and his mother's ratings of his auditory behavior and language abilities from the PEACH had not progressed in a full year. Brandon's mother also indicated that his speech and language scores, obtained as part of the process for transitioning to preschool and an IEP, might help to provide additional information about Brandon's progress in speech and language. Brandon's mother signed a release of information for the audiologist to receive the results of the speech and language assessments from that process.

### *Speech and Language Evaluation Data*

Brandon's early intervention service provider provided the recent results from speech and language assessments completed as part of Brandon's IEP process. Brandon completed a nonverbal test of intelligence, the Wechsler Abbreviated Scale of Intelligence (WASI) (Wechsler, 1999) Matrix Reasoning subtest. Brandon had a standard score of 98, consistent with nonverbal intelligence in the normal range for his age. Brandon was assessed using multiple subtests of the Clinical Evaluation of Language Fundamentals (CELF) (Semel, Wiig, & Secord, 2006). Brandon's composite standard score of the CELF was 76, which was 1.5 standard deviations below the normative mean (100) for his age. Based on these results, Brandon's language skills were poorer than expected for his age, despite the fact that his nonverbal intelligence was within the normal range.

### *Cochlear Implant Candidacy Evaluation*

Given the broad concerns for Brandon's speech and language development, as well as his limited hearing aid use, the potential to have Brandon evaluated by the cochlear implant team was discussed with Brandon's parents. Although Brandon was not considered to be a cochlear implant candidate based on his degree of hearing loss from his audiogram, several other factors supported his potential candidacy. Brandon's limited speech recognition in quiet with his hearing aids suggest that the quality of the signal provided by Brandon's hearing aids, or the function of his auditory system in encoding the acoustic information, might be limited. Brandon's poorer language abilities also may have influenced his speech recognition. His poorer-than-normal scores on auditory development questionnaires, along with his limited language abilities were also evidence that his hearing aids were not providing sufficient benefit. Perhaps the most compelling evidence was the lack of progression in his skills over the preceding year based on the auditory development questionnaire. Based on all of these factors, Brandon's parents decided to proceed with a cochlear implant evaluation. The cochlear implant team reviewed Brandon's progress and outcome measures with his hearing aid, and agreed to approve his candidacy for a cochlear implant in the left ear. Brandon would continue to wear the hearing aid in his right ear after cochlear implantation.

## Case Summary

Brandon's case study highlights one of the key challenges in measuring outcome measures in children who wear hearing aids. Specifically, documenting outcome measures carries the responsibility of changing the treatment approach when there is consistent evidence that an intervention is not working. A cochlear implant is not the only option for altering the intervention approach, though it was the option that was undertaken in this case. In the difficult cases where children with hearing aids are not progressing in terms of auditory development, the presence of additional disabilities or underlying medical conditions should be carefully considered. Sadly, co-occurrence of hearing loss and other developmental disabilities occurs in approximately 40% of children with hearing loss, which could affect their progress. Limited hearing aid use should also not be interpreted as a pure indication of limited hearing aid benefit. A wide range of factors can influence a child's ability and willingness to use their hearing aids that are not related to the benefit that the child receives. Attempts should be made to increase hearing aid use whenever possible. Brandon's parents and early intervention provider did an admirable job of trying multiple strategies to increase his hearing aid use over time. The limited progress in development over the period of a year was one of the most compelling factors to evaluate other treatment options beyond hearing aids. Brandon's case also highlights the importance of audiologists, speech-language pathologists, and early intervention providers working together to get a complete assessment of a child's developmental progress. The use of multiple assessment data can help professionals reach better decisions, rather than relying on one assessment or relying only on parent information. Sharing reports and information can be crucial in responding appropriately when a child's progress with amplification is slower than anticipated.

# CASE STUDY 6: MICHAEL

## Background

Michael was evaluated in the audiology clinic at 5 weeks of age after failing his automated auditory brainstem response (ABR) newborn hearing screening at birth. Michael had an unremarkable birth history and no family history of childhood hearing loss. Michael's parents noted that he startles in response to loud sounds in the same way that his two older siblings had at the same age.

## Clinical Data

Tyampanomery using a 1000 Hz probe tone was consistent with normal middle ear function in both ears. Distortion Product Otoacoustic Emissions (DPOAE) were present from 2000 to 8000 Hz in both ears (Figure 10–10). Because Michael failed an ABR hearing screening in the hospital at birth, a diagnostic ABR was completed under natural sleep.

The stimuli selected for the ABR were clicks in order to assess the integrity of the auditory neural pathways. Clicks were presented in each ear using rarefaction polarity at a level of 90 dB nHL. The ABR response in both ears consisted of an early waveform component within the first few milliseconds, but no repeatable waveform components thereafter. The polarity of the early waveform component reversed when the polarity of the stimulus was changed to condensation. A control ABR recording, with the tubing removed from the insert earphone, indicated no early waveform response, suggesting that the early waveform that reversed in polarity was cochlear micophonic response and not stimulus artifact (Figure 10–11).

The presence of DPOAEs, along with an ABR with a cochlear microphonic and no identifiable waveforms was consistent with a diagnosis of auditory neuropathy spectrum disorder. Because the ABR cannot be used to estimate hearing sensitivity in cases of auditory neuropathy spectrum disorder, hearing aids could not be fitted based on the results. Michael was referred to his local early intervention program, an ENT for medical evaluation, and an ophthalmologist to assess the potential for associated vision problems. Michael's pediatrician also recommended referral to a pediatric neurologist to assess Michael for other potential neuropathies. Behavioral audiological evaluation was recommended at 6 months of age or when Michael could sit up without assistance in order to establish his hearing thresholds and to determine the need for amplification.

## Behavioral Audiological Evaluation

Michael returned to the audiology clinic at 8 months of age for a behavioral audiological evaluation. Since his initial evaluation at 5 weeks of age, Michael's parents had sought a second opinion from another audiology clinic that confirmed the diagnosis of auditory neuropathy spectrum disorder in both ears. Michael's parents also reported that the pediatric neurology evaluation indicated no additional concerns, but that the pediatric neurologist wanted to see Michael back at 18 months of age for follow-up evaluation. Michael's parents expressed frustration at the delay in providing amplification for Michael. Michael appeared to respond to sound normally by his parents' observations, but Michael's parents had talked with another family through social media regarding a child who had auditory neuropathy spectrum disorder who had already received hearing aids by 6 months of age. The need for behavioral assessment to provide amplification was reiterated to Michael's parents.

Tympanometry was consistent with normal middle ear function in both ears. The DPOAE responses were present in both ears at similar levels as the evaluation at 5 weeks of age. Behavioral assessment was completed using visual reinforcement audiometry (VRA) using insert earphones. Air-conduction responses were obtained from 500 to 4000 Hz for each ear in the moderate range (Figure 10–12). Bone conduction assessment could not be completed as Michael lost interest in the task. The results were reviewed with Michael's parents, who agreed to the provision of loaner hearing aids based on the behavioral assessment results. Michael's ENT provided medical clearance for hearing aids. Impressions of both ears were taken for earmolds and a follow-up appointment was scheduled for the loaner hearing aid fitting and orientation within 3 weeks.

Patient: ,
Birthdate:
ID:
Comment:

Ear: Left

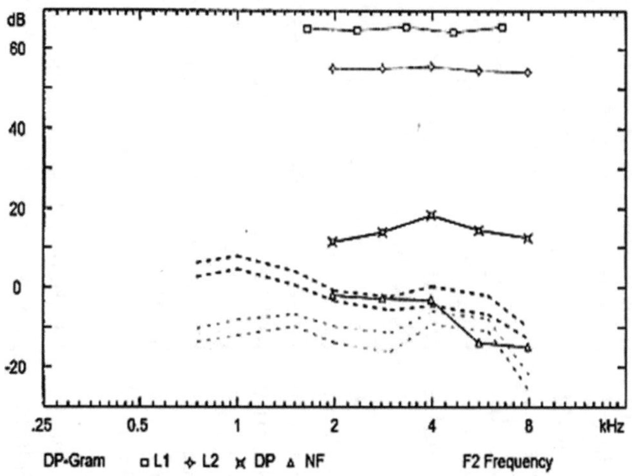


Left: 30-Jul-4: -: 750_8000.lst:

| L1(dB) | L2(dB) | F1(Hz) | F2(Hz) | GM(Hz) | DP(dB) | NF(dB) | DP-NF(dB) |
|---|---|---|---|---|---|---|---|
| 65.6 | 54.3 | 6654 | 7966 | 7280 | 12.5 | -15.0 | 27.5 |
| 64.2 | 54.5 | 4686 | 5623 | 5133 | 14.4 | -14.1 | 28.5 |
| 65.7 | 55.5 | 3327 | 3983 | 3640 | 18.4 | -3.0 | 21.4 |
| 65.0 | 55.1 | 2343 | 2811 | 2566 | 13.9 | -2.9 | 16.8 |
| 65.0 | 55.1 | 1640 | 1968 | 1797 | 11.3 | -1.9 | 13.2 |

Patient: ,
Birthdate:
ID:
Comment:

Ear: Right

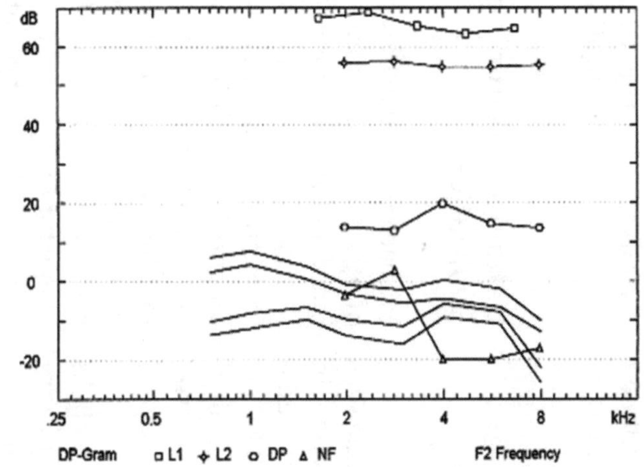


Right: 1-Sep-4: -: 750_8000.lst:

| L1(dB) | L2(dB) | F1(Hz) | F2(Hz) | GM(Hz) | DP(dB) | NF(dB) | DP-NF(dB) |
|---|---|---|---|---|---|---|---|
| 64.8 | 55.5 | 6656 | 7969 | 7283 | 13.5 | -17.4 | 30.9 |
| 63.5 | 54.9 | 4688 | 5625 | 5135 | 14.6 | -20.1 | 34.7 |
| 65.4 | 54.8 | [illegible] | 3984 | 3641 | 19.8 | -20.2 | 40.0 |
| 68.8 | 56.2 | [illegible] | 2813 | 2567 | 13.1 | 2.8 | 10.3 |
| 67.3 | 55.9 | 1641 | 1969 | 1797 | 13.9 | -3.7 | 17.6 |

**FIGURE 10–10.** Michael's Distortion Product Otoacoustic Emission (DPOAE) results from his diagnostic evaluation at 5 weeks of age. The signal-to-noise ratios at each frequency are highlighted within the black rectangles for each ear.

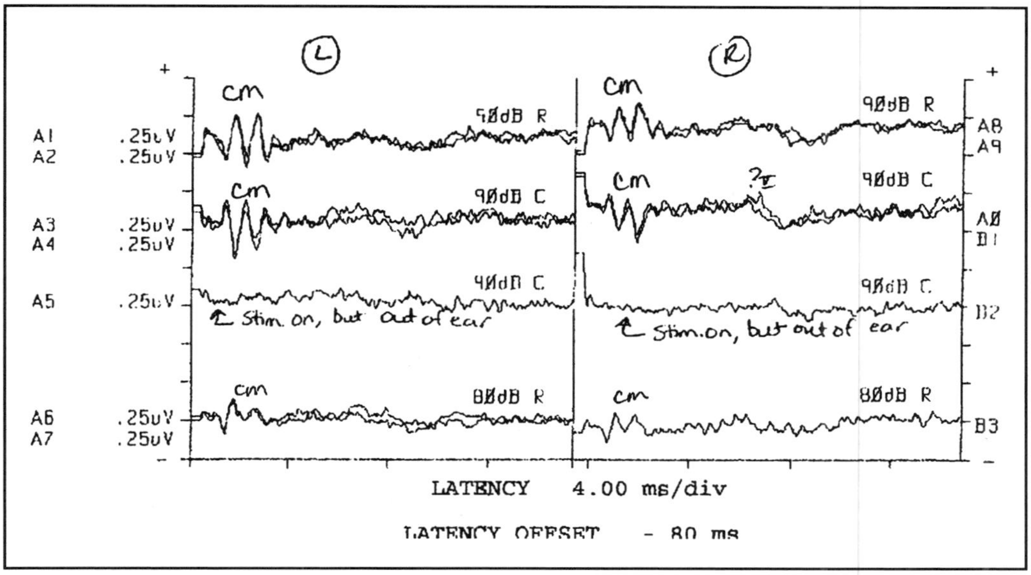


**FIGURE 10–11.** Auditory brainstem response (ABR) responses for click stimuli for rarefaction (R) and condensation (C) polarity in the left and right ear. Cochlear microphone (CM) that reverses in polarity is noted in the early part of the waveform in both ears. Note the control ABR recording without stimulation to the ear where the CM disappears.

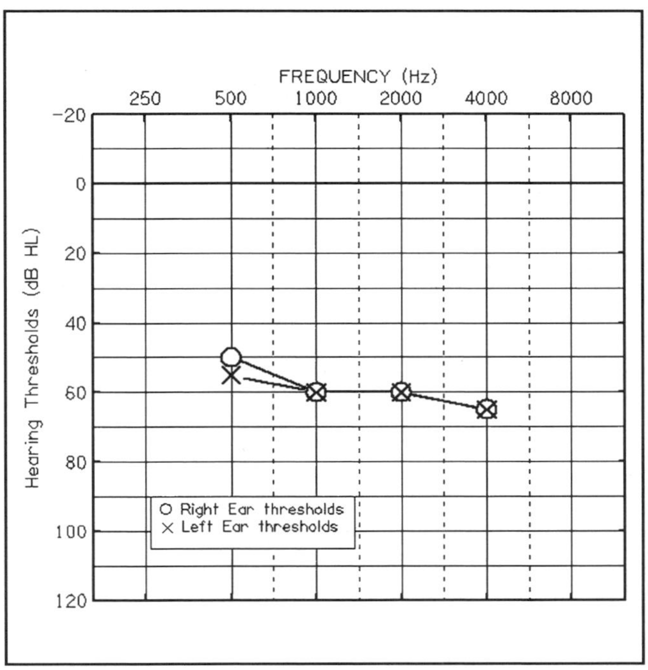


**FIGURE 10–12.** Michael's behavioral audiogram obtained at 8 months of age. The results are consistent with moderate hearing loss in both ears. Bone conduction thresholds could not be assessed at this visit.

## Hearing Aid Fitting

Michael returned to the clinic at 9 months of age for a loaner hearing aid fitting and orientation. Verification was completed with the loaner hearing aids fitted based on the behavioral audiometric results obtained three weeks prior. Results indicated audibility within the normative range for both ears for soft and average speech (Figure 10–13).

Michael's parents were oriented to the care and maintenance of the loaner hearing aid. The LittlEARS Auditory Questionnaire (Coninx et al., 2009) was completed to get a baseline indication of how Michael responded to sound prior to amplification. His mother completed the LittlEARS and his score was 15, which was within the normal range for his age based on the normative data. Michael's parents reported that a recent communication evaluation by Michael's early intervention service provider suggested that Michael exhibited vocalizations and babble that were typical for an infant of his age. Follow-up evaluation to monitor Michael's progress with amplification was recommended at 12 months of age.

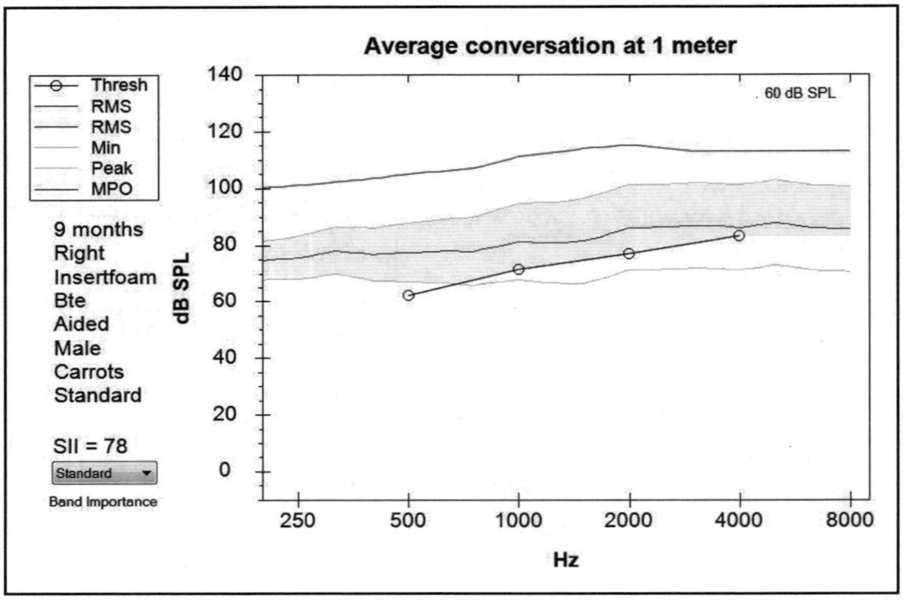


**FIGURE 10–13.** Michael's SPL-o-gram for his right ear at his initial hearing aid fitting at 9 months of age.

## Follow-Up Hearing Aid Check

Michael and his mother returned to the clinic at 12 months of age for a follow-up visit to check his loaner hearing aids and his progress with amplification. An examination of the fit of his earmolds indicated that he was starting to have problems with retention of the earmold in his ears, so impressions were taken of both ears for new earmolds. Michael's mother reported that she felt as though Michael heard better with the hearing aids than before he had hearing aids. She also completed the LittlEARS as part of the appointment. Michael's LittlEARS score was 21, which was an increase from his 9-month evaluation and within the normal range for his age. Michael's mother was offered the opportunity to continue to use the loaner hearing aids or to obtain personal hearing aids for Michael. She indicated that she would like to obtain personal hearing aids and was given information about funding options to help defray the cost of hearing aids, because hearing aid coverage was not part of his health insurance plan. Michael continued to use the loaner hearing aids until his family purchased hearing aids with financial support from a local foundation.

## Case Summary

Management of auditory neuropathy spectrum disorder can be challenging. Michael's case was designed to highlight many of the complications that can affect the ability to provide amplification for children who have auditory neuropathy spectrum disorder. The goal for provision of amplification is within 1 month of confirmation of hearing loss, based on the Joint Committee on Infant Hearing guidelines (American Academy of Pediatrics, 2007). This goal is currently not possible with current diagnostic assessment tools. Unlike children with sensorineural hearing loss, the responses obtained from ABR or auditory steady-state response measures cannot be used to predict behavioral thresholds in children with auditory neuropathy spectrum disorder. Michael's case demonstrates the potential for delays that can exceed months, even in children who do not have additional developmental concerns. For children who have auditory neuropathy spectrum disorder and additional disabilities that delay their ability to complete behavioral audiometric assessment, delays in the provision of amplification can extend even longer. Perhaps one of the most pressing needs in the diagnostic assessment of hearing in infants is the need for tools to estimate thresholds in infants with auditory neuropathy spectrum disorder. As noted in Chapter 2, cortical auditory evoked potential offer some promise in the ability to estimate thresholds in children with auditory neuropathy spectrum disorder, but additional research is needed before these measures can be applied in routine clinical care (He et al., 2013). Until then, behavioral assessment should be undertaken as soon as a child can be evaluated, using a conditioned-response paradigm such as visual reinforcement audiometry, to minimize the likelihood of delays in the provision of amplification.

Another aspect of Michael's case that has been a topic of controversy is the provision of amplification for children with auditory neuropathy spectrum disorder. Many early case reports with children who have auditory neuropathy spectrum disorder indicate limited benefit from hearing aids (see Berlin et al., 2010 for a review), but few of these published cases include information about whether or not children with auditory neuropathy were provided with adequate amplification based on their behavioral thresholds. An evidence-based systematic review by Roush, Frymark, Venediktov, and Wang (2011) concluded that few studies had described whether amplification was provided to children with auditory neuropathy spectrum disorder using methods that assess whether or not hearing aids were beneficial. A recent paper from the Outcomes of Children with Hearing Loss (OCHL) cohort indicated that a subset of children with auditory neuropathy spectrum disorder and aidable hearing achieved speech, language, and auditory outcomes that were on-par with their peers who had sensorineural hearing loss (Walker, McCreery, Spratford, & Roush, 2016). This suggests that some children with auditory neuropathy spectrum disorder can benefit from the provision of well-fit hearing aids. Michael's case is an example based on that subset of children. Children with auditory neuropathy spectrum disorder who do not progress in their communication even with the provision and consistent use of hearing aids should be referred for evaluation by a cochlear implant team. This is consistent with the step-wise management approach described in work conducted at the University of North Carolina, Chapel Hill (Teagle et al., 2010). Loaner hearing aids should be provided for children with auditory neuropathy spectrum disorder to allow time to determine whether or not amplification will be beneficial.

## CASE STUDY 7: LIAM

### Background

Liam is a 7-year-old boy who came to the audiology clinic after relocating to the area with his family. Liam had been diagnosed with mild-to-moderate hearing loss in both ears, and was fitted with hearing aids as an infant at an audiology clinic in another state. Liam's mother reported that he was fairly consistent with using his hearing aids in most situations, but preferred not to use them in specific situations, such as public places where there was a lot of background noise. The family was provided with a frequency modulation (FM) system for home use when Liam was an infant, but the family never established consistent use of the FM system. Liam is a second grader in a mainstream classroom. His academic achievement is near grade level, but his teachers have told his parents that he has difficulty listening in the classroom.

### Audiological Assessment and Hearing Aid Verification

Tympanometry was consistent with normal middle ear function in both ears. Conventional audiometry indicated normal hearing at 250 Hz and mild-to-moderate sensorineural hearing loss in both ears from 500 to 8000 Hz (Figure 10–14).

Hearing aid verification was completed using in situ probe microphone measures. The average root-mean-square error for Liam's hearing aid fitting at 500 to 4000 Hz was 8 dB, with the hearing aid providing less gain than prescribed at nearly all frequencies (Figure 10–15). The audibility provided by the hearing aids was outside of the normative range for his degree of hearing loss.

Liam's mother was informed that the hearing aids were fitted below what would be recommended, and that more amplification should be provided to make speech audible. Liam's mother asked that the hearing aids be adjusted and also commented that no one had ever placed a microphone in Liam's ears to measure the response from his hearing aids. The hearing aid gain was increased across frequencies to match prescriptive targets. The audibility for average speech at 1 meter increased from .79 before the adjustment to .93 after the adjustment (Figure 10–16).

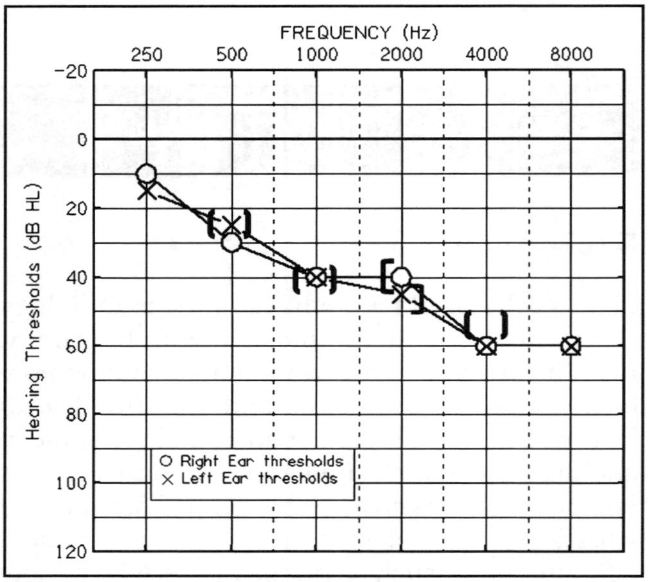


**FIGURE 10–14.** Liam's audiogram at 7 years of age. The results are consistent with normal hearing at 250 Hz and mild-to-moderate hearing loss from 500 to 8000 Hz in both ears.

Liam reported that he could hear more clearly through the hearing aids than before. Aided word recognition in quiet was assessed using the LNT. Liam correctly identified 88% of the words averaged over two lists in sound field at a 60 dB SPL input level. Liam was instructed to return to the clinic for his annual hearing evaluation or hearing aid check the following year, or before that if concerns for his hearing arose.

## Case Summary

Although there are guidelines that outline the appropriate processes for fitting hearing aids for children, Liam's case represents a stunning reality for many children who have hearing loss. These children receive hearing aids, but inadequate or infrequent verification practices limit the audibil-

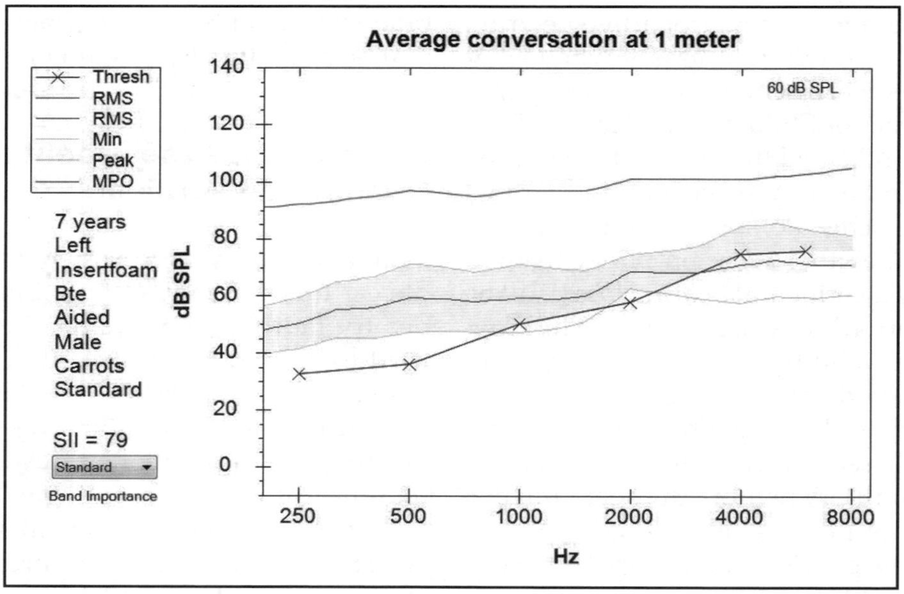


**FIGURE 10–15.** Liam's SPL-o-gram for his hearing aid in the left ear for average speech (60 dB SPL). The audibility is limited by larger deviations from prescriptive target across frequencies.

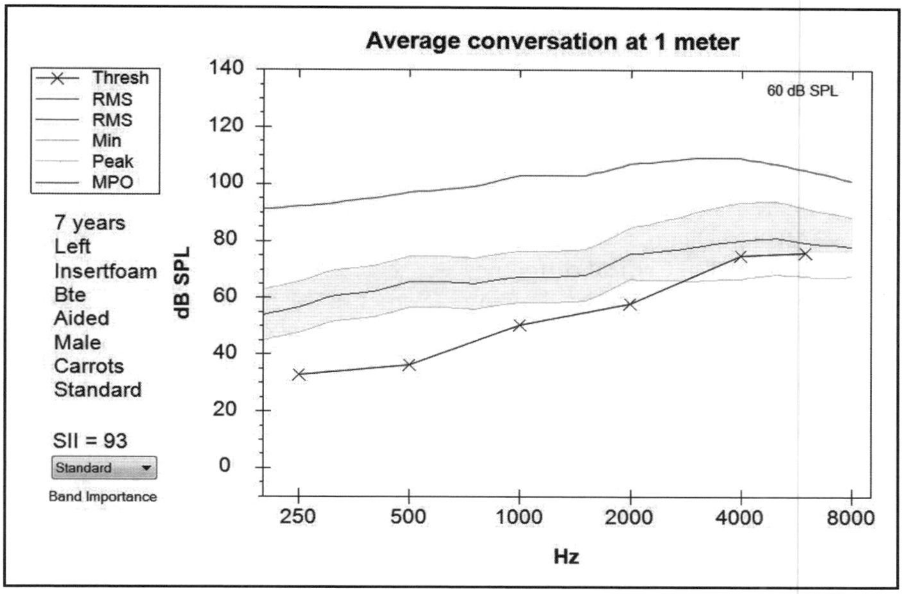


**FIGURE 10–16.** Liam's SPL-o-gram for hearing aid in the left ear for average speech after adjustment to approximate prescriptive targets. Note the increase in audibility for average speech compared to Figure 10–15.

ity that they have through their hearing aids. Our analysis in the OCHL study indicated that more than half of the children in our study had average fitting errors greater than 5 dB in at least one ear for at least one visit during the study (McCreery et al., 2015). The most frustrating aspect of these examples is the fact that they are preventable through the consistent use of probe microphone verification. As in Liam's case, there may not be outward indications that the hearing aid fitting is inadequate unless the fitting provides very limited audibility. In the case of children who do not have adequate amplification, their parents may attribute listening difficulties to the child's hearing loss or simply inattention. Our hope is that examples like Liam's case can be minimized through the consistent practice of hearing aid verification, as outlined in detail in Chapter 4.

## CONCLUSIONS

Each of the case studies were designed to highlight specific concepts that are often encountered by clinicians who fit hearing aids on infants and young children. Our hope is that the case studies can put the information from the previous chapters into an appropriate clinical context and illustrate the challenges and potential solutions that can occur when children need amplification. The process of providing amplification for children with hearing loss is multifaceted, and benefits from the involvement of parents and other professionals. The cases also highlight the current limitations of our diagnostic tools and outcome measures in specific areas of pediatric amplification, including auditory neuropathy spectrum disorder or determining the right time to move from a hearing aid to a cochlear implant. Many researchers are actively pursuing solutions to these challenges to help improve the lives of children who wear hearing aids.

## REFERENCES

American Academy of Pediatrics. (2007). Year 2007 position statement: Principles and guidelines for early hearing detection and intervention programs. *Pediatrics*, *120*(4), 898–921.

Berlin, C. I., Hood, L. J., Morlet, T., Wilensky, D., Li, L., Mattingly, K. R., . . . Shallop, J. K. (2010). Multisite diagnosis and management of 260 patients with auditory neuropathy/dys-synchrony (auditory neuropathy spectrum disorder). *International Journal of Audiology, 49*(1), 30–43.

Boothroyd, A. (1999). *Computer-Assisted Speech Perception Assessment* (CASPA v2. 2). San Diego, CA: Author.

Carney, E., & Schlauch, R. S. (2007). Critical difference table for word recognition testing derived using computer simulation. *Journal of Speech, Language, and Hearing Research, 50*(5), 1203–1209.

Ching, T. Y., & Hill, M. (2007). The Parents' Evaluation of Aural/Oral Performance of Children (PEACH) scale: Normative data. *Journal of the American Academy of Audiology, 18*(3), 220–235.

Coninx, F., Weichbold, V., Tsiakpini, L., Autrique, E., Bescond, G., Tamas, L., . . . Liang, W. (2009). Validation of the LittlEARS® Auditory Questionnaire in children with normal hearing. *International Journal of Pediatric Otorhinolaryngology, 73*(12), 1761–1768.

He, S., Grose, J. H., Teagle, H. F., Woodard, J., Park, L. R., Hatch, D. R., & Buchman, C. A. (2013). Gap detection measured with electrically-evoked auditory event-related potentials and speech perception abilities in children with auditory neuropathy spectrum disorder. *Ear and Hearing, 34*(6), 733–744.

Kirk, K. I., Pisoni, D. B., & Osberger, M. J. (1995). Lexical effects on spoken word recognition by pediatric cochlear implant users. *Ear and Hearing, 16*(5), 470–481.

McCreery, R. W., Walker, E. A., Spratford, M., Bentler, R., Holte, L., Roush, P., . . . Moeller, M. P. (2015). Longitudinal predictors of aided speech audibility in infants and children. *Ear and Hearing, 36*, 24S–37S.

Ross, M. & Lerman, J. (1971). *Word Intelligibility by Picture Identification*. Pittsburgh, PA: Stanwix House.

Roush, P., Frymark, T., Venediktov, R., & Wang, B. (2011). Audiologic management of auditory neuropathy spectrum disorder in children: A systematic review of the literature. *American Journal of Audiology, 20*(2), 159–170.

Semel, E. M., Wiig, E. H., & Secord, W. (2006). *Clinical Evaluation of Language Fundamentals-4*. San Antonio, TX: The Psychological Corp.

Teagle, H. F., Roush, P. A., Woodard, J. S., Hatch, D. R., Zdanski, C. J., Buss, E., & Buchman, C. A. (2010). Cochlear implantation in children with auditory neuropathy spectrum disorder. *Ear and Hearing, 31*(3), 325–335.

Thornton, A. R., & Raffin, M. J. (1978). Speech-discrimination scores modeled as a binomial variable. *Journal of Speech, Language, and Hearing Research, 21*(3), 507–518.

Walker, E. A., Holte, L., McCreery, R. W., Spratford, M., Page, T., & Moeller, M. P. (2015). The influence of hearing aid use on outcomes of children with mild hearing loss. *Journal of Speech, Language, and Hearing Research, 58*(5), 1611–1625.

Walker, E., McCreery, R., Spratford, M., & Roush, P. (2016). Children with ANSD fitted with hearing aids applying the American Academy of Audiology Pediatric Amplification Guideline: Current practice and outcomes. *Journal of the American Academy of Audiology, 27*(3), 204–218.

Wechsler, D. (1999). *Wechsler Abbreviated Scale of Intelligence*. San Antonio, TX: Psychological Corporation.

# Index

**Note**: Page numbers in **bold** reference non-text material.

## B

## D

## I

## J



## K



## L



## M

## N



## O

## R



## S

## T

## U



## V



## W



## Y